The Last Thirty Years in Public Health

First published in 1936, this book is a continuation of Sir Arthur Newsholme's *Fifty Years in Public Health*, and it covers a wide variety of topics in relation to the subject. It is in part autobiographical as the author recollects and reflects upon his experiences of the system. The book is divided into two main periods, 1908-1919, when Newsholme was the head of the Medical Department of the State's Central Health Organisation, and 1919-1936, when he no longer held an official position but had the freedom and time to examine both public health and social activities. Topics explored include the administration of public health, insurance for medical care, child health, The Great War, tropical medicine and American pioneers in public health.

The Last Thirty Years in Public Health

Sir Arthur Newsholme

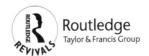

Routledge
Taylor & Francis Group

First published in 1936
by George Allen & Unwin

This edition first published in 2015 by Routledge
2 Park Square, Milton Park, Abingdon, Oxon, OX14 4RN
and by Routledge
711 Third Avenue, New York, NY 10017

Routledge is an imprint of the Taylor & Francis Group, an informa business

Publisher's Note
The publisher has gone to great lengths to ensure the quality of this reprint but
points out that some imperfections in the original copies may be apparent.

Disclaimer
The publisher has made every effort to trace copyright holders and welcomes
correspondence from those they have been unable to contact.

A Library of Congress record exists under LC control number: 37012674

ISBN 13: 978-1-138-90534-4 (hbk)
ISBN 13: 978-1-315-69590-7 (ebk)
ISBN 13: 978-1-138-90537-5 (pbk)

The Last Thirty Years in Public Health

RECOLLECTIONS AND REFLECTIONS ON MY
OFFICIAL AND POST-OFFICIAL LIFE

by

Sir Arthur Newsholme

K.C.B., M.D., F.R.C.P.

*Sometime Principal Medical Officer
to the Local Government Board
Sometime Lecturer in Public Health
Johns Hopkins University*

LONDON
George Allen & Unwin Ltd
MUSEUM STREET

FIRST PUBLISHED IN 1936

PRINTED IN GREAT BRITAIN BY
UNWIN BROTHERS LTD., WOKING

PREFACE

THE cordial reception given to my *Fifty Years in Public Health* has encouraged me to persevere in attempting to sketch my more recent official experiences from 1908 to 1919, and my varied international experiences in the post-official years which have followed. On each of these periods, as well as more generally, it appears desirable to make some prefatory remarks, additional to the outline of events given in Chapter I.

I must deprecate the assumption that this volume, any more than its predecessor, is solely autobiographical, or, on the other hand, that it professes to be a history of the course of Public Health during the thirty years ending in the present year.

In part it is both, admittedly incomplete in both respects. Its reminiscences deal almost solely with the medico-hygienic movements of the last thirty years; but its reminiscent character is retained, for it enables me to avoid the expectation that my history of events will be complete. Notwithstanding many necessary omissions, my historical account of public health developments in my time conveys, I am confident, a true impression of the unfolding of events. But although I think this is so, I realise that many chapters in this volume may appear to be isolated essays on separate problems. They none the less serve to indicate the rapid evolution of public health enterprises, and are really somewhat closely knit together. Through these enterprises there runs the dual theme, that health is dependent very largely on security from poverty, in the sense of privation of essential needs; and that to promote this security, and thereby reduce a large proportion of total poverty, there must be developed a practical intimacy between Medicine and the State, far beyond what has hitherto existed.

My description of events at Whitehall during 1908–19 has been beset with difficulties, as the reader will appreciate. I was precluded from quoting unpublished official documents, an embargo which evidently is in the public interest, but which did not preclude the use of many personal notes made on current events, and happily I have preserved many of these.

The need to avoid criticism, favourable or unfavourable, of the work of other officials or of politicians, except in so far as they are based on public documents, is also a hampering but wholesome condition of official life. But my mainly personal narrative will enable the reader to form valid conclusions on the successive subjects discussed.

In the American and subsequent sections of this volume my account of events has been fragmentary, and my comments on phases of American public life are open to criticism, not only because they are incomplete, but also because they relate largely to the early part of the decade 1920–29. In the last fifteen years there has been a rapid evolution of public health work in the United States.

I may state, however, that my imperfect account of personal observations in the United States has been supplemented by extensive reading of the history of government in the United States.

My American chapters have not been endorsed by any American friends. A similar statement applies to my English chapters. This does not mean that friends have not been generous in supplying facts whenever requested. But I am solely responsible if any statements prove to be inaccurate. Comments and criticisms are entirely my own.

The third part of this volume outlines the facts as to the increasing socialisation of medicine in European countries and in America. Few who have not carefully studied the cumulative evidence, outlined or quoted in this volume and in my *Medicine and the State*, will have realised how very far this responsibility of the State for securing adequate medical care for all has been accepted and met in many countries, including Britain.

ARTHUR NEWSHOLME

June 1936

CONTENTS

Part Two

RECOLLECTIONS OF AMERICAN PUBLIC
HEALTH AND SOCIAL WORK

Part Three

THE INCREASING SOCIALISATION OF MEDICINE

LIST OF ILLUSTRATIONS

DIAGRAMS

PART I
OFFICIAL LIFE IN WHITEHALL

CHAPTER I

INTRODUCTORY

THIS volume is a continuation of my *Fifty Years in Public Health*, and is written somewhat on the same lines. It is in part autobiographical: this is the smaller part; and it is mainly concerned with the subjects in the study of which, and in the realisation of which in social administration, I took a part. I have appreciated throughout that my personal recollections can interest only a few, and that it is the problems in which I have been concerned, and the methods for their solution adopted in my time, that constitute the possible value of what I have written.

In my previous volume I stopped at the year 1908, in February of which year I was appointed Principal Medical Officer of the Local Government Board, the predecessor and chief constituent of the present Ministry of Health. This Ministry was formed out of the Board, with the added work of the National Insurance Commission, work which—had reason ruled instead of prejudice—would have been begun under the Local Government Board in 1911. The Ministry of Health also took under its wing the work of the Central Midwives' Board and of the General Register Office, and (in part) the medical work of the Board of Education.

The present volume divides itself into two periods, 1908–19, when I was at the head of the Medical Department of the State's Central Health Organisation, and from 1919 to the present time, during which I have been free from official shackles and have had opportunities of somewhat detailed examination of public health and social activities in many lands.

A. In the official section of this volume I have said but little of the work of individual colleagues in my official work, for reasons easily divined. Many of them still live, some are still in official life, and if I began to particularise, gaps and omissions might be found in any review attempted by me. Here and there special acknowledgments are made, but it will not be assumed that, in the absence of these, I am lacking in gratitude for the help I received from other colleagues.

Special mention is made of the work of colleagues now departed this life: Drs. Franklin Parsons, Bruce Low, Theodore Thomson, R. Johnstone, H. T. Bulstrode, and Darra Mair, the four last-named of whom died many years before the normal termination of their life work.

The shadow of war was heavy over nearly five of the eleven years of my official governmental life. The Great War impeded much valuable work and it stifled some progressive schemes at their birth, but even during the War great public health work was accomplished in civilian as well as in military life. War in particular expedited increase in special child welfare work, and it had the further advantage of bringing home to the conscience of the people the desirability of greatly increased expenditure on social work.

In my previous volume I sketched, and illustrated from my own experience, the rapidly widening work done in many departments of public health administration, including the earlier developments in public care for individual health, especially in the prevention of tuberculosis, and in the protection of maternal health and still more of that of infants and young children. In these directions, as well as in improved sanitation, and in the treatment and prevention of the acute infectious diseases and of epidemic diarrhoea, notable advances had been made throughout Great Britain. It would, indeed, be a blunder to state that there ever existed a time-limit of demarcation between efforts in environmental hygiene and efforts for advance in personal hygiene; though, as time lapsed, the problems of protection of personal health and of its recovery began to bulk more largely in the programme of public health workers.

With this also went an increasing sense of the importance of social factors in the maintenance of health. In the evolution of my own thought the relation of poverty to disease began, more and more, to engage my attention; and that this was true also of other hygienists is shown in many published papers and reports.

Were I asked to enumerate the most important external

events bearing on the progress of Public Health during the thirty-six years of the present century, and especially in the years 1908 to 1919, while I was in the Government service, I should name three, the second of which, social insurance, while it embodied only slightly the principles of preventive medicine, increased the public willingness to spend money on a more liberal scale for social purposes.

First there came the issue in 1909 of the Majority and Minority *Reports of the Royal Commission on the Poor Laws.* Much of the evidence given before the Royal Commission, and of Sub-Commissioners appointed by it, had already been published, and there followed the educational intensive public agitation in favour of legislation on the lines of the Minority Report.

Next in sequence came the *Passage of the National Insurance Act,* 1911, which in large measure cut across the recommendations of the Poor Law Commissioners, and began a partial attack on the problem of poverty due to sickness and unemployment from a different angle. This most unfortunately was not linked up with already existing machinery to the same end.

The Insurance Act diverted public attention from poor law reform and made legislation impracticable for some years on the lines either of the Majority or the Minority Report on the Poor Law. Then, before the Insurance Act had come fully into operation, there occurred—

The Great War, 1914–18, perhaps the greatest catastrophe inflicted on mankind in the history of the world.

The vast changes in our modern outlook on health problems are closely associated with the three great events enumerated above, and around them can be clustered an account of a large share of public health work in the twentieth century.

Ranking with them and determining immediate lines of administrative reform must be placed the work for the initiation and development of the three new departments of public health work, in whose birth, childhood, and adolescence I was intimately concerned.

These *three new official services* were:

(1) Provision for the *prevention and treatment of tuberculosis*

on a national scale, which was aided and expedited by Exchequer grants made at the time of the enactment of the National Insurance Act;

(2) The similar provision for *the diagnosis and treatment of venereal diseases,* which was completely unrestricted by residential or financial limitations; and

(3) Extensive provision for *the welfare of infants and young children.*

These three new public health services and the three national events previously enumerated, constitute the chief subjects dealt with in the first part of this volume.

I have referred to the War as delaying social reforms already begun; but it had some compensating effects, for it led to the rapid initiation of additional measures for safeguarding public health and welfare. This was especially true of the new work on a national scale for the gratuitous treatment of all applicants, irrespective of their financial circumstances, who were suffering from venereal diseases; it was also true for the redoubled efforts for the welfare of mothers and their children, whose men were at the front. Into this last-named work, the women throughout the land threw themselves with almost feverish energy: and the subsistence allowances for mothers meant that children were as well and often better fed and cared for than under pre-War conditions. The severe restrictions on the sale of alcoholic drinks necessitated by the War were of inestimable service in the same cause.

In this official section of the present volume I have found it necessary to discuss the relation of medical and other technical officers to the secretarial officers in central government departments and have endeavoured to state an ideal, the complete attainment of which would result in maximum efficiency in administration. The complete realisation of this ideal is still in the future; it was only partially realised in my years of office, though in those years its realisation was much more nearly reached than in the earlier history of the Local Government Board.

In order that my subject may be the better understood by non-official readers, I have introduced a short sketch of local and central public health administration and have stated the points in which central administration—in part necessarily—is inferior in method to local administration.

In this first part of my book I realise that I am open to the criticism that too much space has been given to the history of poor-law reform. These chapters may be omitted by those who "do not care for history," but they form an essential part of the story of Public Health, which it is the object of these pages to unfold. Similar remarks apply to the rather full chapters on sickness insurance. Although, as passed through Parliament, sickness insurance was not a public health measure, it opened up great possibilities of preventive medicine, still almost unrealised; but they need not remain so.

B. When I resigned my post in February 1919, a few months after the Armistice and before the enactment of the Ministry of Health Act, I was 62 years old. The last years, during the War, had been characterised by excessive and continuous work with an inadequate staff—a large part of the medical staff was on War duty—and characterised still more by the pertinacious political cross-currents of those later years which rendered it extremely difficult to obtain decisions in accordance with merit on important subjects or even to pursue necessary work. I have copies of minutes and memoranda written during this period, which, if published, would vividly illustrate these cross-currents. In 1918 War calamities were rendered still more terrible by the world-wide pandemic of influenza, which killed more victims than the War itself. Even this uncontrollable pestilence was utilised by agitators, who averred in an important organ of the public Press that one could expect nothing better in the absence of a Ministry of Health!

I do not propose to describe the events leading to the formation of the Ministry of Health. I had repeatedly advocated central, and still more local, amalgamation, under a single authority in each instance, of all divisions of administration concerned with sickness and health, as could be shown by memoranda written by me in the War years and earlier at the time of the passage of the National Insurance Act, 1911. It is only necessary to say here that the bringing of sickness insurance work under the Central Health Authority in 1919 was an important reform; so also was the unification of the school and public health services, to the extent to which it was effected; but these changes had a limited value. The one great reform of unification of poor-law and public health work and of the other local administrative bodies in each area into a local parliament for all purposes of local government, which was urgently needed, was only effected when at long last the Local Government Act, 1929, was passed.

At the time of my retirement from the Board, the cessation of official work was most welcome; and I could not anticipate the rapid succession of adventurous and enjoyable activities in which without personal initiative I became rapidly engaged.

Immediately after the announcement of my retirement, I had a cablegram from the Labour Bureau of the Federal Government at Washington, D. C., to which the Children's Bureau with Miss Julia Lathrop at its head was attached. I was asked if I would take part in a series of conferences to promote child welfare work, which were being held in the chief centres of population from Washington to Seattle and San Francisco, preceded by a conference of several days' duration on the same subject in the Federal capital.

The invitation had an amusing side, which I may be excused for mentioning. It stated that the Bureau would provide me with a private secretary, unless I preferred to bring my own secretary with me. I cabled in reply accepting the invitation on the condition that my wife acted as my private secretary, and she travelled the length and breadth of the States in that not onerous capacity.

Prior to making this engagement I had promised to take part in an International Red Cross Medical Conference at Cannes, having as its object to continue, in peace time, the invaluable work of Red Cross workers in the War. This conference is described in Chapter xxv.

While I was at Cannes my programme of further work was extended. I was asked by Dr. William H. Welch to take part in the initial work of the new School of Hygiene and Public Health at Baltimore, by giving a six months' course of lectures during the coming winter on Public Health Administration. I stayed in Baltimore for a second winter's work, and these two years, both for my wife and myself, formed the high-water mark of our happy life and work together (Chapter XXIX).

During these two years I lectured on public health and medical subjects in university centres and to medical societies in many parts of the States. Some account of this work and of visits to Virginia and New Orleans is given in Chapter XXVI. We returned home in April 1921 with many grateful memories of our American life and more particularly of the friendships we had formed, especially in Baltimore and New York.

In 1926 and 1928 I undertook some special work for the Milbank Memorial Fund (Chapter XXXIV), and this led to my being asked in 1928 to undertake a survey which kept me busy during several years.

The results of this widespread survey were embodied in three volumes, entitled:

International Studies on the Relation between the Private and Official Practice of Medicine with special reference to the Prevention of Disease. (George Allen & Unwin.)

Vol. I. Netherlands, Scandinavia, Germany, Austria, Switzerland.

Vol. II. Belgium, France, Italy, Jugoslavia, Hungary, Poland, Czechoslovakia.

Vol. III. England and Wales, Scotland, and Ireland.

The totality of facts and general conclusions to be drawn from this wide survey were summarised in a further volume, *Medicine and the State,* published in 1932, with a foreword from Dr. William H. Welch.

It would appear that this might appropriately complete my labours; but in 1932 I received an invitation to accompany Mr. John A. Kingsbury, LL.D., the able and devoted secretary of the Milbank Fund, on a similar tour in Soviet Russia, and the results of our inquiries were embodied in a joint volume, published in 1933, *Red Medicine: Socialised Health in Soviet Russia.*

I take leave, for reasons of devotion, to reprint here the dedication to this volume, which was as follows:

To

DOCTOR WILLIAM HENRY WELCH

The Nestor of the Medical Profession in America,
who first suggested the investigation
which is concluded in this volume:

and to

the memory of

LADY (SARA) NEWSHOLME

who gave essential help throughout
its pursuit.

In subsequent chapters will be found a summary of my various itineraries and of various papers and volumes in which the work of this period is described.

When I read over this outline of my post-official activities I recall other events which, although they might have auto-biographical interest, are not primarily concerned with social and public health movements, with which this volume is mainly concerned.

I may, however, be excused for reproducing here an invitation received in 1929 from the newly formed Chinese Ministry of Health at Nanking, inviting me to take part with two other experts (named in the letter) in advising China on the development of its public health work. I append the text of the invitation, and the Chinese inscription accompanying it.

The new Minister of Health, Hsuch Tu-pi, was, as he states in his letter, a layman, but his chief technical vice-minister was Dr. J. Heng Liu, a graduate of Harvard, and the head of one of the departments of the Ministry had been trained in the Johns Hopkins School of Hygiene. So also had Dr. John B. Grant, one of its most brilliant pupils, who was at the head of the great work of the Rockefeller Foundation in China. The acceptance of this invitation would have involved a stay of one or two years, as I was to take up general Chinese problems of administration; and for family reasons I could not accept it.

聘　書

中華民國衞生部聘書

茲聘請

先生為本部名譽顧問此致

紐斯虎先生

中華民國十八年二月一日

薛篤弼

INSCRIPTION OF LETTER TO THE AUTHOR FROM THE CHINESE
MINISTER OF HEALTH
(*Translation follows*)

THE NATIONAL GOVERNMENT OF THE REPUBLIC OF CHINA
MINISTRY OF HEALTH.

NANKING,
January 25, 1929

SIR,

Coincident with the unification of the country under the Nationalist regime, a new era with particular stress on Reconstruction has begun. The importance of Public Health was especially emphasised by the establishment in November 1928 of a Ministry of Health, to which I was appointed the first Minister. Being a layman, I have sought as many specially trained men as I could in the conduct of the work of the Ministry.

But the work is a difficult one, and even the qualified men whom I have in the Ministry are embarrassed by the large size of the undertaking and by their lack of experience in Health Administration. For this reason I have asked permission of the Executive Yuan to establish an International Advisory Council consisting of yourself, Drs. L. Rajchman and Victor G. Heiser as honorary advisers. I am glad to say that the permission was granted on January 22, 1929.

It is our wish that you will give us your advice freely, and that you will be able to accept the invitation to come to China in the near future.

We have known of your great work and your vast experience. Indirectly we heard that you are interested in China and the Chinese. We feel sure that whatever advice you may give us will be most valuable to us.

With kindest regards, I am
Yours truly,
(*Signed*) HSUEH TU-PI,
Minister of Health

SIR ARTHUR NEWSHOLME,
ENGLAND

CHAPTER II

PERSONAL

BEFORE detailing the crowded events of the eleven years during which I was in the service of the Central Government, I must give an account of the events leading to my transfer from Brighton to Whitehall.

My new duties as Principal Medical Officer to the Local Government Board as set out in the official letter to me by Sir S. Provis, the Secretary of the Board, on my appointment were "as the Head of the Board's Medical Department, to advise them on all matters in which medical or public health considerations arise . . . *other than poor-law work* (my italics), to keep myself informed respecting all conditions which, whether at home or abroad, have relation to the public health." There followed reference to dealing with papers referred from other Departments of the Government in connection with public health matters, attendance on international and other conferences, and to optional retirement at age 60, retirement at the age of 65 being compulsory.

I took the place of Sir William Power, who retired at the latter age limit. It will be expected that I should explain how I, an outsider, came to be appointed to succeed Sir William Power. Mr. John Burns had been appointed President of the Board in 1906, and when Sir Henry Campbell-Bannerman, the Prime Minister, made this appointment I had shared the general opinion that "he had done the best day's work of his life"; for John Burns had already made his mark, not only as a labour leader, but also in local health administration as a member of the London County Council, the largest and most important local authority in England. He soon became actively engaged in introducing a more rapid and complete central motivation of public health work. That he was a persistent student of the annual reports of medical officers of health is shown by his public speeches in this period, and especially by his public addresses on tuberculosis and infant welfare work. These fanned the sparks of the child welfare movement already existent in many areas into an active flame, which rapidly became national in extent. They did much also to hasten more general preventive work against tuberculosis.

Quotations from my Brighton reports had appeared in his speeches, and when he visited Brighton in 1907 and had spent the day in studying its public health developments, particularly the provisions made for dealing with tuberculosis, he took me aside, and asked a number of personal questions. Would I care to become an inspector of the Local Government Board? I answered that the only appointment under the Government which I desired was that now held by Dr. Tatham as medical statistician at the General Register Office, although my interest in statistics was almost exclusively as a means of advancing health administration. This post I knew would not be vacant for two years. I had never previously spoken to Mr. Burns, and did not speak to him again more than twice before we met after my appointment under him. Meanwhile he was undoubtedly examining the record of public health work in many parts of the country, a task for which his past long experience as a member of the London County Council exceptionally fitted him. In November 1907, I had a letter from Mr. Burns, saying "without committing myself, may I consider you as one of the candidates for Dr. Power's post?"

Only three days before the official offer of the post was received, Mr. Burns sent me a telegram asking me to call at his home, and after conversation he informed me that I was one of three medical officers of health who were being considered by him! The terms of the official invitation I have given above.

For some time previously my mind had been disturbed by fear of undesirable publicity. This had been increased by a casual conversation with a Brighton lady, a prominent Primrose League dignitary. She had recently met Mr. Arthur Balfour at a reception in London, and, referring to me, he had observed, "but you will not be keeping him long."

It reminded me of a previous occasion (I believe about 1898) when with Dr. Tatham, M.O.H. of Manchester, and Dr. (afterwards Sir) Arthur Whitelegge, then M.O.H. of the West Riding, I was on the list of those under consideration for the succession to Dr. Ogle, who had followed Dr. William Farr, at the General Register Office. One morning I was horrified to see on newspaper posters throughout the town, "Brighton's M.O.H. probably leaving." The local newspaper contained an extract from the *Manchester Guardian*, giving a paragraph by its London correspondent to the effect that of the three candidates for the above-named post, Dr. Newsholme, "whose political colour was that of Mr. Gladstone," the Prime Minister, was likely to be appointed. Dr. Tatham certainly had no responsibility for this paragraph, and, although obviously inimical to my appointment, it may have had no relationship to Dr. Tatham's appointment made a few days later. But rightly or wrongly I have always been tempted to regard that London correspondent as a prince of Machiavellists.

Fortunately no such indiscretion occurred in 1908; but I may be excused for mentioning that when Dr. Tatham retired in 1910, I was asked by Mr. Burns to advise on the appointment of his successor. The medical post in the General Register Office is filled by the Prime Minister, but the President of the Local Government Board is in practice asked who is the best man; and Mr. Burns came into my office to ask me this question. I was in some difficulty, for the best applicant was Dr. T. H. C. Stevenson, who had formerly been assistant M.O.H. with me in Brighton. I told Mr. Burns that I should unhesitatingly have nominated Dr. Stevenson but for this fact. A few days later he was appointed.

I have mentioned Mr. Arthur (afterwards Lord) Balfour, as distinguished in philosophy as in statesmanship. With him I had several contacts based on study of social problems. I had sent him an address on "Social Evolution and Public Health" (see p. 68), and I have before me his letter dated January 22, 1908, just after the announcement of my Government appointment. Referring to my address he said, "I have read it with the very deepest interest. It is an excellent piece of scientific work": and then he added:

May I, as I am writing, offer my congratulations upon your appointment to a post, in which I am confident you will have the opportunity as you will certainly have the capacity of doing great public service.

With this letter he sent me an inscribed copy of his recently delivered Henry Sidgwick Memorial Lecture.

I cannot inflict on my readers extracts from the letters sent by medical confrères all over the country; though the rereading of them when writing this chapter has filled me once more with grateful recollections.

I must mention the congratulations of the Society of Medical Officers of Health. I had been President of the Society in 1899, and prior to that editor for some years of its official journal, *Public Health*. I still retain, along with a silver tray, a large illuminated volume giving the signatures of the President and members of every branch of the Society.

I must not forget to refer to the Brighton Town Council, whose service I left on February 3, 1908, after nearly twenty years of fruitful association. I had been exceptionally fortunate in the degree and extent of the support given me in various new departures in public health work. At that time there was much unemployment in Brighton, and I felt obliged publicly to veto the movement for a presentation which was on foot. There was a banquet, at which I received an illuminated address; and words fail to express my gratitude for an association which had covered so large a part of my working life.

It will save further personal reference if I state here that in 1912 I received the honour of the C.B. and in 1917 of the K.C.B. In this latter year I was elected a member of the Athenaeum under Rule 11,[1] and in the same year I was awarded the Bisset Hawkins Gold Medal of the Royal College of Physicians as a recognition of special work in promoting Public Health. At this time I had a characteristic note from John Burns. "The medal is only the bloom on the peach of service; the latter is the fruit."

The question is still unanswered as to why an outsider was appointed chief of the Medical Department of the Local Government Board, when there were doctors in the Medical Department competent to take on the work. Into this question I cannot enter fully for obvious reasons. The President, I believe, held the view, widely entertained, that there was need

[1] This rule authorises the Committee of the Club to elect not more than nine new persons each year of distinguished eminence in science . . . or for public services.

for "new blood" and for more rapid progress in public health work, especially in its more recently developed branches. I do not suggest that for this lack of progress in some directions, the Medical Department were chiefly, if at all, responsible. Bearing on this point the *Lancet* had a leading article at the time, evidently written with inside knowledge. It included the following pertinent remark:

It would be interesting to know how many schemes of constructive sanitary policy . . . which have entailed endless inquiry and work by Simon's successors, could be unearthed from the Board's pigeon-holes.

Yes: there was the rub!

The highest reputation of the Medical Department was derived from its epidemiological investigations. This important central work had necessarily been pre-eminent. Locally small sanitary authorities were the rule, England was then more rural than it became, and county councils, especially on the medical side, had not yet become fully effective. Even in many large towns medical officers of health were too often being paid poor and unattractive salaries. For these reasons and others, on which further light is shed in later chapters, there had been inadequate advance in central public health administration and in the closer linking of local and central public health work.

One reason actuating an outside appointment of a new chief, was the fact that the two next after Mr. (soon afterwards Sir) William H. Power in seniority were Dr. Franklin Parsons and Dr. Bruce Low, both due shortly to retire under the age limit. I received from these two distinguished civil servants and from other members of the Medical Department invaluable help.

CHAPTER III

PREVIOUS MEDICAL OFFICERS OF THE LOCAL GOVERNMENT BOARD

BEFORE discussing the methods of central administration in medical and public health matters which held good when I began to take part in it, and the changes in methods and scope which gradually evolved during my term of office, it is appropriate to devote this chapter to some recollections of my predecessors at the Local Government Board. These personal recollections cannot entirely be separated from official considerations, but they are in the main personal and necessarily biographically incomplete.

The office of Medical Officer to the Local Government Board had been held in succession by John Simon, C.B. (after retirement K.C.B.), 1871–76; Dr. E. Cator Seaton, 1876–79; Dr. George (later Sir George) Buchanan, 1879–92; Dr. Richard Thorne Thorne, K.C.B., 1892–99; Dr. William Henry Power, K.C.B., 1899–1908.

SIR JOHN SIMON

In my previous volume of earlier recollections I have outlined the main features of Simon's life-work. It is only necessary here to add that after being M.O.H. of the City of London for the seven years, 1848–55, he had been Medical Officer to two departments of the Government; first to the General Board of Health and then from 1858 to 1871 to the Privy Council which exercised some central control of sanitation and disease prevention.

Simon's appointment to the Privy Council was made under the Public Health Act, 1858, which authorised inquiries by the Council into any matters concerning the public health, and required its Medical Officer to report to the Privy Council in relation to such matters.

The fourteen annual reports written by Simon as Medical Officer of the Privy Council embodied much of the history of public health work during these years. Associated as they were

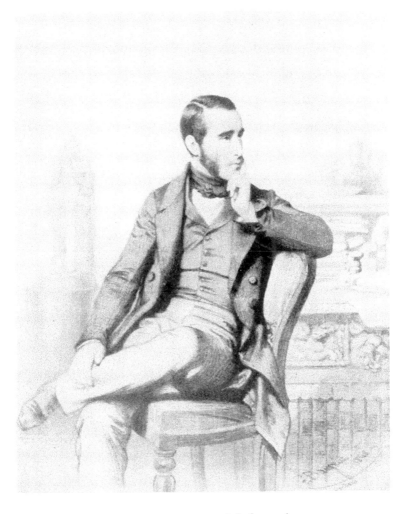

JOHN SIMON, F.R.S. (1816–1904)
(*From a Portrait taken in* 1848)

Reproduced by permission of the Royal Sanitary Institute

with expert inquiries on health problems as they arose, they recorded "increasing applicable knowledge," which was available as the scientific basis for improving sanitary legislation and administration. In 1860 Simon, in connection with the approaching census of 1861, persuaded the Registrar General to arrange for the preparation of accurate general and specific death-rates for each registration district in England and Wales. Thus was begun that series of decennial supplements to the Registrar General's reports which have proved of immense value in the local and occupational study of the incidence of fatal disease.

In 1866 an extended Sanitary Act was passed, its passage being aided by the "moment of popular piety towards the cause of sanitary reform" produced by fear of an invasion of cholera. In Simon's graphic words, under this Act "the grammar of common sanitary legislation acquired the model virtue of an imperative mood," in connection with the duties of local sanitary authorities. The passing of this Act was regarded by Simon, who had already on his staff several medical inspectors, as making it increasingly the duty of the Medical Department of the Privy Council to carry out inquiries into local health administration throughout the country, ready to give skilled advice where ignorance or neglect existed, and ready in the last resort to enforce the law. As an aid to these inquiries the Registrar General, after hearing Simon's plea, began quarterly returns of local incidence of fatal disease, thus giving a further step forward to that knowledge of the incidence of disease which renders effective preventive work practicable.

In 1871 a Royal Sanitary Commission recommended that the administration of the laws concerning the public health and the relief of the poor should be presided over by one Minister; and that for this purpose a new department, the Local Government Board, should be formed. It was also recommended that the work of the new department should be directive only, interference with the actual work of local government being avoided. (See also p. 48.)

The circumstances leading to Simon's retirement in 1876 are stated in my earlier volume (p. 79). His successors inherited the limitations of utility incorporated in the working of the Local Government Board, and so did I, as the last of these, to an extent which, in the progression of public opinion on health matters, had been much reduced. Satisfactory work was still, however, hampered by the unsatisfactory relationship between the Poor Law and Public Health Divisions of the Board.

DR. EDWARD CATOR SEATON

Succeeded Simon on his retirement in 1876. Dr. Seaton had long been associated with Simon in his work and had been distinguished for his special knowledge of the problems of vaccination. But as Simon has put it (*English Sanitary Institutions*, p. 392), even Dr. Seaton's experience . . . "could not bring into much effectiveness the very circumscribed office to which he had been called." His health soon failed, and in 1879 he died.

Fortunately, Dr. Buchanan was already on the medical staff, and he was appointed in succession to Dr. Seaton.

SIR GEORGE BUCHANAN (SENIOR)

As I had repeated opportunities of seeing and being advised by Buchanan, my recollections of him are more personal than of his successors. He was born in 1835 and died in 1895. He held the post of Medical Officer from 1879 to 1892. His death on May 5, 1895, followed a serious operation, which he had postponed to enable him to complete his work as chairman of the Royal Commission on Tuberculosis.

Early in that year I had applied for the advertised post of Examiner in State Medicine at the University of London (I was appointed in the following year); and Buchanan in this connection wrote me a personal letter dated early in April 1895, including the following statement, which I quote here as showing his foresighted appreciation of the scope of State Medicine:

We shall never get a proper recognition of Medicine by the State if we continue to limit "State Medicine" to the area of a statutory health officer's business; and we shall continue to confuse, as we do now in a programme which lies before me, "sanitation" with privy arrangements. . . .

At present the statutory health officer has no concern with crime and its punishment, with insanity and other matters that are dealt with by other departments of the State than the Local Government

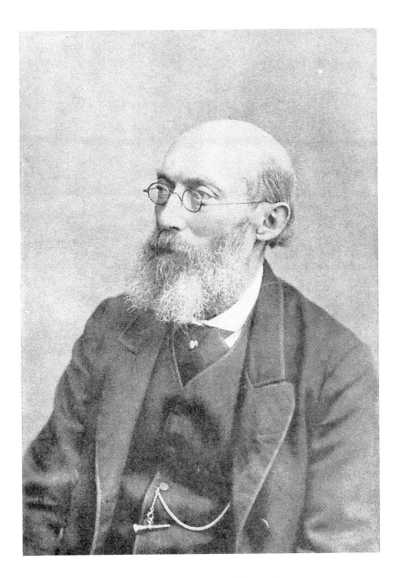

GEORGE BUCHANAN (1835–95)

Board. He may have something to do with diseases of animals, but certainly he is looked on as transcending his province if he says anything about them. I have come to see this from my place in the Tuberculosis Commission. Such a Commission ought not to have been wanted if there had been a medical department *of the State* to guide in the medical business *of the State.*

This is a striking statement, when we bear in mind that it was made when modern advances in the synthesis of treatment and prevention had not emerged above the horizon.

Soon afterwards he wrote again to the effect that I had been recommended by the Senate for the above-named examinership. This was followed almost immediately by a further letter saying he had blundered, and no change was to be made until next year. He added would I refrain from writing for a week and then say I forgave him! My letter of appreciation never reached him for the operation intervened!

I relate this incident as showing Buchanan's exquisite kindness.

He was greatly beloved. His work was marked by scrupulous accuracy, and there was in it an entire forgetfulness of self. He was frank in his statements in official papers; and I wish I could quote some of these statements which I subsequently read in official files. There was a pungency and causticity in some of them, which evidenced the "stone walls" by which he sometimes found sanitary effort blocked.

Buchanan had the supreme advantage of previous experience as a M.O.H. before his appointment as medical inspector with Simon under the Privy Council. I have read some of his reports as M.O.H. of St. Giles's Parish, London. These show the intensive study, both by field work and by statistical examination, which he gave to all local problems, including the endemic typhus fever of the district. His reports on the influence of sewerage in reducing the death-rate and on the apparent association between phthisis and dampness of soil are still landmarks in epidemiological and sanitary research.

SIR RICHARD THORNE THORNE

Born in 1841, Thorne succeeded Buchanan as Principal Medical Officer of the Local Government Board in 1895, and held the post until 1899, when he died suddenly at the age of 58. I shall not forget the painful impression produced by the announcement of this fact at a preliminary meeting of the British Congress on Tuberculosis in that year.

At the time (*Public Health*, January 1900) I wrote as follows:

His high ethical standard was not inconsistent with a diplomatic ability and urbanity which ensured for him and his department a favourable hearing from those high in the councils of the State.

I used the same opportunity to emphasise the high literary value of Thorne's reports, as also those of his predecessors, which were always enlightening, without being verbose and journalistic.

It is not without importance that those who have held the post of Principal Medical Officer of the Local Government Board should all have been able to make their contentions more impressive by the literary form in which they were set forth.

Thorne, and Power who succeeded him, had not been administrative local medical officers of health, and this appears to me to have tended to place them at some disadvantage when concerned with the difficulties and defaults of local officers and local authorities, which Simon held (p. 49) was to be a main subject of the activities of the Medical Department of the Board. But this is a minor point; the substantial difficulties in the way of urging and initiating reform were never in the Medical Department, but in the Board as then constituted, and in the lethargy of Parliament, as representing public opinion.

Thorne's name is especially associated with his reports on Isolation Hospitals, which did much to ensure their general provision. Medical requirements and administrative difficulties were intermingled in this provision. Had there been governmental insight and driving power, many of the ridiculously small administrative units for which isolation hospitals were needed would have been merged into larger administrative areas; but the country blundered on, while its advisers failed to put first things first; and thus multitudes of expensive and relatively inefficient isolation hospitals were built and maintained, instead of the hospitals for larger areas which "thinking through" the

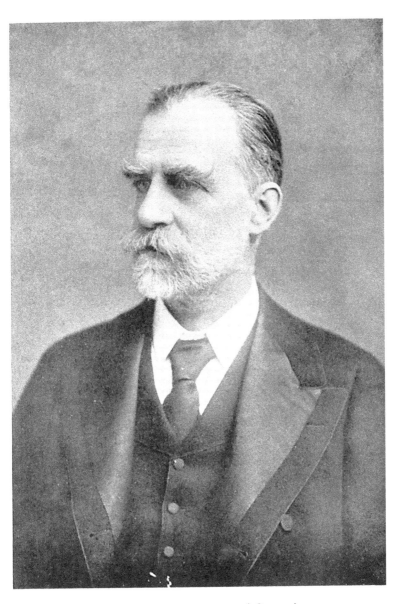

RICHARD THORNE THORNE (1841–99)

problems and acting accordingly would have provided, had Parliament and the Central Government been ready for this.

When Thorne wrote his report, and for years afterwards, the significance of the inevitable incompleteness in notification of infectious cases and delays in notification had not been appreciated. Furthermore, the occurrence of exceptional cases of protracted and recurrent infection described on p. 183 of my earlier volume had not been verified; nor were "carrier cases" as yet recognised. Extended knowledge has placed the provision of hospital isolation in an altered perspective.

Thorne introduced the hypothesis of the "progressive development of the property of infectiousness" in diphtheria, a useful conception in the study of epidemiology. His views on tuberculosis have already been given in my earlier volume (p. 185). Like most of his contemporaries he stressed bovine as a source of human tuberculosis, and objected strongly to the compulsory notification of human tuberculosis.

I remember that his cross-examination of my evidence before the second Royal Commission on Tuberculosis was directed towards establishing the value of fresh air and ventilation, rather than of considerations of direct infection from cow to cow.

Thorne's work in international conferences on public health work greatly helped in promoting the practice of international hygiene and in the abolition of measures of quarantine.

SIR WILLIAM H. POWER[1]

Power had been on the staff of the Privy Council when Simon with his staff, including Seaton, Buchanan, Thorne, Radcliffe, and Ballard, was transferred to the Local Government Board. He succeeded his colleague, Sir R. Thorne Thorne, in 1899 as Principal Medical Officer. His reputation as an epidemiologist was already established.

Other important epidemiological investigations stand to his credit, as well as the two outlined below, with which his name is usually associated.

It was a great event in public health history when Dr. Michael Taylor of Penrith in 1858 first drew attention to contaminated cows' milk as causing fever. In 1870 Taylor gave the first

[1] No photograph of Sir William Power is obtainable.

recorded account of an outbreak of scarlet fever due to milk; and in the same year Dr. Edward Ballard demonstrated that an outbreak of typhoid fever in Islington was due to a particular milk supply. In 1878 Power traced an outbreak of diphtheria to infected milk. His further inquiries led him in 1882 to advance the hypothesis that the harmful attributes of a given milk supply might be "an affair of the very system of the animal furnishing the milk," and not the result of contamination from a human source of infection. Investigations on the milk supplied from a farm at Hendon to certain metropolitan districts led him to conclude that the outbreak of scarlet fever among the consumers of this milk "depended on the diseased condition of certain milch cows at the farm, a condition first introduced there in the previous month by some animals newly arrived from Derbyshire"; also that personal infection of this condition occurred from cow to cow. He showed also that the distribution of the scarlatiniform disease followed the distribution of the milk from the newly involved sheds. Here there seemed to be a close analogy with the relationship between bovine and human tuberculosis, accepted at a later date, and with that still more recently found to exist between an infection causing abortion in cattle and undulant fever in man. Since Power's original investigation, outbreaks of septic throat with or without septicaemia have been traced to milk from cows having diseased udders, and furthermore doubt has been thrown on the exact specificity of scarlatinal infection. Nevertheless it cannot be said that the evidence connecting a special disease of cows with human outbreaks of scarlet fever has gone beyond hypothesis; and experience has shown that in the majority of milk-borne epidemics of scarlet fever a human source of infection of the milk can be detected.

Power's investigations on aerial convection of smallpox infection have already been mentioned in my earlier volume (p. 134). These investigations must have occupied years of work both by Power and by several members of the medical staff of the Local Government Board. They led to important changes in the policy determining the site of smallpox hospitals. I may recall that when large capital expenditure beyond local competence was required by any sanitary authority, the consent of the Local Government Board was required before a loan for the purpose could be obtained, and this gave the Central Board much control in determining local expenditure, on sewerage, on town halls, parks, etc.; for consent to a loan could be withheld if the local plans were regarded as unsatisfactory. This power was rigidly exercised in regard to smallpox hospitals. The Board laid it down that such hospitals must be remote from an inhabited district, and must not be in the same curtilage as pavilions for the treatment of other infectious diseases. As a result, all smallpox hospitals were removed from within London; and this measure, and the ancillary precautions taken in connection with the removal of patients, doubtless were an important factor in minimising the spread of smallpox. But the practical value of the measures taken in consequence of Power's investigation does not compel one to accept the hypothesis that the risks of smallpox hospitals were other than those of maladministration and resultant personal infection from the staff of these hospitals, and that the infectious material, in the absence of more appreciable and "close-by" infection from person to person, could be carried a quarter or half a mile by currents of air from the hospital which had in it a few cases of acute smallpox.

In 1881 a Royal Commission, chiefly of distinguished doctors, investigated this problem. They did not commit themselves to support or rejection of the hypothesis of distal aerial convection of infective matter; but wisely recommended the discontinuance of hospitals in populous districts.

In the preceding paragraphs I have mentioned only two of the great epidemiological problems with which Power's name is associated; but his influence in activating researches in which his name never appeared is well known to all who have had an inside view of his work. In my second annual report as Power's successor was included the following testimony.

His period of office had been brilliant in scientific advancement and marked by great sanitary amelioration throughout the country. . . . His influence both in initiating and in inspiring work of far-reaching scientific and practical importance impressed itself in every branch of the Board's medical administration.

CHAPTER IV

LOCAL ADMINISTRATION OF PUBLIC HEALTH

MY own experience during eleven years of public health administration from the centre followed on some twenty-three years of local public health administration. Thus I have taken a protracted part in administration from each of these related viewpoints, and can write with a large background of experience of their respective merits and interrelation.

For the convenience of readers who have not taken part in official administration it is, perhaps, desirable to set out briefly the conditions of health administration in England, with some remarks on their steady approach towards completeness and satisfactory working. Evidently I cannot do more in this chapter than indicate salient features.

England has, since 1835, been a country of local self-government, in which the degree of independent local self-government and of what is sometimes called "domination" from Whitehall has varied to a remarkable extent. The need to bring about the disappearance by fusion of the large number of the small local authorities whose continued existence meant defective public health administration was the repeated subject of comment in my annual reports to the Local Government Board. Thus writing in my Annual Report (1907–08, p. viii) on extreme instances of small local authorities I commented:

Local self-government in such districts is both extravagant and inefficient. There is an unnecessary multiplication of officers, who cannot be paid sufficiently to devote themselves without distraction to the public interests; on the part of the sanitary authorities of paltry districts like these, local and personal considerations too often outbalance the public interest, and the multiplication of small areas is a serious obstacle to an efficient and economical settlement of problems of water supply and sewerage in which neighbouring districts are mutually concerned.

In giving evidence before the Royal Commission on the Poor Laws (Vol. IX of their Report) in 1908 I had similarly drawn attention to the fact that the average sanitary district

tion with the Central Government is also great. This has been recognised especially for education, which even before 1870, when the first great National Education Act was passed, was receiving from the Central Government small subsidies for local work. These subsidies in recent decades have vastly increased.

The central subsidisation of certain branches of public health work has been of more recent origin; but nevertheless long before "Grants in Aid" of anti-tuberculosis work by public health authorities began in 1911, of maternity and child welfare work in 1914, and of anti-venereal work in 1917, central funds for many years had been devoted to paying half the salaries of local medical officers of health. Poor-law work for many years also has been supported in large part by the Central Government, and in recent years unemployment allowances have been made largely from central funds. The final results, both in vast expenditure (much of it investment) and in the change of proportion of the cost of total local expenditure borne by local funds (rates) and by the Government (general taxation), is seen in the statement that while in 1884 total local official expenditure in England and Wales was about £54 millions, in 1932 it exceeded £500 millions; and in the further fact that in 1884 the central exchequer supplied 12·4 per cent and now supplies about half of the total expenditure by local authorities.

Every one of the central grants towards local expenditure has been accompanied by some measure of control by the Central Government of the method of expenditure of the grant; and if these grants increase, central control must also increase. This accords with the principle that "who pays the piper calls the tune," but the extent of central control thus exercised has varied greatly, and it need never go beyond insistence on standards of administration. Police and educational services have had largely centralised control; in poor-law administration the Boards of Guardians abolished by the Local Government Act, 1929, were controlled rigidly, and not always intelligently or with realisation of the possibilities of their work in the prevention of sickness and destitution. But some Boards of Guardians succeeded in doing admirable work, and it must be

recalled that even to the wisest among us the preventive conception of each branch of social work has only in relatively
recent years started fully into life.

The grants given for local work done in the three special
branches of public health (tuberculosis, venereal diseases,
maternity and child welfare) necessarily meant some control by
the Central Department of Health over their expenditure. This
was a willing partnership, rapidly increasing in efficiency and
extent.

When in 1929 the grants given for these three specialised
public health services were replaced by "Block Grants," allowing more local option in their expenditure, central approval of
detailed expenditure was no longer required. It appears
doubtful whether these Block Grants, especially in the smaller
units of administration, will secure as efficient local service in
these three departments of work as grants previously based on
the needs of the community concerned, and there may arise
the temptation to save local rates at the expense of these special
services and of their improvement. This will be ascertained by
inspection by skilled officers of the Ministry of Health, but
coercion if needed is always a less potent agent than the per-
suasion constituted by the sharing of expenditure. Long
experience has shown that the direct coercive power of the
Central Government is almost negligible.

This brings us to the relation between the Government and
local authorities in the performance of their multifarious
duties. It has steadily become one of partnership in a large
business rather than that of an overlord insisting on quasi-
military conformity to central demands, and I was fortunate in
seeing much of this change from overlordship to partnership.

RELATION OF CENTRAL TO LOCAL AUTHORITIES

The relation between central and local governing bodies has
often been a source of controversy. It was a chief subject of
investigation by the Royal Sanitary Commission of 1869. Each
local authority already had a medical officer of health and an
inspector of nuisances in the excessive number of small areas
into which the country was divided for local administration;
and the Commission in their report laid it down that the

central authority "must . . . avoid taking to itself the actual work of local government," only exercising *direction*.

The same Commission recommended that health officers should only be removable with the sanction of the central authority, an important recommendation, not made fully effective until recent years.

The consultation and co-operation between central and local authorities steadily improved in each succeeding decade. The central authority had, furthermore, always been able to exercise some control over local expenditure in several ways.

(*a*) There is the initial limitation constituted by the fact that expenditure must come within the scope of the various Public Health Acts.

(*b*) Local authorities are controlled financially not only because their expenditure must relate to objects comprised in their statutory powers, but also by the fact that if the expenditure is so great that payment for it needs to be spread over a series of years, the consent of the central authority is required before the loan is obtained for this purpose. Furthermore, total borrowing must be kept within a definite relationship to rateable value. These are valuable checks on local extravagance. In regard to urban and rural districts and county councils their value is increased by the annual independent auditing of local expenditure by the central authority.

(*c*) There is the further indirect check on the action of local authorities other than county borough councils formed by grants from the exchequer via county councils of half the salaries of health officers, and by the special grants in aid of expenditure on maternity and child welfare services, and on the treatment and prevention of tuberculosis and of venereal diseases. These, prior to 1929, more than since that year, were conditional on the maintenance of a certain standard of efficiency, as education and police grants continue to be. They have given an important impetus to local expenditure on satisfactory lines.

OCCASIONAL CENTRAL BLOCKING OF LOCAL LEGISLATION

The large municipalities, sometimes with a population approaching a quarter of or even a complete million, and the county councils which came into existence in 1888, have sometimes found that their efforts at progressive work are impeded by inadequate legal powers. Hence the promotion of local Bills in Parliament by these larger local authorities. The case for the added powers is stated on behalf of the local authority before the Police and Sanitary Committee of the House of Commons; expensive counsel are retained for and against the proposed powers, especially if they infringe on local vested interests, expert witnesses are called, often medical officers of health, and I have several times given evidence in such cases and witnessed short-sighted opposition to useful proposals of local authorities (see for instance *Fifty Years in Public Health*, p. 209).

The Local Government Board was officially represented at the hearing of these cases; and the legal official of the Board who held a watching brief was heard by the Committee with respect. His advice or hints occasionally led to refusal to confer the powers desired by the legal authority and thus valuable local experimentation has frequently been inhibited or delayed. The usual plea was that if the powers were to be conferred they should be given by general and not by local legislation, and this plea when accepted meant indefinite and prolonged delay. There was often lack of central consultation with the medical department before the hearing of the case, illustrating the evil on which Simon animadverted and on which more is written in Chapter VI.

I had the chagrin in several instances of not being consulted on proposed local legislation which I favoured, and of receiving expostulations from the local medical officers of health concerned on the assumption that I had been consulted. But I was the victim, as had been my predecessors, of the assumption of secretarial and legal omniscience, and in these cases vigorous protests on my part did not secure adequate consultation. In my view much wider latitude should be given to local authorities for local experimentation in improved sanitary administration, so long as general principles of good government are not contravened.

CHAPTER V

CENTRAL ADMINISTRATION OF PUBLIC HEALTH

THE department of the State which was most closely related to and was responsible for supervising and regulating the work of local governing authorities was the Local Government Board until 1919, when it was renamed the Ministry of Health, and was given some further powers (p. 53).

The Local Government Board was formed in 1871, and to it were transferred the poor-law functions hitherto exercised by the Poor Law Board, and the public health functions of the Privy Council. Its first President was J. J. Stansfeld, a man of high character with much anti-medical bias; and the new Board's chief officials were derived from the Poor Law Board, with its extremely centralised methods of administration. Successive Presidents were J. J. Stansfeld (1871–74); G. Schlater Booth (1874–80); J. G. Dodson (1880–82); Sir Charles Dilke (1882–85); Arthur Balfour (1885–86); Joseph Chamberlain (1886); J. J. Stansfeld (1886); C. T. Ritchie (1886–92); and in more recent years H. H. Fowler (1892–94); G. J. Shaw Lefevre (1894–95); Henry Chaplin (1895–1900); Walter Long (1900–5), Gerald Balfour (1905); John Burns (1905–14); Herbert Samuel (1914–15); Walter Long (1915–16); Lord Rhondda (1916–17); W. Hayes Fisher (1917–18); Auckland Geddes (1918–19); C. Addison (1919–21).

The last-named became the first Minister of the Ministry of Health constituted in 1919. This change of name for the Local Government Board, with added functions, did not alter the fact that it remained that department of the Central Government which was concerned with the affairs of local government, and that these were then and remain now of much wider scope than can be included under the name of Ministry of Health. The title is acceptable, if this fact be remembered.

Dr. Addison was succeeded by Sir Alfred Mond in 1921, when the Government realised and decided on drastic reduction of the vast sums spent on post-bellum housing with inadequate results. Then followed G. Boscawen (1922–23); Joynson Hicks

(1923–24); John Wheatley (1924); Neville Chamberlain (1924–29); Arthur Greenwood (1929–31); Sir Hilton Young (1931–35); followed by Sir Kingsley Wood in 1935.

The impression given by this list is one of fugitiveness. Relatively few Ministers have stayed long enough to learn their job, too often the President or Minister being a pawn in the rapid changes of political appointments. In 1914–19 there were six presidents within six years.

Although chiefly advisory, the Local Government Board did much initiative work, and exercised a valuable influence in stimulating the activities of local authorities. On the public health side there was abundant expostulation with negligent local authorities; medical inspectors' reports showing local sanitary defects and defaults were followed by letters from the Board urging reform; and although the powers of the Board to act in default of these local authorities were clumsy and almost unworkable, much good was done by this central supervision. Did space permit I could illustrate these statements from printed reports of many of my colleagues in the Medical Department. But, in the main, coercion has wisely not been greatly utilised either by the Local Government Board or the Ministry of Health, and with advance in public opinion the need for it has greatly diminished.

The effective head of the Local Government Board was its Permanent Secretary, and he and the secretarial staff under him were almost all-powerful. Sir Samuel Provis was Secretary when I joined the medical staff of the Board, but I knew slightly his predecessor, Sir Hugh Owen, the son of a distinguished father in the same service.

Sir Hugh was an astute and able lawyer and for years held his post with supreme ability. When I became an official of the Board in 1908, the following lines were current:

> Said Sir Hugh, "In this case I confess
> Some reasons weigh more and some less;
>   And the case being so
>   We can hardly say 'No,'
> Yet I hesitate much to say 'Yes.'"

To assume that to shelve an awkward problem was Sir Hugh's

general practice would, however, be erroneous; for sometimes wisdom lay in delay.

His successor, Sir Samuel Provis, was a past-master in similar suspension of decision, when from his viewpoint this was desirable; and I have seen a photograph of him at his desk, showing the piled-up files on his table surrounding him on three sides and almost concealing him as in a zareba.

I take this opportunity to state that I had no real difficulty in consulting the Secretary and the President when I desired this; the difficulty was to know beforehand when important public health matters—sometimes they arose out of my own minutes— were under discussion between the President and Secretary, and thus to secure a voice in the final discussion before decision. A similar difficulty applied to the Medical Officer's relation to Assistant Secretarial officers. These corresponded to the two or three Assistant Medical Officers in my own department, and these Assistant Secretaries decided matters occasionally without re-reference to me when differences of opinion arose, especially when proposals had been put forward by an Assistant M.O. This general difficulty is discussed on p. 62.

The essential vice of the Local Government Board appeared at its birth, and was a long time in dying. Readers of John Simon's *English Sanitary Institutions* will only need to be reminded of a few inherent administrative errors. As Simon states (p. 355 of the above book), "the new Office started virtually as a continuance of the old Poor-Law Office," its President and Secretaries coming from this source. The fact that these secretaries might act in sanitary business "unlimited by any condition" that these acts "must have the sanction of skilled concurrence" implied a dangerous discretion, and under-lying it appeared to be the assumption that "mere clerkship was meant to be the Office's sanitary strength." Thus secretarial officers formed the inner circle in the Sanitary Councils of the Board, while technical officers, as, for instance, medical and engineering, were left in an outer circle, and their voice might be unheard in the final discussion of problems of administration. There can be no doubt as to the wisdom of Simon's remark:

Reasonable principles would have been, that so far as the Office was to transact sanitary business, and to deal with questions of sanitary policy, the Secretaries and the Medical Officer should be regarded as one consultative body advising the Minister.

Simon resigned in 1876, because of his dissatisfaction with the poor-law-secretarial exclusive management of sanitary affairs, and although the Old Adam was much shrunken when I went to the Board and shrunk still more during my time, one may doubt whether even now adequate arrangements are made for consultations when differences on points of policy arise. The necessity for this ideal of policy applies at each stage of consideration of administrative problems. A recent statement of a Minister of the Crown that scientific advice should "be on tap and not on top" is profoundly foolish. The dictum assumes a relative position which is fanciful. The relation of the secretary to the expert should be that of *primus inter pares*.

THE MEDICAL DEPARTMENT'S WORK

A few paragraphs are needed to indicate the scope of the activities of the Medical Department of the Local Government Board.

During the year ending March 1908–09 the central work of the Local Government Board on its medical side was carried on by Dr. Franklin Parsons and Dr. Bruce Low, the two assistant medical officers of long experience and by myself, with the occasional help of a medical inspector at office. We dealt in that year with some 13,000 papers chiefly relating to current administrative questions.

In addition, day by day, there were numerous interviews with local medical officers of health, and with representatives of local authorities and others seeking counsel concerning difficulties in current local administration.

More formal conferences with local deputations were also numerous by appointment. If the problem was one of hospital construction or housing, one of the Board's architects or other non-medical expert, along with a secretarial officer, would be present, and these conferences constituted one of the most important and influential divisions of the work at the centre. With the development of maternity and child welfare schemes, and of local tuberculosis and venereal work, conferences greatly increased, and there was seen at its best the close relationship between local and central public health work and the co-partnership between secretarial and expert representatives of the Board.

In September of the year 1908, I represented the Government at the Washington International Congress on Tuberculosis, along with Mr. Macdougall, C.B., of the Scottish and Dr. Stafford, C.B., of the Irish Local Government Board. In that year also the late Dr. Theodore Thomson had been in very efficient charge of the international part of the Government's health work, Dr. Darra Mair had been engaged as chairman of a Departmental Committee on the use of intercepting traps in house drains; and in view of the appearance of cholera in Russia, a cholera survey was undertaken throughout the coastline of England by some of the Board's medical staff.

I might continue this annual review for subsequent years: but my annual reports give full details, and I must content myself with the general statement that the medical inspectors were engaged in inquiries directed to the control of epidemic diseases and to the improvement of local sanitary administration, even though by so doing I am obliged to omit or give only scanty reference to much valuable work undertaken by my senior colleagues, of whom Dr. Monckton Copeman, F.R.S., and Dr. S. W. Wheaton still remain, but others have died.

When, too soon after my appointment, Drs. Franklin Parsons and Bruce Low retired, under the official age limit, Dr. Theodore Thomson, C.M.G., became assistant medical officer. He had already done distinguished public health work, especially in international hygiene. His health ere long failed, and his death followed in a later year. He was succeeded by Dr. George Seaton Buchanan, the son of a former medical officer of the Board (p. 34), for whom I had profound admiration; and with him was associated Dr. R. J. Reece, a most painstaking officer, who, like Dr. (afterwards Sir) George S. Buchanan, did distinguished work during the Great War.

Among other colleagues who did distinguished work for the Board, and have since died, was Dr. Ralph Johnstone. He made early investigations on carrier cases of typhoid fever and wrote a report on venereal diseases, which partially anticipated the conclusions subsequently reached by the Royal Commission on Venereal Diseases (p. 156). His life ended prematurely; and the same remark applies to Dr. H. T. Bulstrode. Before 1909 the latter had completed an elaborate review of the tuberculosis and sanatorium problem, written from the earlier somewhat conservative point of view. His reports on the relation of shell-fish to disease and on plague in Suffolk were valuable contributions to public health. (See Chapter xxv of my *Fifty Years in Public Health*.)

I have previously referred to my senior colleagues, Dr. Franklin Parsons and Dr. Bruce Low. They were devoted public servants, both with great knowledge of administration and epidemiology, and their relation to one who came to the office from outside was always cordial.

Reference should be made to the Foods Subdivision of the Medical Department, which had been formed by my predecessor, soon after the revelations as to Chicago meat. It was placed under the charge of Dr. (now Sir) George S. Buchanan, who was followed by the late Dr. MacFadden, C.B. It did much to advance protective health measures as to imported meats and other foods. A mere enumeration of the sanitary inquiries made by the Board's medical inspectors on the efficiency of work by sanitary authorities, on problems of water supply and sewerage, on defective sanitary administration especially in smaller districts, on the carrying out of the vaccination laws, on epidemics of various diseases, and on excessive infant mortality, would occupy many pages, and I cannot attempt it. But it was good work, even though the means for making it effective in local reform were clumsy and only partially successful.

More general inquiries and the greater problems of public health administration will receive fuller notice in subsequent chapters; but inadequate notice of the work in the many branches of the medical inspectors' activities indicated above must not be allowed to create the false impression that this was of poor quality. Reference to my annual reports in which many of the reports of medical inspectors are included will disprove any such view.

REVIEW OF CENTRAL PUBLIC HEALTH WORK

A fuller account of the unavoidable sharing of public health work by several Government Departments is given in my *The Ministry of Health* (Putnams, 1925). Some parts of central public health work are not included in the work of the Local Government Board or its renamed successor the Ministry of Health, and some of these will never be so included. Thus the sanitary work of our Defence Forces must always form part of the general administration of these Forces. Nor is it likely that much of the medical and sanitary work of the Department of Mines as to mines and of the Home Office as to factories, will ever be administered by local health authorities, although both locally and centrally some readjustment is desirable.

The Board of Agriculture and Fisheries again is concerned with health problems, as, for instance, the interrelation between human and animal diseases and the quality of milk and meat supplies. The Board of Trade is concerned with the health of the mercantile marine, and in my time had inadequate skilled advice on these subjects. And in other Government Departments health functions intrude, and only by friendly co-operation with the Ministry of Health can the public welfare be promoted.

But the Local Government Board, since 1871, and the Ministry of Health, since 1919, have been the special Central Health Authority for most purposes. Neither of these names is altogether happy. Their chief merit is their shortness. Necessarily they have both dealt also with administrative problems, which can only indirectly be considered as health problems— finance, order, amenities of life, parks and pleasure grounds, and many others—and these duties as related to central administration could not find a better home.

Since 1919 sickness insurance has come under the administrative care of the Ministry of Health. Non-contributory old-age pensions, payable at age 70, were administered by the Local Government Board from 1908, when they were initiated by Mr. Asquith. They came automatically under the Ministry of Health in 1919. Contributory old-age pensions and widows' and orphans' pensions became law in 1925, and are administered by the Ministry of Health.

Much of the medical work of the Board of Education has already come partially under the Ministry of Health, and this work of the two Departments should be more completely fused (see discussion in Chapter XLI of my *Fifty Years in Public Health*); this fusion has been much more nearly effected for the medical work of local Education Committees.

The preceding instances illustrate the complexity of public health administration. They also point to the conclusion that public health administration can never be completely separated from other problems of central and local administration. A "Parliament" centrally and a general local authority for all public purposes in each large area, with committees for branches of work, constitute the arrangement which best secures that every branch of administration is satisfactorily placed and interrelated.

This is illustrated best of all, and with maximum social importance, in the relationship between Public Health and the Relief of Destitution; and with this subject much of the present volume is concerned.

CHAPTER VI

SECRETARIES AND TECHNICIANS IN THE GOVERNMENT SERVICE

My reading of Simon's *English Sanitary Institutions* had prepared me for such difficulties as I experienced at the Local Government Board. It gradually became clear that the problem was one affecting more or less the whole range of the Government Services; and I propose to set out in this chapter considerations arising from mature consideration and frequent consultations with well-informed officials in other Departments of the civil, military, and naval services. Unfortunately I am unable, for obvious reasons, to fortify my comments by adequate illustrations.

I preface this statement by an expression of my conviction that an impartial and thorough inquiry as to whether in each Government Department the relation between secretarial and technical officers is as conducive to the public interest as it might be made to be, would be more fruitful in public good than any one of the numerous Royal Commissions and Departmental Committees of investigation which have reported on governmental problems. And I would place on that *Committee of Administrative Investigation* men of eminent business capacity not holding any official post, as well as secretarial and expert technical representatives of great local authorities and of the Central Government.

RELATION OF SECRETARIAL TO TECHNICAL STAFF

I use the word technician to denote officials appointed because of their special professional skill in medicine, veterinary medicine, architecture, engineering, and in electrical or other specialist avocations. I omit legal advisers from my review, as every Government Department adopts precautions to protect itself from accusations of acting *ultra vires*, and when there is doubt obtains a special opinion from the Law Advisers of the Crown. I omit also actuaries from my review. The growth of insurance problems has made the work of actuaries extremely

important, and the special actuarial department possesses, I
believe, satisfactory independence. Other technical appointments are made, as those of accountants and auditors, and it
should be added that many of the general secretarial staff of a
Government Department possess technical skill as well as
their general ability on points of policy. To use a municipal
analogy, the clerk of a large city or of a county council and the
clerk of an Education committee can make valuable comments
on the technical as well as on the general-policy aspect of the
problems coming before any committee of the council. But on
the other hand, no self-respecting technician can accept the
assumption which underlies much official procedure, that the
acquisition by long training of his specialist skill has deprived
him of such common sense and business judgment as he previously possessed; and no such technician—unless merely called
in on an isolated technical problem—can be contented to be
regarded merely as an expert, and can be satisfied if he is not, at
least partially, in executive charge of the work for the initiation
of which he was responsible. He is indeed the chief, and may be
the sole available, possessor of the technique needed for successful administration. In public health work this is especially
evident. In local administration the M.O.H. is always entrusted
with the full control of the daily work of his department. Indeed,
years ago I have known instances in which too much executive
work was piled on some M.O.H.s, as for instance the direction of
household scavenging.

THE POSITION OF THE M.O.H. AS AN ADMINISTRATOR

I set out at this point the admirable position of the M.O.H. as a
health administrator (as well as adviser); for this brings out the
contrast between local and central methods of administration.
The difference is especially well seen when a new proposal is
advanced by the M.O.H.; it may be a new departure in disinfection, in hospital provision, in child welfare or anti-tuberculosis
work, or in some other branch of his work. His proposal is
brought before the Public Health or Child Welfare or other
Committee, as the case may be. The Committee comprises a
tenth or more of the total members of the local Parliament or
Council, stiffened perhaps by one or two aldermen, who are

not subject to re-election every third year by the ratepayers. After discussion the proposal is accepted or rejected or postponed. A majority vote of the Committee decides. Before the Committee decides, and especially if legal or financial or other considerations arise, the Town Clerk or County Clerk and the Treasurer or Accountant are heard. These are analogous to the secretariat in Central Government. Thus general policy as well as the technical recommendation of the M.O.H. has an adequate hearing, and no single officer has the last word.

If the M.O.H.'s proposal is rejected by the Committee he may realise that it needs modification; he appreciates that he has had an adequate hearing; and if he is a "bonnie fechter" he knows that after judicious delay he can again put his proposal forward with good hope of success. Every M.O.H. knows that time is an important factor in reform.

But the Committee's positive decision does not determine immediate action. Their approval must be confirmed by a majority of the entire Council; and prior to the meeting of the Council extracts from its agenda are noted in the local Press, and there may be public agitation for or against the M.O.H.'s proposal. The stability of decisions of local councils, except sometimes as regards scales of relief for the necessitous, is evidence of the value of these democratic methods of government. In my view these methods are sound and practical. I say this though sometimes as a M.O.H. I have been fretted by delay in securing reforms on which I had set my heart. Local government depends directly on local public opinion; and the M.O.H. knows that he can only be completely successful in his life-work, when he adds to competence in his specific work the ability to "educate his masters," and to instil into them some of the enthusiasm he himself possesses.

Contrast this with what happens in the taking of decisions on the many technical problems in Central Government. Except by written "minutes," the reading of which for a Parliamentary chief or even for a secretary is a heavy burden, there may be no systematic pooling of experience and knowledge between technicians and secretaries. In my governmental experience office conferences were sometimes held between myself and the secretary or an assistant secretary of the Board;

and there were frequent conferences between one or several members of the medical staff and myself. But conferences between the expert and the secretary, when desirable, were not always held; and the procedure satirically described in the late Lord Sydenham's remarks in a discussion in the House of Lords on anti-bombing precautions, has held good not infrequently in civilian government:

It should be an axiom in government administration that no one should be permitted to have anything to do with any question on which he could not bring special knowledge to bear. This axiom prevailed in all well-managed private businesses. But his own experience, in some Government matters, had been that one had to fight for a necessary improvement through an ascending series of officials, each knowing less than the last, until one reached the deciding authority, who knew nothing at all. This was euphemistically called the "chain of responsibility."

In discussing, in my *The Ministry of Health* (Putnams, 1925), this picture of the "ascending series of officials," I expressed in the following words my modified agreement with Lord Sydenham's criticism, which must have been based on vast experience of Indian and of Army administration:

I would add that not only "special knowledge," but also the critical opinion of the trained non-expert, is necessary before important administrative action is undertaken. Nevertheless, the quotation aptly states the "snowing under" of expert advice which sometimes occurs probably in all Government Departments.

CENTRAL MEDICAL ADMINISTRATION

The quotation from the *Lancet* given on page 31 gives a glimpse of what prior to my appointment had been happening in the Medical Department of the Local Government Board. Although my experience became relatively more favourable, similar difficulties emerged from time to time.

MR. JOHN BURNS'S WORK

Two years before I went on duty, Mr. John Burns had been appointed President of the Board, and his appointment introduced a wholesome and activating breeze from without. The results were soon visible in the Local Government Board. He did not content himself with receiving abstracts of reports and recommendations from various divisions of the Board's work; he was also a frequent visitor in my own room and doubtless in the rooms of other officials.

But even though, as indicated above, there was exceptional activity and some discussion between secretarial and technical officers, I cannot regard the methods of central administration as satisfactory, when I compare them with my experience during more than two decades under local sanitary authorities. Although in many sanitary areas there was often delay in carrying out necessary work, the M.O.H. always had the satisfaction of knowing that delay and opposition to reform occurred only after ample discussion between expert and non-expert officials and between them and the elected representatives of the ratepayers; whereas there was no certain guarantee of similar systematic "exchange of values" in central administration.

I found each President of the Local Government Board under whom I served wishful to give a hearing to professional advice. The difficulty was that the opportunity for this did not arise as often as was desirable, in the absence of the system which I advocate on page 64. The possibility that the President could, if he wished, read my minutes on a given subject, and could, and probably did, hear the Permanent Secretary's account of them is not contradictory of this statement.

As already indicated, the Parliamentary Head of each Department is chosen by the Prime Minister from his own party majority and his duration of office depends on political exigencies. Swapping of offices, apart from electoral misadventures, occurs and an inexperienced Parliamentary Head then replaces one who is relatively experienced. This goes far to explain the great weight which a Permanent Secretary properly exercises in carrying out the national government.

Obviously—I do not speak from personal experience—the Minister may be complaisant and easy-going, accepting the summary of each problem given by his secretary; or he may—as I have experienced—read carefully the minutes giving the technical and non-technical aspects of the particular problem; or he may then—as I happily often found—insist on an interview with the principal medical officer in the presence of his non-technical secretarial adviser. When in major problems the last-named procedure is followed, the technical adviser cannot complain if his proposals are not accepted.

It is not surprising that in hurried circumstances—alas! sometimes when no urgency existed—the last-named action has been neglected; and this fact led me to make the following request at my first interview with Mr. Walter Long, when he became President in 1915. He at once asked me if I had any special wish. My answer was that I had only one: that if any proposal of mine came before him and he was advised secretarially that action was inopportune, he would see me personally before making his decision. He at once promised this, and kept his promise.

Before stating how, by the adoption of the rule stated on page 64, the occasional unsatisfactory position of the technician in government would be remedied, I must attempt further to indicate improvements in procedure needed in the public interest.

DEFECTS IN CENTRAL ADMINISTRATION

The need for improved procedure is not limited to any one Government Department. My personal experience, and evidence collected from various Government offices, showed that an administrative vice existed throughout, though it may be agreed that, with advancing public appreciation of science, the scope of vicious methods has been gradually restricted.

There are obvious difficulties in furnishing illustrations; and as my experience of Government service ended in 1919 it may be assumed that with lapse of time methods have still further improved. I believe this is so; but I doubt if it is even now generally true that the necessary condition for balanced decisions set out on page 64 always holds good. If it does, then the contents of this chapter have historical interest and no more.

I have before me as I write details of lamentable defects due to past neglect of scientific advice in several Government Departments which I have decided not to set out at this point.

An instance of this on an interdepartmental scale occurred

in the preparation and passing through Parliament of the National Insurance Bill, 1911, for which Mr. Lloyd George, then Chancellor of the Exchequer, was responsible. More is given on this in Chapter XIII.

An unsatisfactory position arose in 1871 when the supervision and control of local Boards of Guardians, hitherto exercised by poor-law lay inspectors under the Poor Law Office, was transferred to the Local Government Board, and these inspectors were renamed "general inspectors," and took on much public health supervision in addition to their poor-law work. (On these, see also p. 92.)

The secretariat of the Local Government Board was recruited by examination chiefly from University graduates, who join it in early adult life, and who subsequently had no experience of the various branches of local public services, beyond what is acquired by reading the Board's correspondence and the minutes of their seniors, with occasional interviews with local officials and councillors. They gradually acquired in these ways wide knowledge of what may be called the anatomy of local government, but often without that knowledge of its physiology and pathology which is only acquired by taking part in or inspecting local work. Their experience was primarily paper experience, supplemented by occasional conferences with local delegations; and they were dependent chiefly on the field staff (medical, engineering, lay) of the Department for complete knowledge of local conditions. It is the staff with this lack of experience of local work which was responsible for most ultimate decisions of the Department.

I do not maintain that if this knowledge of local sanitary work and technical skill in it were available in every instance, the result would always be satisfactory; but I have no doubt that the risk of wrong or obstructive decisions would be greatly reduced, as would also the waste of specialised knowledge which has been so serious in the past.

In the final issue, under *any* administrative system of health government there will be relative inefficiency with delay in reform, if on one hand there should be a secretarial staff not interested in or actually inimical to social legislation and administration; and if on the other hand there should arise a chief medical officer of the central department who is ignorant of the health problems concerned in securing advance in public health administration, or who does not trouble to master these problems. Nor will an active and intelligent President entirely compensate for either of these contingencies, though he can do much in that direction. The chief remedy in such circumstances will consist in still further independence of central control in local activity.

In my own experience most instances of neglect of technical advice arose from two factors:

First, there was honest belief, common to many Government Departments, that technical advice is advice which is not to be given until called for by the secretariat who, it is assumed, are entirely competent to decide whether such advice is needed.

Second, when such advice is on record, it is assumed that it can safely be reapplied in what are regarded by the secretariat as analogous circumstances.

When technical advice has been given and is on the "minutes," there is the further occasional great defect that—

Third, the Secretary of the Department, or in major instances its Minister, may decide contrary to expert advice, without having heard personally the statement and arguments of the expert adviser.

Were it practicable to collect the testimony of experts employed in Government Departments there would, I am confident, be general agreement that most of the anomalies and defects of central administration come under the above three headings.

These general statements do not imply disparagement of the secretaries of the central departments of Government. In my own experience it would be difficult to find more courteous, intelligent, and painstaking chief secretaries than the late Sir Samuel Provis, K.C.B., and Sir Horace Monro, K.C.B., with whom I was concerned during my eleven years of official life. But the above-named defects existed, though to a diminishing extent, and will I fear continue in some measure unless the procedure suggested on page 64 is universally adopted.

As regards the first of these causes of unsatisfactory central administration its folly is not unlike that constituted by refusing a sick man medical advice or in addition a skilled medical consultant except at the request of the family lawyer.

As to the second source of official inertia, it will be recalled that a vast number of papers came daily before me and my medical colleagues at office, and that in the settlement of any moot point, a precedent of action in like circumstances in the past was a valuable time-saving provision. By means of such precedents the inconsistencies which so easily arise when a considerable and varying staff are called on to advise on a given problem are minimised. But the use of precedents may be misleading when not backed by the technician's knowledge, giving warning against their use in altered circumstances. I recall an instance of this in hospital administration, in which my attention was drawn to the fact that I had advised contrary to precedents. I answered:

These points do not alter my advice or give any substantial reason for altering my draft letter. . . . But the course of these precedents illustrates very well the unintentional evil resulting from the extension of a precedent, especially an old one, to medical circumstances other than those under consideration when the precedent was established.

To ensure safety in this instance, I had the final draft letter once more referred to me before dispatch. Difficulties under the three headings already enumerated decreased with time, and especially in War circumstances, 1914-18. This was due in part to the widening public appreciation of public health work; but it resulted much more from the fact that during my tenure of office three great additional national medical services were initiated and developed—largely by the aid of Treasury subsidies.

Maternity and Child Welfare Schemes.
The Tuberculosis Medical Service.
The Special Service for Venereal Diseases.

All of these necessarily were medically initiated, Mr. (later Sir) Frederick Willis, C.B., K.B.E., and the staff of his division working cordially with their medical colleagues in the framing and development of these services. Central financial grants to local authorities were given on work done under each heading, and these new services formed good illustrations of the value of combined secretarial and medical administrative skill.

I have mentioned the uniform courtesy of Sir Horace Monro, the Secretary of the Board during the greater part of my tenure of office. I had from the beginning of my official work protested when medical advice that ought to have been called for had not been asked, and when after it had been proffered it had not been acted upon (without re-reference to or consultation with me). In a courteous letter of his sent in answer to my expostulation on a particular omission he said: "I feel sure that there is no intentional ignoring of you or avoidance of reference to you in matters of importance," and he continued that he was anxious to know if some rule could be devised to avoid recurrence of this in future. I answered substantially on the lines set out in the next paragraph.

THE PRACTICAL REMEDY

There still remains the question what I should regard as a satisfactory method of central administrative control, giving due weight to secretarial and technical skill respectively.

My answer is that there should be an approximation toward the methods of the best local authorities. Apart from minor matters no proposal on which medical or other technical advice is given should be disposed of without the Departmental Minister having heard the technician on the subject, *whenever secretarial advice is against the proposal*. This is essential in major problems; and in minor matters the technician should have a personal hearing by the Minister if he (the technician) asks for it. These are the essentials. I am aware that in the formation of the Ministry of Health, its chief medical officer was given secretarial rank; and it has been suggested that this fulfils the needs. In experience it fails of effect, except when the medical officer's recommendations are accepted, if in fact he is not present when important ministerial decisions on medical and public health matters are about to be made. It fails also if in public health and medical matters his contribution as a medical administrator is not heard at the final stage in all instances in which there is secretarial intention to act or to advise contrary to his advice.

In setting out the preceding proposal, I have had in view my own central administrative experience. The arrangements in other departments of central public health administration varied, and doubtless they have gradually become more satisfactory. Through my friend the late Sir Leslie Mackenzie, the medical member of the then Scottish Local Government Board, I heard much that was unfavourable of the working of a Board of three or four, of which he was one; but the circumstances were special, the Parliamentary Head of the Department being in London, while official work was centred in Edinburgh.

In other Government Departments periodical or occasional round-table conferences have been held, in which each officer can explain his own proposals. But if he is not present when subsequently the Parliamentary Head decides *against* his proposal, his due weight in the decision may still be lacking. I have not claimed that the expert's views should preponderate. Other than expert considerations—monetary or political—may call for postponement or rejection of his proposals. All that is claimed is that—as in local official life—his expert views should be adequately expressed up to the moment of decision.

CHAPTER VII

POVERTY IN RELATION TO SICKNESS
THE CHIEF PROBLEM OF PUBLIC HEALTH

IT is difficult for the generation younger than my own to appreciate how far poverty—in the sense of privation of one or more of the necessities of well-being—has been regarded in the past fatalistically or even with complacency as being in the natural order of things. Voluntary charity and the official poor-law organisation have been busy in relieving already existent destitution and its effects; but this assistance has been associated with partial blindness to the possibilities of removing the conditions favouring destitution, still more to the greater possibilities of prevention of its origin. It is in this failure to study means for preventing destitution that there has been the greatest default. It was early sanitary reform, directed specially to the prevention of epidemic diseases, that first opened out one efficient means for reducing poverty and dependence. The etiological conception has now spread over the whole range of destitution with its multiform causation, and first place in bringing about this more general result must be given to the inquiries and reports of the Poor Law Commission, which reported in 1909, and which initiated and compelled extended inquiries as to preventive measures against poverty, and rendered inevitable an organic fusion between official agencies for the prevention and the treatment of sickness, and of destitution however originated. In clearly teaching this doctrine and in compelling uninterrupted action for the prevention of destitution, a specially distinguished place must be given to Mrs. Beatrice Webb.

She was not the only woman member of the Royal Commission on the Poor Laws. Miss Octavia Hill and Mrs. Helen Bosanquet were also on it. They took the individualist point of view, while Mrs. Webb was a Socialist. I had been an admirer of Mrs. Bosanquet's writings, especially her *Strength of the People* (Macmillan, 1902). Miss Hill's equally strong views as to the need to avoid giving help which would tend to undermine individual or family responsibility are well known (see, for instance, p. 164 of my *Fifty Years in Public Health*).

I had myself expressed similar views in a paper written over forty years ago. In this paper I began by stating a sound principle. The family being the unit on the integrity of which the welfare of the community depends, "the question as to what is the most advantageous relationship between it and communal organisations is of prime importance to the social welfare." I committed myself too sweepingly to the view that "when the community has attempted to share or supplement the responsibility of the parent, the practical consequence has been that it has been compelled to assume almost the full burden." This being so the test to be applied in regard to new reforms was, "will the reform tend to weaken or strengthen the bonds of family life?" This evidently was the view for which Miss Hill and Mrs. Bosanquet stood. At the same time I justified public health reforms which diminished family responsibilities in that they were called for in the interest of the community.

I described the Poor Law as "amongst the earliest developments of State Socialism": for

it ensured that no person need die of destitution, and no family need be without medical aid when the bread-winner of the family is moneyless,

Adding a statement of my recently acquired realisation of

the large share which the provision of indoor medical relief in workhouse infirmaries has played in reducing the amount of consumption (phthisis) in England,

I concluded that this indirect benefit to the community, uncontemplated when indoor Poor Law relief was more generally insisted on, illustrated how measures for the benefit of the family and the individual may "in unexpected ways cause even larger aggregate benefit to the community."

After claiming that the early recognition and subsequent treatment of communicable diseases at the cost of the State "constitutes the payment of an insurance premium against the infection of the community with disabling and impoverishing attacks of the same diseases," I asked "may not the same principle be claimed to cover the cases of the non-infectious diseases, which diminish personal efficiency and are likely if long continued to bring a burden on the rates?" Unfortunately, I then regarded acute infectious diseases as in a distinct category, because their occurrence meant immediate risk to the community; and that in other cases of sickness the worker should provide for himself by co-operative means, evidently referring to the medical care given in "sick clubs." Thus in some measure I then endorsed the "deterrent principle" of the Poor Law Act, 1834.

I view with dismay the strict Charity Organisation Society views which I then expressed: but I confess them as illustrating the views then generally held and the rapid emergence from them.

The one sentence in this paper on which I can look back with satisfaction is the following:

> I lay stress on . . . the more permanent and substantial uplifting, which is practicable by means of religious and moral teaching in our schools, and by the teaching in them of domestic economy, cooking, hygiene, thrift, and temperance.

My next attempt to discuss the social economics of destitution was in an inaugural address to the York Medical Society, at its meeting on October 21, 1904, which was published in the *Lancet* of November 12th in the same year. Its subject was "Social Evolution and Public Health." This has already been quoted in my *Fifty Years in Public Health*, page 407. I quote here some comments bearing on the subject of this chapter.

"The health of a community usually varies with the material well-being of its members"; in confirmation of which statement I quoted an analysis made by me of the 1901 census and death returns for each district in London (*British Medical Journal*, March 2, 1902), which showed

> that the order of health of the several districts as measured by their general death-rates and their phthisical death-rates was approximately the same as that of the proportion of houses in each district employing domestic servants.

This I regarded as an index of sanitary circumstances and of social status. I stressed also the truth, that "improved health permits the means of prosperity to be earned and contrariwise failure in health brings a large proportion of the population below the 'poverty line.' "

I emphasised the point that "most poverty is a symptom of disease and not a disease in itself." Historically this confusion between symptoms and disease has been rampant in the practice of medicine, through lack of scientific knowledge; and both medicine and our past social treatment of poverty

illustrate the mischief and the hindrance to real progress which are caused by adopting an empirical treatment of symptoms instead of a scientific treatment of disease.

Prior to 1835 official Poor Law charity meant that in many places subsistence from poor-rates was more easily obtained than by labour. The Act of 1834 secured a severe reversal of earlier policy; but the symptomatic treatment of destitution except in regard to fevers unhappily continued till recent years. In the same address I advocated contributory old-age pensions.

I may pass on to the next stage in my own mental evolution as regards the relation of sickness and poverty. It is illustrated in two papers read by me to two different societies in 1907, and by the evidence which I prepared for the Royal Commission on the Poor Laws. I summarise these here, as showing the development of ideas, in my own mind and I think the evolution in the minds of many others, on this subject.

The interrelation between poverty (destitution) and disease was more intensively studied in these contributions, which showed also an appreciation of the unscientific and incompetent manner in which sickness on a national scale was being treated.

I was especially interested in the interrelation of poverty with tuberculosis and typhus fever, on which more in a later chapter. I devoted my Presidential Address to the Epidemiological Society to this subject at its first meeting in 1907 (it had recently become a division of the Royal Society of Medicine); and quote from the preliminary paragraphs of this address here, as stating much of what I now wish to write on this general subject:

Poverty and disease are allied by the closest bonds, and nothing can be simpler and more certain than the statement that the removal of poverty would effect an enormous reduction of disease,

Adding that:

The diseases which would be reduced by this means include not merely those which physicians treat, but many moral diseases which persist because they are only to be avoided by the poor through the exercise of discipline and self-restraint far beyond what is practised by the average person in classes not subject to poverty.

It was clear that the work of both the central and local guardians of the poor failed in many respects, but especially in those stated in the following extract from my *The Ministry of Health* (Putnams, 1925, p. 163).

Poverty being a symptom complex, it is most important that in every case we should *seek to divide the consideration of poverty into that of its component parts.*

Investigation on these lines enables us to particularise in our preventive efforts, while remaining confident that each set of measures will help towards reducing poverty: it further promotes confidence, which is needed for complete success, in the efforts of others who are devoting themselves to other factors of poverty than the particular one in which we may have special concern.

.   .   .   .

The *importance of a careful analysis* of the circumstances of poverty is particularly great *when sickness accompanies it.* In such a case the interest of the community as well as of the family in question can only be met by sparing no medical or nursing or material assistance which will conduce to early restoration to economic and social efficiency. This point is essential and it is one on which poor law administration in the past has partially failed.

In the 1907 addresses already quoted I admitted that although Public Health activities had reduced poverty and would as they became more efficient reduce it even more, especially when they included medical aid for the sick,

there will still remain a cruel residuum which can be attacked in no other way than by the removal of poverty, or by the removal from poverty of the elements of personal privation which affect the public health.

And at this point I emphasised what has always impressed my mind:

in prophylaxis it is supremely important to know the relative value of every weapon that is available against disease.

The remainder of this Presidential Address was concerned chiefly with the contrasted historical experience in England and in Ireland of typhus fever and tuberculosis, as illustrating the need for such specific measures against illness as are best calculated to produce the greatest effect in reducing both poverty and sickness.

Before summarising what I wrote in 1907, I may make the following further remarks.

Destitution evidently has a varied causation. It may be the result of misfortune, and this again may be caused by moral incapacity or idleness associated commonly with ignorance. It is still oftener the result of economic evils for which the sufferer is totally irresponsible; and until old-age pensions were given on a national scale, destitution was the common lot as age advanced.

But apart from unemployment and underemployment and unpensioned old age, sickness is the most abundant cause of destitution, either by disabling or killing the wage-earner, or by weighing him down with expenditure beyond his means.

This was fully realised by Edwin Chadwick and Southwood Smith. They directed their attention to the prevention of the devastating "fever" rampant in their time. It was not until the earlier years of the twentieth century, however, that there was general practical realisation of the fact that sickness, whatever its causation, is a general and terribly prevalent cause of poverty.

Among sicknesses "clearly phthisis is the most convenient mirror of poverty" (Niven). I may quote here Niven's further dictum—which coincides with my own experience—that "the relatively high incidence of phthisis in males in Manchester is, for the most part, not due to the housing conditions." The difference between Niven's opinion and mine in regard to phthisis in the poor consisted in the greater importance attached by me to the segregation of consumptives during a large part of their sputum-discharging lifetime, and the greater importance attached by him to malnutrition as favouring phthisis. Whether prevention results from improved nutrition or from diminution of the opportunities for spread of infectious discharges, or whether—as alone is wise—we assume that both are important, the conclusion is reached that poverty and tuberculosis are very closely associated.

In the year 1907 I had already become convinced that in the interest of the community and as a means of preventing both poverty and continued sickness, *free medical aid should be given at the communal expense to all who lacked it*. The first draft of my views on this subject was given in opening a discussion on Free Medical Aid to the Brighton Problem Club on May 14, 1907. They are also set out in a Presidential Address given in the section of State Medicine at the Annual Meeting of the British Medical Association at Exeter in July of the same year. The title of the address was "The Co-ordination of the Public Medical Services" (*British Medical Journal*, September 14, 1907). In this address I emphasised the point that each year the scope of preventive medicine becomes wider; for it is concerned not only with the prevention of infection, but also with the removal of the conditions favouring infection; and its scope is not even thus limited, for its ultimate scope must include any disease or stage of a disease which can be prevented, or its duration curtailed. In this paper I do not appear to have gone beyond this: though elsewhere I emphasised the importance of the physiological side of hygiene, and also of efficient treatment of all diseases.

I placed on record once more my conviction that in the relation of poverty and disease, "disease much oftener causes poverty than poverty disease."

That poverty and disease work on each other in a vicious circle is obvious. But this circle has the quality of its defect, for the circle can be broken at any point; and the practical problem for us is that of the means by which it may be possible to stop people from becoming poor by preventing them from becoming sick. I do not say that this is the only way in which the problem of poverty can and ought to be attacked. But it is a way which has not received the attention that it deserves, and will yield a higher and a quicker return for the energy and money required than others which at present are more in the public eye.

This address at Exeter was important, because my views were, I think, representative of the growing enlightenment of the medical profession and of its public health members, and these views had further importance in view of my promotion a year later to the chief position in the Government Medical Service.

I then recited some of the chief forms of communal provision against disease, by official and voluntary agencies. I cannot afford space to give full quotations; but must content myself with a mere enumeration of some of the many directions in which the State was already making medical provision. This enumeration relates to the year 1907; it would now need to be greatly expanded. Each local authority provided gratuitous isolation accommodation for the chief infectious diseases, arranged for gratuitous disinfection, and there was some medical inspection of contacts. The M.O.H. often acted as a gratuitous consultant in infectious diseases. Diphtheria antitoxin, both as a prophylactic and as a curative agent, was beginning to be provided gratuitously for doctors. Occasionally nurses were being supplied to help in infectious cases treated at home. Some local authorities had begun to train and treat cases of pulmonary tuberculosis, and provide spit-cups and handkerchiefs for patients. Free bacteriological diagnosis of tuberculosis, diphtheria, and typhoid fever was being given. Some local authorities paid the fees of doctors called in by midwives. Gratuitous primary vaccination was available for the entire population. Workhouse infirmaries were becoming State hospitals for many forms of disease. Already some school doctors had been appointed, and treatment given for scholars suffering from contagious skin diseases. A few authorities had started municipal milk depots.

The above enumeration does not include the vast amount of treatment being given in voluntary or charitable hospitals. Evidently patients were being provided with medical treatment to a rapidly increasing extent at the expense of the State, the rates, or some other non-personal organisation, and I urged that it was important to consider whether the expense thus incurred gave a satisfactory return. The necessary test was that the return of service for expenditure should be the maxi-

C*

mum possible; and judged by this standard, and whether viewed from the standpoint of patients, of the medical practitioner, or of the public health, "the present state of medical service must be condemned as inefficient. Unhappily a far less exacting standard would exhibit its insufficiency and its extravagance."

I particularly stressed the difficulties of medical practitioners. I said:

Doctors have never been doing so much and such good work on behalf of the public as at present; but this work is being done under conditions involving the petty worries of fee-collecting, the stress of competitive commercialism, the strain of work which for most doctors is excessive in order to secure a "living wage," and the "sweating" of the medical profession by hospitals, friendly societies, and similar organisations. The doctor earning his livelihood among the artisan and labouring classes not only has to do excessive work under harassing conditions without leisure, but he is in a large measure cut off from consultation with doctors having special knowledge in the very considerable proportion of complicated cases which come under his care. To the patient in the same classes the conditions are equally unsatisfactory. His limited means necessitate delay in obtaining medical aid until compelled by urgent symptoms, and necessitate dispensing with this aid at the earliest possible moment.

I concluded by citing some of the principal respects in which failure occurred:

1. *Diagnosis is belated.* This is inevitable for the largest proportion of the population under circumstances which involve payment of a fee or seeking for a hospital letter, and then waiting several hours in an out-patient department. The dangers of delaying diagnosis are too well known to need detailed consideration.

2. *Treatment is curtailed* and its efficiency diminished by similar considerations of expense.

3. When patients are treated under present circumstances in dispensaries and in out-patient departments the *waste of time* involves a serious economic loss to the community.

4. There are no co-ordinated arrangements for *medical consultations* in all difficult cases.

5. *Valuable information as to the incidence of disease* is wasted under the present conditions of medical service. . . .

6. There is *a great waste of information as to the existence of conditions conducing to disease* which might promptly be removed under more systematised conditions of medical attendance.

The position evidently was transitional. That it rapidly became less unsatisfactory is shown by the initiation of the school medical service, of the insurance medical service for a third of the population, and of the special medical services for maternity and children, for tuberculosis and venereal diseases, and lastly in 1929 by the provision made for transfer of the medical work of Boards of Guardians to the public health committees of the largest Public Health Authorities.

But the position in 1907 justified my statement that:

At the present time the co-existent but unco-ordinated systems have failed lamentably to provide what the health of the community requires—means for ensuring effectively the early recognition and proper treatment of all disease.

I added my belief that "what had been done already towards securing this end is merely a phase in the evolution of the system which will attain it ultimately."

I am glad to be able to add a further quotation, indicative of an improved personal vision.

I see no reason to expect that such a medical service, whether partial or general, would tend to deprave any part of the community morally, any more than the system of free (that is tax-paid) education has tended to pauperise the parents of the children who benefit by it. There would be, I think, no difficulty in proving that each additional form of medical aid officially given up to the present time, so far from undermining self-help, has imposed new duties and responsibilities on the recipients of such help; while in the aggregate these measures have been largely instrumental in securing the immense improvement in the public health already realised.

It will be convenient to state later the evidence I gave before the Royal Commission on the Poor Law (p. 87).

CHAPTER VIII

THE INCREASING HUMANITY OF DESTITUTION AUTHORITIES

As an interested observer of the progress towards replacing the conception of relief of those already necessitous by the higher conception of the prevention of destitution, it devolves on me to sketch the administrative changes as I saw them, which resulted from the altered viewpoint, illustrated in Chapter VII. In doing so, I must go somewhat further back in history. The essential difference consists in a partial—even now not complete —change from what with some exaggeration may be described as post-mortem or post-sickness first aid, and the work of the physician and the hygienist who seek to curtail as well as alleviate existing illness, and still more aim at preventing its occurrence or recurrence.

EARLIER EFFORTS TO RELIEVE

It is undesirable, I think, to inveigh against those who in these earlier days were mere alleviators. All of our predecessors were alleviators, and some of our contemporaries are still so; and the change in our attitude towards destitution and sickness is part of the advance in sanitary education, and in the wider realisation of cause and effect, which has come with increasing knowledge of the laws of life and health. This increased knowledge has embraced more humane economics and a higher moral standard with a more tender social conscience as well as the increased application of physiological science and better sanitation and housing.

The change can be followed in the Reports of many medical officers of health, of the Royal Commission on the Poor Laws, and more clearly in Sidney and Beatrice Webb's writings, especially in their *English Poor Law History*, 1929, which is utilised in this elementary sketch.

RETREAT FROM THE "PRINCIPLES OF 1834"

Gradually the rigid conditions of poor-law relief initiated by the Poor Law Amendment Act, 1834, were relaxed, as humanity and increasing medical knowledge demanded; and from 1871 when the Local Government Board was formed, and public health and poor-law concerns became contiguous in one central though bifurcated supervising authority, changes and some improvement became visible. Although I am chiefly concerned in the gradual medical ameliorations which occurred, it is impracticable to separate these from other branches of poor-law administration.

With the increasing departure from the rigid system of Poor Law administration, the relief work of Boards of Guardians was supplemented to an increasing extent by relief work undertaken by voluntary bodies and by statutory authorities other than the Poor Law, and especially by the help in sickness given by voluntary hospitals and dispensaries. This was seen especially in dealing with unemployment. In 1886 Mr. Joseph Chamberlain, then President of the Local Government Board, emphasized the need for providing paid employment for able-bodied persons out of work, not by Boards of Guardians, but by municipalities, and in subsequent years similar efforts by these two local bodies acting in concert were urged by later Presidents of the Board.

The position of the children of the necessitous became more and more a subject of anxiety. Poor-law schools were made separate from workhouses, and "scattered homes" began to replace the "barrack schools." The treatment of the sick is dealt with later. The treatment of the old and infirm became gradually more humane, though most of these continued to be massed in workhouses and infirmaries. In earlier years they were compelled to come into these institutions; but in 1896, Mr. Chaplin, then President of the Local Government Board, sent a circular to Guardians reminding them of the recommendations of the Royal Commission on the Aged Poor to the effect that:

in the administration of relief there should be greater discrimination between the respectable aged who become destitute and those whose destitution is distinctly the consequence of their own misconduct,

the former being given home relief, when they lived under decent conditions.

For the old in workhouses "deterrent discipline" was gradually withdrawn. Thus a weekly screw of tobacco might be allowed, it was centrally said in 1892. In 1894 the property qualification of a member of a Board of Guardians was removed, and this, it was said by a conservative official, "opened wide the door to the demagogic dispensation of relief." For other inmates of workhouses dietetic improvements appeared in the General Order of 1900, and even earlier, sanitation and cleanliness, clothing, and some efforts at classification of inmates received attention. These items give but a faint indication of the spirit of mercy and pity, of human regard, that was gradually finding an entry between the rigid ribs of official deterrence. That the "principles of 1834" were in partial flux was seen also in the very varying degree of rigidity in union regulations in different parts of the country. Although theoretically it continued to be assumed that the recipient of relief must be less favourably circumstanced than the labourer engaged in actual daily work, this began to be subject to the condition that certain minima of tolerable life must be given.

In 1904 the direction of public opinion was clearly shown by the passage of the Medical Relief Disqualification Act, which excepted medical relief from electoral disqualifications. In the same year also it was enacted that Guardians in giving relief were not to take into account sums up to five shillings received from a Friendly Society by the recipient of relief.

For the sick, for children, and for aged persons in particular less severe conditions were imposed than for others requiring relief. When the Royal Commission on the Poor Law was appointed in 1905, the problems with which Boards of Guardians were concerned had become also the concern of other Local Authorities, especially of Sanitary Authorities and School Boards; while voluntary hospitals and other voluntary agencies continued to busy themselves in supplementing the blanks left by official charity.

Chaos of administration naturally followed on this diversity of effort; agencies of relief overlapped and yet serious omissions to meet the needs of misery and reduce its amount continued to exist. The elements of chaos can best be realised by reading the account of the investigations and the reports of the Royal

Commission on the Poor Law, but the summary in the last chapter of my paper written in 1907 shows that, especially on the medical side, the vast overlapping and the still gaping hiatus in provisions for the welfare of the necessitous were already being realised. The doctrine of *laisser-faire* had steadily declined in favour, and the sentiment gained impetus that even public efforts which might tend to inhibit personal endeavour were preferable to doing nothing to relieve social misery.

But until these influences became very effective, an earlier statement made by me was approximately accurate: "The ideal of poor-law relief is to do as little as possible, as late as possible, and for as short a time as possible."

CHAPTER IX

THE INVESTIGATIONS AND REPORTS OF THE
ROYAL COMMISSION OF 1905-9

REASONS FOR THE ROYAL COMMISSION

The appointment of the Royal Commission on the Poor Law in December 1905 by a Conservative Government, shortly before its sensational defeat at the hustings, was an event of great importance. Royal Commissions have sometimes been a device for shelving for awhile remedial action in respect of a crying evil, but not in this instance. The object was to secure a thorough examination and display of the problems concerned. Such an examination prevents hasty legislation, based on inadequate knowledge, and public opinion—without which laws are apt to be still-born—is educated and prepared for action.

When this Royal Commission was appointed, there was widespread dissatisfaction with the work of Boards of Guardians, and especially with their care of aged persons and young children. The medical services they supplied were disliked, and the poor often accepted them only when their need was extreme; and even when efficient medical help was available in more enlightened areas it was not fully utilised. The bad odour in which poor-law provision was held must have been an important factor in inducing the Prime Minister, Mr. Balfour, to appoint the Commission. This bad odour was persistent and insistent, and when Mr. Lloyd George's Insurance Bill was under discussion, the medical institutions of Boards of Guardians were specially excluded from use for providing Sanatorium Benefit for the tuberculous insured, except to a partial extent in London. In London, hospital provision was under the Metropolitan Asylums Board, and this treatment was expressly stated by statute not to be parochial or pauper relief. This political necessity meant that a great public health possibility of hospital reform had been missed.

The existence of two schools of thought on relief of the necessitous was another reason for the appointment of the Royal Commission. On one side activities within and outside the Poor Law to maintain those out of work, to aid the aged, and to provide for children, and especially the sick, were often regarded as undermining the manliness and self-reliance of the nation; while on the other side the inadequacy of these attempts to alleviate distress, and the need for greater and better co-ordinated activity both within and without the scope of the Poor Law, was becoming widely appreciated.

DEVELOPMENT OF ITS INQUIRIES

But whatever the motives leading to the appointment of the Royal Commission, an exhaustive investigation of methods of relief was carried out by it; and, what was even more important, the inquiries of the Commission led up to an investigation of the causal factors in human misery, and an attempt to establish prevention as the ideal, and not merely to continue the allevia-tion of already established misery.

Two elaborate reports were published in 1909 by the Royal Commission, and it is regrettable that the recommendations common to the Majority and the Minority Report did not form the subject of early legislation. Had this been secured, more complete and more secure medical treatment under the National Insurance Act, 1911, would have been available, and the creation by this last-named Act of one more independent medical service—in addition to the medical services under Boards of Guardians, Public Health Authorities, and School Authorities—would have been avoided. Only very partial legislation resulted from the work of the Poor Law Commission prior to 1929.

COMPETING MEDICAL SERVICES

The evidence given before the Poor Law Commission was supremely interesting. Both reports brought out the facts that the "principles of 1834" had been more and more discarded, and that there had grown up "an array of competing public services." These competing services may be said to have had one object in common, to prevent the misery and destitution which ends in pauperism: whereas the Poor Law as it worked, waited for destitution and then proceeded to alleviate its results, with an uncertain admixture of curative, especially medical curative, effort at this advanced stage of misery.

The Majority Report was signed by the Chairman, Lord

George Hamilton, by Sir Samuel Provis, and Sir Henry Robinson, secretaries respectively of the English and Irish Local Government Boards, by Mr. Patten-Macdougall, c.b., a member of the Scottish Local Government Board, also by Sir Henry Davy of the English Board; by Miss Octavia Hill and Mrs. Helen Bosanquet, and by Rev. L. R. Phelps, Mr. F. H. Bentham, Sir C. S. Loch, secretary of the Charity Organisation Society, and Mr. T. Hancock Nunn (the last named with a reservation pressing for increased and more systematic use of voluntary agencies for social service); the Minority Report was signed by Mrs. Sidney Webb, Mr. Chandler, Mr. Lansbury, and Rev. Russell Wakefield, afterwards Bishop of Birmingham.

The evidence heard before the Commission, as it appeared in the Press, deeply interested me; and in particular I was soon concerned in contributing to the volume of evidence on "sickness as a cause of pauperism," which gathered like a snowball, and on which Mrs. Sidney Webb, a member of the Commission, concentrated her wonderful energy. Special inquiries by selected sub-commissioners were organised by the Commission itself, and the members of the Commission found themselves "more and more minimising lax Poor Law administration as the main cause of pauperism." Very wisely the inquiry ceased in large measure to be one into the causes of pauperism (in the official sense), and became one into the causes of destitution. And out of the inquiry came an increasing urge for Old Age Pensions, which were given in 1908, on the initiation of Mr. Asquith.

UNCONDITIONAL HOME RELIEF

One great result of the Commission's inquiries was the revelation of the vast amount of relief which was being given to the necessitous in their homes, without any attempt to regulate unsatisfactory though remediable conditions of life. No attempt was being made to raise either the material or the moral condition of the recipients of relief. Dr. J. C. McVail, a medical officer of health of high repute, appointed by the Royal Commission as a special medical investigator, said:

the worst kind of public policy is that under which an Authority representing a community confers personal benefits without any accompanying requirement of good order or obedience.

And after giving a number of medical illustrations he concluded—

it is not worth while entering on any reform of the Poor Law unless this policy is changed. Beneficiaries must be compelled to obedience alike in their own and in the public interest. (Appendix, Vol. xiv, Report of R.C. on Poor Law.)

But the medical aspect of the Commission's inquiry must be given a whole chapter to itself (p. 87).

Before stating the medical side of the Report it is convenient to summarise here the Majority and Minority conclusions of the Royal Commission.

The summary given in the reports is too long to be given in full, and I therefore utilise and quote the summary prepared by Sidney and Beatrice Webb (*English Local Government. Part II: The Last Hundred Years*, 1929), which is quoted by them from a statement by Sir C. S. Loch, who for many years was the head of the Charity Organisation Society, and a signatory of the Majority Report.

SUMMARY OF MAJORITY REPORT

"The Commission aim at unity in the administration of relief." They deprecated the new separate existence of various forms of statutory relief, as for instance for unemployed workmen and in the provision of meals for school children.

They desired the provision of large means of variation in the treatment of the destitute, with separate provision for the unemployed, for the aged, the sick, and others.

They urged a change in administrative machinery, making the county or county borough the area for institutional treatment and for the general supervision. Thus:

1. The treatment of the poor applying for public assistance should be adapted to the needs of the individual.

2. There should be co-operation between public administration for relief and local and private charities.

3. Public assistance should include processes of help which would be preventive, curative, and restorative.

4. The instincts of independence and self-maintenance of the assisted should be encouraged by steady effort.

It was proposed also:

1. That out-relief should, except in sudden emergencies be given only after thorough inquiry;

2. That it should then be adequate for the needs of those receiving it;

3. That the persons assisted should be supervised, and the case-paper system should be everywhere adopted for this purpose, the purview to include the moral and sanitary conditions under which the recipient is living, and voluntary agencies being utilised as far as possible for this purpose.

This meant that Outdoor (that is, home) Relief would thus become conditional.

An increase in the staff of central inspectors was recommended; and a Public Assistance Committee of the County or County Borough Council was to undertake the main work, the *ad hoc* elected Board of Guardians being abolished. It was recommended that half the members of the Public Assistance Committee should be "persons qualified for membership on the ground of experience," and chosen from outside the ranks of members of the Council.

In large measure these recommendations amounted to a denunciation of a deterrent Poor Law.

SUMMARY OF MINORITY REPORT

The Minority Report was based on a consideration of "the dominant facts of the situation" which may be thus summarised from their report.

(1) There is overlapping confusion and waste owing to the relief of the poor being undertaken in the same district by two, three, or even four local authorities, as well as by voluntary agencies.

(2) This unco-ordinated rivalry of indiscriminate, unconditional, and gratuitous provision is producing demoralisation of character and slackening of personal effort.

(3) Means for securing prevention or cure of distress should replace in so far as practicable mere relief.

It evidently was impracticable to oust the various specialised local authorities which had grown up since the Boards of Guardians were established, and "there remained only the alternative . . . of completing the process of breaking up of the Poor Law, which had been going on for the last three decades."

This meant that, leaving out the treatment of vagrants or able-bodied, the provision for

(a) Children of school age;

(b) The sick and permanently incapacitated, children under school age, and the aged needing institutional treatment;

(c) All mental defectives; and

(d) The aged to whom pensions are awarded should be removed out of the Poor Law and given to Committees of the County and County Borough Councils, namely:

(a) The Education Committee,
(b) The Health Committee,
(c) The Asylums Committee,
(d) The Pensions Committee, respectively.

The Minority recommended the establishment of a national authority for the unemployed, and this was carried partially into effect by the National Insurance Act, 1911, which was on a contributory basis.

The proposals of the Royal Commission, imperfectly summarised above, included a unanimous recommendation that larger authorities should be entrusted with the administration of relief, the Boards of Guardians being abolished. The need for prevention as well as amelioration of symptoms was acknowledged, and the Commission (the Minority more than the Majority) endorsed the relaxation of inhibitory conditions for relief which successive Presidents of the Local Government Board under public pressure had already initiated. This, as is remarked in Sidney and Beatrice Webb's work (op. cit., p. 548),

fundamentally came back to the discovery by Charles Booth that, although the Poor Law Statistics might register only two or three per cent (of the population) as applying for Poor Relief in any one year, as many as thirty per cent of the total population were always living under conditions that involved the majority of this considerable section passing, at one or other period of their lives, at least temporarily into the pauper class.

Thus without, as well as within, the usual purview of the Poor Law Authorities, there was a vast mass of social misery —always present though in varying bulk—which needed scientifically applied amelioration before the help of the Poor Law Authorities was at last sought. Such help might in some respects then be characterised as belated ambulance work, for its prevailing characteristic was that it began when little more than palliation was possible.

A few months ago I read the life of the late Canon Samuel Barnett of Toynbee Hall (see Vol. ii, p. 286) and can appreciate and endorse his expression of appreciation of the Royal Commission's Report. The whole report, he said, was "an answer to disbelievers in progress"; and he further emphasised—as I have always felt should be done—that the points of agreement between the Majority and Minority Reports were more striking than their points of disagreement. Both reports agreed that Boards of Guardians as hitherto constituted as *ad hoc* bodies should be abolished; that relief for the sick, for children, and for the infirm and old should be adequate; and that adequate preventive and remedial measures should be taken to remedy the unsatisfactory position of vagrants and of the unemployed.

CHAPTER X

MEDICAL CARE UNDER THE POOR LAW

RESUMING discussion of the relation between Poverty and Sickness, which in Chapter V I have described as the central problem in Public Health, I propose to discuss it in this chapter as an administrative problem; continuing and expanding what has already been written in the latter part of Chapter VII.

Like some other medical officers of health I was asked to prepare a draft of the evidence I was prepared to give before the Royal Commission on the Poor Law. On April 9, 1907, I received a printed copy of my proposed evidence which now lies before me. It has been published in one of the Appendices of the Report of the Royal Commission. I was not called to give evidence until February 3, 1908, the day before I was due to commence my new duties as Principal Medical Officer of the Local Government Board. In view of my prospective altered position, I had written to and subsequently conferred with Mr. John Burns, President, and Sir Samuel Provis, Secretary, of the Board, as to whether it was still open to me to give evidence based on my statement already in print and in the possession of the members of the Commission. At this Conference it was left to me to decide, and I then wrote to Mr. Burns that I would present myself for examination, while stating that if any modification arising from new official knowledge were called for, this would be intimated to the Commission. The need for this did not arise. My evidence followed the lines already indicated on pages 70 *et seq.*, and I need only quote a few sentences.

In every branch of medical practice among the poor the arrangements for diagnosis are wholly insufficient. . . . Similar remarks apply as to belated and inadequate treatment. The conclusion at which I have arrived is that it is impossible under any practical or conceivable application of the existing systems (of administration) to secure complete co-operation, to prevent overlapping, and to provide medical aid which shall be "generally sufficient for the health of the community"; while the wider application of the

principles of preventive medicine would enable this to be done. . . .
*It is in the highest degree desirable that the existing medical services,
together with additions . . . should be placed under one control . . .*

It seems to me necessary for the maximum economy, as well as
efficiency, that *every man should have the right to call for gratuitous
diagnosis, treatment, and provision of medicine*. . . . The real difference
between this system and that towards which our institutions seem
trending of their own accord at the present time is the provision of
gratuitous treatment; and from the standpoint of preventive medicine
that provision is an essential part of the needs of the public health.

At the time when the above paragraphs were written, contributory sickness insurance with medical attendance had not
appeared above the horizon as a half-way house.

I added that I assumed that

medical aid is to be regarded as entirely separate from other aid,
thus avoiding altogether in my belief the possible demoralising
effect of gratuitous relief.

I further emphasised that the recipients of medical aid should
not be passive in their acceptance of advice and treatment:
there should be demanded from them

habits of life and even sacrifices of personal taste in the interest of
the health of the community, their families and themselves, which
would leave them conscious of a sensible discharge of duty in return
for the attention which they received . . . Such a system would
require the medical aid to be in the hands of the public health
department, while the poor-law function of the Board of Guardians
might be taken over by the Municipality, perhaps with co-opted
members, as in the case of the Education Committee.

I yield to the temptation of adding a further quotation from
my evidence, which it will be seen foreshadowed in some
respects the governmental action taken in the year 1929.

The public health department would take over the present parochial medical officers . . . All new district medical officers should
be required to be trained in public health as well as in clinical
medicine. In small districts the district medical officer would likewise be the medical inspector of scholars, in larger districts these
medical officers would be separate; but their work would be co-
ordinated by the medical officer of health, and the information

obtained by either would be at the disposal of the other. The work-house infirmary buildings would be utilised in most cases as municipal hospitals.

To complete this personal aspect of evidence before the Poor Law Commission, I should add that when I assumed my work at the Local Government Board I found an outstanding reference from the Royal Commission to the Board's medical officer desiring his opinion on the question which had been raised as to

whether the powers and duties of Poor Law Guardians in connection with medical relief should be severed from those in connection with ordinary relief and transferred to the existing sanitary authorities.

The phrase "existing sanitary authorities" tied my hands to some extent in the memorandum (quite separate from my evidence already submitted) which I then prepared; for it was notorious that many of the smaller sanitary authorities which had been allowed to be created were hopelessly inefficient. I pointed out that sanitary authorities included bodies charged with the health of as few as 219 and of more than 700,000 persons.

I stated, however, that there was no inherent impracticability in the suggestion to unify the medical services for the poor, and I gave reasons for concluding that the present division of medical duties was gravely mischievous to public health.

Writing of the evidence given by many poor-law medical officers and medical officers of health Sidney and Beatrice Webb (op. cit., p. 514) said:

The evidence of these medical witnesses transformed the outlook of the Commission.

This evidence went far to disprove the contention advanced in favour of rigid poor-law administration that medical relief was "the first step to pauperism." Dr. McVail, in his protracted inquiry, could not find an instance in which pauperism began as out-medical relief. The evidence disproved the pernicious notion, still applied until recent years in much of the poor-law medical service, that the treatment of the sick poor should continue to be inferior to and less merciful than that for others. I had no difficulty in testifying that the giving of medical aid to the poor patient "has undoubtedly increased the patient's duties and responsibilities." (Appendix to R.C. Report. Vol. IX.)

Dr. McVail had been specially appointed by the Commission to report generally on conditions of medical relief, and his evidence was convincing.

He described poor-law medical relief as

a cripple supported on two crutches, the general (voluntary) hospitals on one side and gratuitous medical work (by private practitioners) on the other,

and had no doubt that the whole system would break down if it were not thus supported.

He especially emphasised the need for making monetary relief conditional, giving many illustrations, the purport of which can be gathered from the following enumeration—delirium tremens, gonorrhoea in a prostitute, child-birth of a feeble-minded mother, a case of consumption in a crowded home.

The medical treatment given by Boards of Guardians was partly domiciliary, partly institutional. There was a parochial medical officer for each parish or union. In England they numbered over 3,400, and the standard of medical work varied greatly. It was practically unsupervised and uncontrolled, and it had fallen into disrepute, relatively few of the poor availing themselves of it. On the other hand, the outpatient departments of voluntary hospitals and dispensaries were commonly crowded.

The institutional treatment of the sick poor varied enormously in quality. In a few large towns it was of high quality; more generally poor-law infirmaries were inadequately staffed, nursing was unsatisfactory, and there was a dearth of skilled consultatants, or they were entirely lacking.

The work of the medical staff of these institutions at the time the Royal Commission reported was almost completely unsupervised. This is the more astonishing, because in questions of finance and of general administration all forms of relief were rigidly controlled by the Local Government Board. The position as regards central medical inspection of poor-law work at that time is given in Chapter XI.

DIFFICULTIES IN INITIATING ORDERLY REFORM

In my critical remarks in Chapter VI on the relation between secretarial and technical (especially medical) officials in central administration, I did not discuss the difficulties arising from supervision of medical work by laymen. In this chapter, which deals with several similar problems, this difficulty is considered historically. It is important, because of the obstructive influence on progress in public health administration exercised by this undue lay supervision in the past.

THE BOARD'S GENERAL INSPECTORS

When I entered the Government service, as already indicated, some unsatisfactory arrangements dating from 1871 existed, the year in which the Local Government Board took over public health work from the Privy Council and poor-law work from the secretarially much better organised Poor Law Board. The eyes and ears of the Local Government Board were a staff of general inspectors transferred from the old Poor Law Office. These were intermediaries and interpreters to Boards of Guardians of the will of the Board, and, beyond this, they exercised a beneficent influence on the Guardians by controlling extravagance and guiding good general management.

It could not be expected that they would secure satisfactory administration in all districts; nor would any inspector appointed by the Government have had full success. But these general inspectors were open to Simon's weighty criticism that the Board in its iron control over the finance and general administration of Boards of Guardians, always "relied very unduly on the sufficiency of non-medical officers in these relations."

There were two medical poor-law inspectors, one (Dr. Fuller) for the whole of provincial England, and one, Dr. (afterwards Sir) Arthur Downes for the metropolis. They were physically unable to accomplish the gigantic amount of medical inspection crying aloud to be done: and their activities were further sterilised by the fact that, expecially in the provinces, the medical inspector visited poor-law medical institutions chiefly when such a visit was asked for by the general inspector of that particular area. Imagine this! It is difficult to suggest an illustration which will bring out the absurdity of the situation; but it may be compared to a patient who requires a skilled consultant, this consultant only being called in when the family lawyer has decided that this help shall be sought.

Sir Arthur Downes was a member of the Royal Commission on the Poor Law, and signed the Majority Report, but he appended a memorandum dissenting from the Majority and the Minority Reports, in their proposal to hand over the administration of relief to the largest public health authorities. He urged the retention of *ad hoc* relief authorities, and suggested that existing poor-law units should be grouped rather than that county and county boroughs should become the units of administration. Some such grouping of Relief Areas would have been desirable, but subject to the condition that each of them would be administered by a committee under the County Council for all the Areas in a given county.

DUAL MEDICAL INSPECTORATE

In May 1909, I was instructed by the President of the Local Government Board to report on the recommendations of the Poor Law Commission so far as they could be carried out without legislation "in matters affecting the Medical Department," and I give here a summary of a memorandum prepared by me in that month.

It will be remembered that when appointed my functions had been limited as set out on p. 27, so the instruction to report on this subject may be regarded as indicating the Board's willingness to consider the abolition of its dual medical arrangements. The following pages paraphrase some parts of my memorandum.

The memorandum was in two parts, the first giving the results of my study of the Royal Commission on the Poor Laws, and the second setting out the past views and policy of the Local Government Board in regard to medical inspections to be undertaken by it.

The Royal Commission emphatically disapproved of the almost

complete lack of expert inspection of poor-law institutions, and the absence of inspection, either lay or medical, of the conditions of domiciliary relief. Dr. McVail in his report to the Royal Commission also strongly urged the need for regular and systematic inspection by medical inspectors from the Local Government Board of all local indoor and outdoor medical relief.

As regards the past attitude of the Board itself to this subject, I found that so long ago as January 10, 1873, Sir J. Lambert, then Secretary of the Board, quoted with approval the following extract from the Report of the Royal Sanitary Commission:—

"We deprecate the maintenance of parallel inspectorates of Sanitary and Poor Law Administration under the same chief minister, not only on the ground of waste of powers, but still more of probable conflict,"

and Sir John commented that Poor Law medical questions should, according to his view, be remitted to the Medical Officer of the Board.

He urged, furthermore, that in the medical business in connection with poor-law administration he did not see how the Board could avoid resorting to the Medical Department for all such assistance as they might require; and he commented on Mr. Simon's position which, as stated by Sir J. Lambert, was one of treating this business as foreign to what should devolve upon him. [It appears to me that Lambert shared the erroneous view that a medical man, because he is a medical man, must be competent to advise on *any* medical problem. This view is still a long time in dying.]

The exact position as between Simon and Lambert is difficult to state, for about the same time Simon was stating: "I have been strongly impressed with an opinion that workhouses universally ought to be under systematic medical visitation by the Board." Evidently the failure at that time to secure central unification of medical work arose in large measure from the Board not agreeing with its Medical Officer as to the conditions of this work. Two Poor Law Medical Inspectors for Poor Law purposes were subsequently appointed: and these appointments called forth the following comment in the final paragraph of a report of a Treasury Commission:—

"We venture to suggest that whenever opportunity serves the present arrangement should be reconsidered with a view of remedying the anomaly to which we have drawn attention by placing all the Medical Inspectors under one department."

A second attempt to remove this anomaly was made by the Board in 1892. Sir Hugh Owen, then Secretary of the Board, Mr. Knollys, then Assistant Secretary, and Sir R. Thorne, its Medical Officer, agreed in Conference to a provisional arrangement "in case it should be decided that the Poor Law" medical work of the Board is to be placed under the Medical Department.

In a further minute dated November 3, 1892, Sir R. Thorne, however, asked the Board to hesitate before casting upon the Medical Department the great responsibilities connected with poor law medical administration.

The proposal then fell through.

I cannot give fully the reasons which led Thorne to withdraw from a fusion which in itself was desirable. There were perhaps reasons of personnel. One cannot assume Thorne was wrong in withdrawing from the proposed amalgamation of staff. Viewing the matter in 1936, from an evolutionary standpoint, one must remember that poor-law administration was then tight bound in central secretarial red tape, while specialised public health work was progressing rapidly. One must recall also that in 1892 public health work was regarded as chiefly concerned with sanitation and the prevention of epidemic diseases; and no accusation of lack of vision can attach to Thorne and his colleagues, if they shared the views on this point held by intelligent doctors and laymen throughout the country. The realisation of the importance of treatment in illness as a means of prevention of disease had scarcely risen above the national horizon.

In my memorandum written in 1909 I set out in detail my reasons in favour of a *unified* central medical service. The recent Royal Commission on the Poor Laws had emphasised the disadvantage and wastefulness of overlapping local medical administration. The immediate difficulties in reforming local administration did not exist in regard to central administration; and in view of the extent in which the problems of medical aid, especially in relation to such diseases as puerperal fever, phthisis, and in regard to infant mortality, and the provision of nurses, midwives, and health visitors, and district nurses, are also problems of public health, it was, I stated, important that the Board should focus under one head all the medical guidance needed by it in poor law and public health administration.

I then gave a detailed statement of how combined public health (including vaccination) inspections might be combined with inspection of the general sanitary work of the same district.

The preceding statement gives in part the history of the dual medical department in the Local Government Board.

For some years no practical action was taken on my recommendation of a unified central medical service, and up to the time of my retirement in 1919, there had been no increase of the central medical poor law inspectorate, which had been urged by the Royal Commission on the Poor Law. But the special circumstances must be remembered. During the years 1914–19 the Board's work was carried on under the shadow of war; even the special public health work under my supervision suffered from a heavily depleted staff, and it was difficult to entertain advances in administration, beyond the three new medical services which were initiated during this period— child welfare, tuberculosis, and venereal diseases. It is striking enough that in war circumstances these three services were born and rapidly developed with great success.

Similar remarks may be made respecting other branches of poor law reform. But the War was not the only circumstance which prevented the adoption of the poor law reforms common to the Majority and Minority Reports of the Royal Commission.

DIFFICULTIES IN INITIATING REFORM

When the drastic recommendations of the Poor Law Commission came to be considered by the Board there were grave difficulties in promoting immediate legislation to carry them into effect, even had Mr. Burns and his secretarial advisers considered this gigantic task desirable. For such legislation called for a drastic reconstruction of the entire organisation of local government throughout England and Wales, a difficult and intricate task, as it proved in 1929; and there was the great preliminary difficulty of deciding between the conflicting proposals of the Majority and Minority Reports. This might have been accomplished had not only the Local Government Board, but also the entire Government as represented by the Cabinet, been unanimous on the subject, and had the Board immediately put forward legislative proposals based on a synthesis of what was common to the two Reports.

THE BLOCKING OF POOR LAW REFORM BY THE GOVERNMENT

But these conditions were lacking; and action on the then possible lines of much needed reform was soon blocked by alternative insurance proposals put forward by the Chancellor of the Exchequer (Mr. Lloyd George) (see Chapter XIII). These "gave the go-by to all the proposals of the Royal Commission," while they left almost untouched the essential evils of the Poor Law. I write "untouched" advisedly, even though Old Age Pensions and contributory sickness Insurance for a third of the population markedly diminished the burden of poor-law administration, by putting many outside its scope.

Although the proposals of the Royal Commission, especially of its Minority Report, received enormous publicity, there was too little driving power behind them. The Government and the country generally became absorbed in the agitation against the veto of the House of Lords which followed Mr. Lloyd George's Budget of 1909, and everything else was put aside for the next two years. It would be incorrect to say that the agitation for poor-law reform was useless. It had a valuable educational influence, and—allowing for the latent period which almost inevitably elapses between first attempts at reform and their realisation—it may be said that the efforts then made led up to the Local Government Act of 1929.

Meanwhile Mr. Burns at the Local Government Board was actively engaged in introducing poor-law reforms which could be effected without new legislation. These may be described almost in the words of Sidney and Beatrice Webb (*op. cit.*, p. 723). An important circular was sent to Boards of Guardians in March 1910 on outdoor relief. It condemned indiscriminate or unconditional grant of this relief, and emphasised that, when given, relief should be adapted to the needs of the case and adequate in amount. In the following year a consolidating Order on outdoor relief was issued. In a further circular special measures were recommended for children. More trained nurses were recommended for workhouse nurseries. The need for close supervision of the home into which outdoor relief is received was emphasised; and a further circular advised that this relief should be given on the basis of "the normal standard of income on which a woman may reasonably be expected to bring up her family." This, I think, implied an abandonment of the old poor-law principle that the family should be relieved on a standard lower than that of the lowest paid independent labourer.

A further important principle was definitely enunciated by the Board.

As the Board has frequently stated, a person may be entitled to relief although not destitute in all respects, nor entirely devoid of the means of subsistence . . . and in the case of widows with children, who will obviously require assistance from the Poor Law in the near future, the Guardians will not only be within their rights, but would be acting with wisdom and foresight, in affording relief before the family resources, such as the stock of clothing, bedding, etc., are so depleted as to render it impossible afterwards to deal with the case without making good the deficiency.

In regard to Poor Law Institutions a new Order issued in 1913 restricted the age at which children could be retained in a workhouse, and recommended a number of other reforms, including the provision of trained nurses for all the sick and infirm inmates. This was largely acted upon.

The general effect of the Reports of the Royal Commission and of these official circulars and orders was to put the Boards of Guardians "on their mettle," and to make them desire to justify their continuance.

I cannot follow all phases of the improvement which occurred. It was seen in the treatment of the sick, and especially of tuberculosis.

Mr. Bagenal, one of the ablest of the lay (general) inspectors of the Board, wrote wisely in 1911:

A vast majority of cases of tuberculosis that come under the administrative control of the Poor Law are hopeless cases: it follows therefore that the main task of Boards of Guardians must be to benefit the community by diminishing the centres of infection . . . by the treatment of the bedridden consumptive.

But although this was a statesmanlike remark as concerns the classes of cases with which Boards of Guardians dealt, and showed also appreciation of the public health value of this work, it also pointed to the need to make one authority responsible for the care of the whole of a consumptive's life, and of measures of prevention at all stages of the disease, as well as in its advanced stage.

Subsequent events are discussed in later chapters. Of the special forms of preventive and curative activity initiated between 1908 and the present time, especially the work begun during the eleven years of my work at the Local Government Board, two—the rapid development of school medical work, and the initiation of insurance medical treatment—were outside the range of the Local Government Board, while the three special new medical services for mothers and their children under school age, and for the treatment and prevention of tuberculosis and of venereal disease, occupied a large and almost a predominant part of my eleven years' official work at the Board.

RECOMMENDATIONS ON WAR AND AFTER-WAR PROBLEMS

I conclude this chapter by giving the substance of recommendations on War and after-War problems written by me in January 1917, as they are concerned chiefly with what was still medical work under the Poor Law, and show that even during the War, recommendations were being made by me directed to some of the reforms which eventually fructified in the Local Government Act, 1929.

The following reasons indicate the desirability of detailed early consideration of the problem of providing medical assistance at the public expense:—

(1) The great displacements of population, which are likely to persist to some extent after the War, mean that the present institutional facilities for the treatment of disease by Poor Law and Public Health Authorities are unequally distributed.

(2) A large proportion of the inmates of workhouse infirmaries

have been displaced by military patients; and before they return, it is desirable that effort should be made to classify patients *by* institutions as recommended by the Poor Law Commission, as well as to classify them *in* institutions.

(3) Many temporary military hospitals have been erected, and their possible utilisation after the War needs consideration.

(4) The National Insurance Commission just before the War had important proposals for the appointment of consultants and referees and they had also considered the setting up of Treatment Centres for insured patients. These provisions cannot be made economically and satisfactorily unless existing Poor Law and Public Health arangements are utilised.

(5) The provision of nurses both for insured and non-insured patients needs consideration.

These were the recommendations:

A. *Recommendations as to Institutional Treatment*
(Residential and Non-Residential).

1. That the medical work of Boards of Guardians should be transferred to County Councils and County Borough Councils in order to give an adequate basis for classification of institutions, as well as classification in institutions.[1]

Difficult cases, where a Poor Law Union is in more than one County or County Borough, to be referred to a Boundary Commission.

2. That all officers at present employed in the medical work of Boards of Guardians should be taken over by the new Authorities.

3. That the Registrar-General's proposals as to registration be incorporated in the proposed legislation.

4. That the present Boards of Guardians remain as Committees of the County Council or County Borough Council, power being taken to co-opt other members.

5. That the present arrangements for domiciliary treatment of necessitous persons by the 3,400 district medical officers of the poor law might remain under these Committees until combined arrangements with the National Insurance Commission become practicable.

6. That the first duty of the County Council or the County

---

[1] If it is found impracticable to divorce medical from other institutional work, the question of entire transfer of poor law work to the larger Councils will require to be considered.

Borough Council after the transfer of institutions has been arranged should be to make a survey of institutional provision within their area, with a view to its efficient classification and utilisation.

The Board might give a time-limit for reports as to this, offering to arrange conferences between the local authorities and inspectors of the Board at an early date.

The survey should include possibilities of utilising temporary military hospitals.

The question of extending this reference to isolation hospitals of Local Authorities should be considered.

7. That Sec. 133 of the Public Health Act, 1875, should be incorporated in the proposed Bill, to enable all Local Authorities to provide institutional medical assistance for all the poorer inhabitants of every area; and non-institutional treatment with the consent of the Board.

Personally I should greatly prefer that this power were not limited to the "poorer" inhabitants; or at the least that these should be defined to include all who come within the terms of the National Insurance Act or their dependents for domiciliary treatment.

B. *Domiciliary Treatment.*

It is, of course, desirable that the arrangements for domiciliary treatment under the Poor Law should be combined with those under the National Insurance Act; but to do this at the present stage would involve immediate discussion with the National Insurance Commission and change in the present arrangements of the latter. It may be preferable to settle plans for institutional treatment first. For this reason I have made the suggestions 4 and 7 under A.

CHAPTER XII

INSURANCE FOR MEDICAL CARE

HAD those recommendations of the Royal Commissioners on the Poor Laws on which there was unanimity been promptly followed by legislation to secure their practical adoption, a firm foundation would have been laid on which a satisfactory system of medical care for the necessitous part of the population of Great Britain could be organised. And this could have served for a larger proportion of the total population than is ordinarily included in the word "necessitous"; for destitution in the sick is rightly defined as existing when there is inability to secure the particular treatment demanded by the patient's condition.

That the statement in the first sentence of this chapter is correct can be shown by extracts from the Recommendations of the Poor Law Commissioners.

Thus the Majority Report:

Medical treatment should be more readily accessible to all who are in need of it. (Part v, chap. 2 (186).)

Domiciliary medical assistance should be conditional on the maintenance of a healthy domicile and good habits (176).

Immediate steps should be taken for the organisation of a satisfactory system of nursing or attendance for the outdoor sick poor (169).

Medical assistance should be made available for all, and it should be reorganised on a provident basis.

The Minority Report stated:

We agree with the evidence given by medical representatives of four Government Departments that "the defects of the existing arrangements" are ascribable "to the lack of a unified medical service based on public health principles." This does not necessarily imply the gratuitous provision of medical treatment to all applicants.

The Majority on the Commission had differed from the Minority in not wishing to transfer all treatment provided at the public expense to the Public Health Committees of the larger Public Health Authorities. According to their recommendation the Public Assistance Committee of each of these larger Authorities would have this work, and the nascent school medical work would also be undertaken by the Public Assistance Committees, while the Public Health Committee of these Authorities would continue such share of publicly provided treatment as they were already undertaking. There was thus an important difference between the conclusions of the Majority and the Minority on the principle of unification of administration of provision for the sick, though both agreed in recommending the abolition of the Boards of Guardians and the transfer of their work to the Councils of Counties and County Boroughs, to be undertaken by Committees of these bodies, a reform which at last was secured by the Local Government Act, 1929.

CAUSES OF DELAY

This long delay resulted in part from cross-currents of political activity. These wrecked any immediate hope of action on the lines common to the two Reports. The responsibility for this delay need not and possibly cannot be completely identified or stated; but the circumstances leading to it throw light on the subsequent course of events.

(1) The problem of medical aid was entangled with that of general destitution, and remained so until a very recent year; while the difficulties of the underlying problem of unreformed local government favoured the pushing forward of social insurance, admittedly a beneficent provision, with which this chapter is concerned. True, it meant building a house without a ground-floor, and, as a consequence of this, there was created an additional medical service unrelated to the existing medical services of the State, conducted respectively by Poor Law Guardians, Public Health Authorities, and Education Authorities. It cannot be doubted that the complexity of the local services concerned in medical and other assistance for the people led to the shirking of the fundamental need for radical reform of local government. A large share of this reform would have been secured had the Government, as a preliminary to insurance, carried out the unanimous recom-

mendations of the Poor Law Commission to abolish the Boards of Guardians and transfer their duties to the Councils of County Boroughs and Counties. Already in 1908 Public Health Authorities were doing much of the medical work which previously, though in a hesitant manner and on a restricted scale, Boards of Guardians had undertaken. Public Health Authorities had taken over most of the work of hospital isolation of the chief acute infectious diseases, as well as similar work on a smaller scale for tuberculosis, venereal diseases, and puerperal and other forms of sepsis. Education Authorities were just beginning, as authorised by the Education (Administrative Provisions) Act, 1907, to search out illness in children in elementary schools and arrange for its treatment. Already much work in infant hygiene was being done by Sanitary Authorities (see *Fifty Years in Public Health*, Chapter XXXVII); and in the prevention of tuberculosis they had also become active (*op. cit.*, Chapter XXX). In a few instances Sanitary Authorities had even provided hospitals for accidents and general diseases.

Furthermore, there had already occurred marked encroachments on the non-medical work of Poor Law Guardians. The feeding of some school children who lacked food was being undertaken by voluntary agencies, aided or authorised by Education Authorities, and soon expenditure by these non-poor-law authorities for the same purpose was authorised.

As to medical aid, the facts discovered in school medical inspection gave additional impetus to further medical aid for infants and pre-school children; and this extension to earlier life meant that medical work for children had gradually come to partake less of the character of discovery and treatment of "end products."

The above-named and allied medical services, although in 1908 they were in their infantile stage, supplemented the corresponding work of Boards of Guardians to an important extent, and they differed from poor-law work in that it was no part of the duty of poor-law officers, medical or non-medical, to search out disease, and there was little or no attempt to correlate the health problem of the patient with his social conditions.

The efforts of the many voluntary agencies, as well as of Sanitary and Education Authorities, were, in fact, evoked in the attempt to fill the terrible gaps in the work of the destitution authorities—gaps which were inevitable in view of the constitution of these authorities and of the deterrent principle at the core of their work.

(2) But although Sanitary Authorities were attempting in many instances to undertake the work of relief authorities, the small areas served by many of them led to hesitation and ofttimes refusal to undertake new work. The existence of these too numerous authorities and the difficulties associated with the urgently needed reform of local government, doubtless were a factor in inducing politicians in the Government to indulge in the *ad hoc* vice of following the easier but, nevertheless, mischievous alternative, of creating a new authority to undertake a new job, that of social insurance, regardless or ignorant of the fact that it could not be carried out efficiently and economically except through the existing general local authority for other purposes. I can best sum up this important problem in government in words I wrote in 1932 (*Medicine and the State*, p. 241, George Allen & Unwin).

I emphasise the necessity in social improvements of building on and extending from what already exists, and of not multiplying machinery whenever a new or added need arises. In Britain . . . this creation of new and independent machinery whenever a new need emerges has been the bane of satisfactory and economic progress; and the Insurance Act as administered is the great example of this evil. Now, happily, the trend is back to intelligent co-operation and combination in the administration of all public medical services.

During the later stages of the Great War and afterwards, reform in local government came within practical range. In 1917 a special Committee, with the late Sir Donald Maclean as its chairman, and with the chief previously opposing members of the original Poor Law Commission among its members, unanimously confirmed the previous recommendation of this Commission for the abolition of the old Poor Law, and the allotment of medical aid to Committees of the larger local councils, the Public Health Committee for infants and the aged, and for institutions, the Education Committee for children at school, and a special Committee for the mentally defective.

The Government formally committed itself to reform in these directions "as soon as possible," and in 1929 this promise was redeemed.

(3) A public agitation in favour of the adoption of the Minority Report had, as already indicated, great influence in educating public opinion as to the importance of this social problem. But this agitation excited a counter-movement on the part of the Boards of Guardians, who hastened—many of them—to adopt such reforms as were practicable without legislation; and similar activity prevailed in the central governmental department responsible for poor-law activities (page 97). Although three members of the staff of the Local Government Board had been members of the Poor Law Commission, and had signed the report recommending the abolition of the Boards of Guardians, the Board proceeded—no other course was open, when the National Insurance Bill became the adopted policy of the Government—to initiate such reforms as were practicable without legislation. Nor can the value of these be minimised. I cannot detail them here: but the student should refer to pages 723 *et seq.* of Sidney and Beatrice Webb's *English Poor Law History: Part II, The Last Hundred Years,* which gives a full account of these administrative reforms.

(4) The "prepossessions of the Liberal Cabinet" (S. and B. Webb) were doubtless the main cause of delay in legislative reform of the Poor Law. It was the alternative proposals for a vast scheme of sickness insurance, and for an initial experiment in unemployment insurance, which as is stated in the above volume

gave the go-by to all the proposals of the Royal Commission (and) presently absorbed the whole attention, not only of the Cabinet and the Legislature, but also of the public. All the steam went out of the movement for extinguishing the Boards of Guardians. . . .

This diversion of political and social energy is not altogether surprising. The German system of insurance against sickness was becoming widely known and appreciated: and for some years agitation in favour of pensions for the aged poor had been spreading.

OLD AGE PENSIONS

Several committees had already sat on this subject, and in 1908 Mr. Asquith, the Prime Minister, introduced the first scheme for giving old age pensions to persons aged 70 and over on a non-contributory basis, subject to certain income limitations. This was the first considerable supersession of Poor Law relief. The weekly pensions increased in subsequent years, and finally in 1925, old age pensions were grafted, on a contributory basis, on to the National Insurance Act, and thus became—with insurance in other respects—an additional form of compulsory thrift. This meant, incidentally, that employers paid a quota towards support of their former employees when they reached a pensionable age.

Mr. Lloyd George, then the Chancellor of the Exchequer, had already in 1909 made some inquiries into the German system of sickness insurance. Sickness insurance of the mass of the people opened up many possibilities of improved health as well as monetary and medical aid during sickness. But Mr. Lloyd George was out of touch with the Local Government Board and with local governing bodies, and partly for this reason, and partly because the majority of politicians, not having had experience of local government, are ever apt to rush towards a special *ad hoc* machinery when initiating a reform, he and his advisers—many of whom were inexperienced in English methods of local administration—ignored the urgent necessity of preliminary reform of local government if a national scheme of insurance administration was to function economically and efficiently. Had this preliminary work been first done, a thoroughly sound and much more complete medical insurance provision could have been made, and the voluntary insurance societies already giving benefits could have been made to arrange their work geographically, so that it would coincide with the areas of authorities of local government which provided institutional treatment. Without this, insurance administration still remains unsatisfactory in its separation in practice from efforts which prevent sickness. Thus it fails to accomplish the great public health work which with reformed functional methods will, I am convinced, hereafter become its supreme value for national well-being. Meanwhile, the important public good secured by sickness insurance is shown in the following chapter. I emphasise at this point its value in securing better domiciliary medical treatment for a third of the total population, freed from the inhibition resulting from the system of payment on the basis of attendance. This was a great public gain, and the present arrangements are capable of being extended so that each medical practitioner having the medical care of an insured person, can become in substance the health officer for the family to which the patient belongs in all matters affecting personal hygiene.

CHAPTER XIII

NATIONAL SICKNESS INSURANCE

THE history of the enactment of insurance against sickness forms an important chapter in the social history of Britain. I watched the stages of its initiation and can write with some knowledge of the politics of its enactment. The system is described rather fully in Chapter VII of my *Medicine and the State* (George Allen & Unwin, 1932), and I can therefore curtail the present sketch. Its chief aim was by means of regular contributions during health (aided by concurrent contributions from the insured person's employer and from the State) to supply medical and financial aid during sickness. The underlying desire for security has led most European countries to adopt systems of social insurance, giving financial aid during sickness and unemployment, and provision for old age, and giving also medical care during illness.

In words which I may quote from page 148 of my *Health Problems in Organised Society* (P. S. King & Son, 1927):

> The haunting fear of disabling sickness or of being "out of work" at any time on a week's notice is a condition of affairs the malignity of which others than those concerned find it hard to realise; but that it is felt keenly by a large proportion of manual workers is beyond doubt. It is a demon which can only be exorcised by some system of insurance against the casualties of life.

As regards sickness there are two approaches to this problem: by the *prevention of illness*, or by *insurance* against monetary loss and lack of medical care while the bread-winner is ill. As not all sickness is preventable or in practice prevented, both measures are necessary if social effort is to be complete. The immense superiority of prevention, when practicable, over insurance against loss for non-prevented evil is beyond dispute; but our knowledge and the willingness on the part of many to live hygienically being restricted, insurance has an important place in our armamentarium of social welfare. For many years, Friendly and Trade Union Societies already had systems of voluntary sickness insurance, before the National Insurance Bill, making this compulsory for a third of the total population, was introduced. In 1883 Germany first introduced the principle of compulsion into social insurance, and extended its application to wider circles in 1911. In the latter year Britain followed Germany's example and took the lead in initiating also Unemployment Insurance for certain sections of the population. Parliament accepted readily the principle of compulsion, and the public fell into line. The problems associated with compulsion are discussed by me on page 113 of my *Medicine and the State*, and more fully in *Health Problems in Organised Society* (P. S. King & Son, 1927), Chapters XI and XII; but briefly it can be said that in the modern mind liberation from unfair conditions has become the social desideratum more than liberty, in the sense of freedom from communal restrictions. This liberation with its necessary compulsion (to ensure universal adoption) can only succeed as a permanent measure when it continues to be desired and sanctioned by a large majority of the community.

The national insurance scheme was not national in the sense of applying to the entire nation; for, in fact, it was limited almost entirely to the industrial classes. This selected population became insured, and the State's contribution to the insured was to a partial extent at the expense of the uninsured portion of the population. The same criticism applies to British unemployment insurance, and to insurance for old age and for widows' and orphans' pensions. It also applies to municipal housing schemes (page 163 of *Fifty Years of Public Health*), and is justified by wider considerations.

BENEFITS OF THE SICKNESS INSURANCE ACT

This Act undoubtedly secured important help to the insured, both monetarily and by means of its provision of the domiciliary care of a medical practitioner for every insured person, who could promptly be consulted without fee for each attendance. The maternity benefit for wives of insured persons and for insured women gave financial aid when aid was specially needed, though the benefit would have been more valuable had medical and nursing attendance been given in addition to or even in place of a financial benefit.

THE DEFECTS OF THE INSURANCE PROVIDED

Some of these defects were obvious from the first, and arose largely from the lack of early consultation with central and local health authorities and with the medical profession, without whose co-operation medical benefit was unworkable.

Mr. Lloyd George was in early touch with the Friendly Societies of the country who were administering benefits under voluntary sickness insurance schemes. But the methods of administration of these Societies were disadvantageous for a national scheme. Most of those voluntarily insured belonged to Societies scattered throughout the country, and even now the failure to provide for administration of insurance on a geographical basis means that in England statistics of incapacitating sickness based on certificates of incapacity are not generally available for administrative areas, and thus cannot be utilised as the basis of investigation directed to prevention of sickness.[1] Although I do not here enlarge further on this point, I regard it as a blot on our insurance system.

The medical notions of the Friendly Societies were imported into the Insurance Bill, and although through the persistence of the doctors themselves a medical service was secured which was superior to that previously available for Friendly Societies, there still remained many defects of the past, especially the notion that a "bottle of medicine" is needed whenever a doctor is consulted. But this, of course, is not special to insurance medical practice. I refrain from comment here on the fact that sickness insurance—unlike such insurance in other countries—is limited to the worker, his dependents being outside its scope.

So far as the insured themselves are concerned, the system fails to provide the medical care which, when needed, is most difficult to obtain. There is scanty provision for consultants

---

[1] The records of illness have been stated to have little value for statistical purposes; this may be partially so for certified causes of incapacity, but comparative investigation of local incidence of total incapacity would be of immediate value.

when in doubtful or serious illness these are desirable; no provision for examination of pathological material (but see p. 121, where it is shown that a large amount of this work is done gratuitously by Public Health Authorities); no nursing provision (in most instances): and for most patients no provision of hospital beds when these are required, and only limited dental treatment. Some of these deficiencies are being increasingly met. There is an official Regional Medical Staff, who are available for consultation as to diagnosis as well as on the question of doubtful incapacity. In 1933 (Annual Report C.M.O. Ministry of Health) a million and a half sterling was spent on dental benefit in England, and about £350,000 on ophthalmic benefit. But for many medical needs, necessitating exceptional skill or hospital treatment, the insured sick still have to depend chiefly on voluntary or official charity or personal means apart from insurance.

Had the reform of local government which took place in 1929 preceded the national health insurance system, the way would have been open for meeting these essential needs. Already the Sanatorium Benefit (in 1921) has been placed outside the scope of the Insurance Act, and is now provided by Public Health Authorities (p. 142). Eventually medical attendance will likewise cease to be a benefit under Sickness Insurance, which will then be limited to financial benefits. Then a National System of Medical Aid provided for—in part at least—out of local and general taxation will take its place, and will be linked up with the services rendered by voluntary as well as official hospitals. This more complete medical service may be provided on an insurance basis, or the means of each family can be assessed and payment required according to means at the time when medical care is needed. This subject is further discussed in Chapter XLV. But as matters now stand the medical service supplied under the British Insurance Act is more incomplete than that provided under the national insurance schemes of the chief European countries.

At the initiation of the British Scheme the Chancellor of the Exchequer availed himself of advice obtainable from Friendly Societies and from the less desirable industrial insurance societies, which unlike the smaller Friendly Societies had no real self-government by the insured. But until the Bill had been framed, there had been no adequate consultation between the Local Government Board, with its unique knowledge of local administration, and the Chancellor, or apparently between him and the British Medical Association, as representing the general medical practitioners of the country. For these mistakes the country has had to pay dearly. The British Medical Association were well aware that a scheme of Sickness Insurance was being incubated, and their Council had been steadily studying the subject and formulating a policy for medical practitioners. When they were consulted, they were able to insist on the adoption of nearly all the cardinal points which they had adopted as their considered policy.

As the Bill passed through the House of Commons, one saw lightning changes in it almost day by day. Mr. Lloyd George had courage and resource, great persuasiveness, and daemonic drive. It was a marvel to see the passive House adopt changes or modifications, some of which, it might almost appear, he had not considered until prompted in the middle of a speech! The Bill passed through the House of Commons, many clauses without discussion. Few opposed it, perhaps from fear of unpopularity; but one must also remember that the Prime Minister, Mr. Asquith, had recently secured a redoubtable victory limiting the power of veto of the House of Lords, and opposition was thus largely sterilised.

Had the National Insurance Bill after its introduction been referred to a Committee of persons expert in local administration and in public health and medical work, along with insurance representatives, it would have benefited immensely, and much extravagant expenditure might have been saved. As events went, when the Bill became law, and Sir Robert Morant was placed at the head of the National Insurance Commission, with the task of putting it into operation, it required all his great driving power, aided by some of the best brains of the Civil Service working with him, to make the insurance system work. But it was made to work, and it is certain that great good has been achieved through it.

The defects in the structure of the Insurance Act are not

exhausted in the preceding sketch. Its chief defect was the failure to bring Public Health Authorities into functional relation with the new insurance scheme. There was no co-ordination with existing preventive machinery. The machinery of the Act was rapidly improvised, and the intervention of the Local Government Board and some local authorities to improve this machinery only became possible at a late stage and was then relatively ineffective. I refrain from quoting official memoranda written by me during the progress of the Insurance Bill through the House of Commons in which some of its defects were plainly indicated.

I must, however, animadvert further upon the failure of the Act to realise the principles of practical administration of health problems. Mr. Lloyd George had probably been influenced in deciding not to entrust the administration of medical insurance to existing public health authorities, because the medical profession as voiced by the British Medical Association did not favour this, and perhaps it was feared that insured workmen would suspect that insurance money might be used to relieve public health and poor-law authorities of some of their existent medical work.

A clause was inserted in the Insurance Bill providing that an Insurance Committee or an Approved Society might claim compensation from a Sanitary Authority or other Body when through its default or action excessive sickness occurred among the insured.

When watching the discussion on this clause from the officials' "pew" in the House of Commons I expressed my conviction that the House of Commons would not endorse a proposal so unworkable, and if attempted to be worked, so contrary to continuance of co-operation between Sanitary and Insurance Authorities. A distinguished Treasury official disagreed, and we bet a pound on the event. I lost, for the House of Commons was as ignorant or careless of the principles for promoting good local government as was, in this instance, the Chancellor of the Exchequer himself. The powers thus conferred were never acted on, and they were "dropped" when some years later the Insurance Act was revised.

Writing in 1936, it can be said that the belated reform of

sanitary authorities is rapidly progressing, their medical work being now entrusted only to the largest local authorities, and that thus the way is open for much closer co-operation between insurance and public health.

The medical arrangements made for attending all sick insured persons were made by the Government on behalf of all insurance societies. Thus local difficulties in negotiations were avoided. Every medical practitioner was entitled to place his name on a "panel," and thus each insured person, except in some rural areas, would have a choice of doctors on whose list he could be placed. This point was only reached after much difficulty.

At first doctors regarded contract practice under the Act as abhorrent and even degrading, and the measure providing for this as "constituting a deadly threat to the work of the profession." Soon, however, they were reconciled to contract practice, subject to the medical arrangements being entirely uncontrolled by the Friendly and other Societies, through which insurance worked on its monetary side. The struggle on this point was severe and in retrospect is amusing. The medical practitioners were able to drive a hard bargain with Mr. Lloyd George, and secured their freedom from the thraldom they had previously experienced in "club practice," Insurance Committees on which doctors were represented being formed, whereby an independent hearing of medical disputes was secured. Without following more closely the course of events it may be stated briefly that medical objections to insurance medical practice have disappeared; it has been found to be financially a highly satisfactory part of general medical practice, and in recent years the British Medical Association have officially given it their blessing, and have advised its continuance and its extension to the dependents of the insured. Were this done it would imply that about 80 per cent of the total population will be medically attended under the conditions of contract practice, so far as this work is within the competence of an average general practitioner of medicine. It may be noted that already contract medical practice is extending with the approval of the British Medical Association among the non-insured.

SUMMARY ON SICKNESS INSURANCE

The English system is in reality a combination of true insurance effected by those who will benefit, aided to more than one half of the total cost by contributions from the employers of the insured and by taxation.

In its working there is still very imperfect co-ordination with the work carried on by Public Health Authorities for prevention of sickness and enhancement of health. Some imperfect arrangements have been made in the insurance system for health propaganda, but these are fragmentary. The insured patient can change his doctor when not satisfied with the doctor's services, and an insured person can lodge a complaint against his doctor or pharmacist and require that his complaint shall be heard in accordance with the procedure set up for this purpose. He can also complain against his Approved Society.

The great accomplishment of sickness insurance on its medical side has been that so far as nearly half the domiciliary medical work of the country is concerned, medical aid has ceased to be given under conditions which encourage, and often necessitate, delay in obtaining it, thus rendering early recovery less likely.

This replacement of medical practice paid for by direct fees by contract medical practice is a great gain in social medicine; and the way is open for repairing the defects of insurance medical service and bringing it much more closely into functional relationship with the public medical services for the prevention of disease. Some indications of the means by which these further ends can be accomplished are given in later chapters. Meanwhile it is a great fact that prompt medical care has been made available for the insured· part of the population, while the intimate personal relationship of the private medical practitioner to his patient has been left unbroken.

It will be noted that the Insurance Act, on its medical as well as on its non-medical side, is contributory in character, direct contributions being required both from the worker and his employer, the State also contributing a quota. As already mentioned old-age pensions similarly are now given, chiefly on a contributory basis (p. 107). Unemployment insurance is also on a contributory basis, although in recent years the State has been obliged to take the place of the unemployed in enabling them to remain eligible for benefits. Theoretically, there is objection to the incidence of contributions of employers, in view of the fact that in some industries large numbers and in others very few workers are employed for a given "turn over." In the Soviet republic there are no direct contributions by workers, as there are no private profit-making employers in Russia.

In Public Health, administration for sickness provision is made mainly at the expense of local and national taxation, and a vast amount of hygienic and medical care is given on this basis. The future of these two parallel British methods of providing medical care, extended as they will be, remains to be seen. There need be no rivalry between co-existent systems of care provided partially at the expense of the insured, and care provided for him by the community out of taxation to which as a rate-payer and tax-payer he has indirectly contributed. But as already stated, it is likely that ere long the separate existence of those two systems will cease, and the medical care of the insured will be undertaken, whether on a contributory basis or not, by "panel doctors"—as the present insurance doctors are commonly called—working in a great unified system of national medical service, which will include complete medical care of the insured, of all poor persons, and will incorporate the many branches of medical care undertaken, now or in the future, by Public Health Authorities.

Meanwhile it can be said that both unemployment insurance and sickness insurance in this country have done magnificent service in steadying public opinion in times of adversity, in mitigating social misery during years of unemployment on an unexampled scale, and in maintaining the well-being of those who without insurance would have suffered very seriously.

This conclusion was arrived at by a Royal Commission on British National Health Insurance which sat and reported early in 1926; and my statement as above is in accord with their finding on this important point. They concluded that the difficulties of a completed medical service based in part on insurance funds and in part on Government grants and local taxation—financial, administrative, and social—were so great, that "it would be difficult to retain the insurance principle," and that the ultimate solution would lie in the divorce of the medical service from the insurance system, and in the support of the medical service from the general public funds. (On this and other points see McCleary's *National Health Insurance*, Lewis, 1932.)

As to the sanatorium (tuberculosis benefit) under the Insurance Act, and the encouragement given under it to medical research, see Chapters XIV and XV.

CHAPTER XIV

PROVISION FOR RESEARCH. INVESTIGATIONS ON TUBERCULOSIS

In discussing the national health insurance system I have omitted, so far, reference to its two most beneficent provisions, which, apart from all other provisions, entitle it to be regarded as rendering important service in aid of socio-hygienic progress.

One of these was the allotment for the organisation of research of a penny annually from the insurance fund accruing to each insured person; and the other was the provision made for a special "Sanatorium Benefit." This benefit was backed up by a grant of 1½ million pounds sterling from National Funds for building sanatoria in Great Britain for insured and non-insured, and by the decision to pay half the total approved expenditure incurred by local Public Health Authorities in the treatment and administrative control of tuberculosis in the entire population.

I may first briefly outline the provision for research in this country. On such research medico-hygienic progress is largely dependent; but although this general statement in the long run is correct, one needs always to remember that at any given time our knowledge of preventive medicine is greater than our actual practice of it.

RESEARCH

Research is a word perhaps too widely employed. In a sense every medical practitioner, if he is worth his salt, is engaged in a diagnostic research when first consulted by a patient; and, if we except the failure to cure resulting from the patient's delay in consulting the doctor, the latter's failure to make this research is a chief reason why much illness has been unsatisfactorily treated.

In my experience at the School of Hygiene, Johns Hopkins University (1919–20), I was impressed by the value of the association of advanced public health teaching with research on the subjects being taught; and in 1927, in *Health Problems in Organised Society*, I expressed my appreciation of this association in the following words:

The professor whose whole time is occupied in teaching is likely to lose freshness and to become a non-inspiring guide for his students. A University is the seat of many allied branches of learning, and thus the valuable help of other workers can easily be obtained. From such institutions as . . . the Medical Research Council in England we may confidently expect to receive new light on the dark corners of preventive medicine which remain. The problems of cancer, of the prevention of catarrhal infections, of means for reducing the fatality of pneumonia, at once occur to the mind, as among the regions in which we still grope in almost medieval darkness.

MEDICAL RESEARCH COUNCIL

The funds for this bye-product of national insurance, as already stated, were supplied by a toll of 1d. per annum per person from the total annual contribution given by the State, the insured person's employer, and the insured person. This sum at first brought in approximately £60,000 a year; but by means of further Government grants it had become £165,000 in the financial year 1934–35. During the sessions of the Departmental (Astor) Committee on Tuberculosis in 1912 there was some difference of opinion as to the extent to which research expenditure should be centralised in a single institution; but when the National Research Committee (later Council) got to work, with Dr. (later Sir) Walter Fletcher as its energetic and able secretary, it organised extensive and far-reaching research, some of which was centralised at the National Institute for Medical Research at Hampstead and its farm laboratories (£58,500 in 1934–35), while the larger moiety was paid to promote various researches by the Industrial Health Research Board and at a number of University and other centres (total £97,000 in the same year). It is impossible to enumerate here the many branches of physiological, pathological, and clinical researches, also statistical investigations, carried out year by year; the aggregate result of this work is one of the most satisfactory of the bye-products of national insurance.

It will not be assumed that no other researches are being

undertaken by other bodies. The volume and value of investigations to find out the further secrets of health have been held back by the sparsity of adequately trained workers to undertake them.

Prior to this relatively munificent official endowment of research, the only annual grant systemtically given for the investigation of health problems was an annual sum of £2,000 administered by the Local Government Board. When I came to the Board this sum had been reduced to £1,900, because in a preceding year the total of £2,000 had not been expended! The Treasury condition of completion within the year of allotted expenditure did not fit in with the exigencies of scientific work. The subjects investigated under this small fund over a long series of years can be seen as summarised in successive reports of medical officers of the Local Government Board.

PERSONAL INVESTIGATIONS ON TUBERCULOSIS

As I am reviewing investigations from a personal angle, I now briefly outline my investigations, undertaken prior to 1908, into the causes of the decline in the incidence of tuberculosis, as bearing on future administrative control of this disease. The great historical influence of partial segregation of consumptives does not seem to have been generally accepted as a principle, though adopted in actual practice. It is therefore incumbent on me to state the general argument in the light of maturer experience. These investigations led me to the conclusion that, in producing the past reduction of tuberculosis, segregation of advanced and especially of bed-ridden cases of tuberculosis played a large and even a predominant part. At this point let me emphasise what is common ground in practical public health administration. In every public health district throughout Britain local authorities are actively engaged in measures directed to the prevention of massive or frequently repeated infection from open cases of tuberculosis, especially by the treatment of vast numbers of open and advanced cases of tuberculosis in institutions; but although this is so, not a few public health administrators continue to doubt or deny that this work, now regarded as an intrinsic and indispensable part of the anti-tuberculosis fight, *has in the history of tuber-culosis been largely responsible for its decline.*

At the risk of being tedious, I propose briefly to outline the stages of the inquiries which led me to conclude that, in the history of the past decline in tuberculosis, segregation and allied measures of human intervention by diminishing the spread of infection have played a predominant part. In doing so, I utilise the special papers enumerated at the end of this chapter, and my successive annual reports to the Local Government Board, 1908–19.

In my earlier *Fifty Years in Public Health*, I have discussed the relatively small share borne by bovine tuberculosis in producing fatal human tuberculosis. Tuberculosis of bovine origin is important in relation to tuberculosis in children, and it can be brought peremptorily to an end when we decide to allow only pasteurised cow's milk for human consumption. I need not, then, discuss milk as a cause of tuberculosis, except to comment that, as regards bovine tuberculosis, we all of us concentrate on infection as the chief enemy needing to be attacked, though we do not leave out of consideration measures for increasing the resistance of children to infection.

In a report presented to the International Congress on Hygiene and Demography, Brussels, 1903 (*Journal of Hygiene*, Vol. III, 1903), I set out the general position as regards mortality from tuberculosis in England. The recorded death-rate from phthisis (pulmonary tuberculosis) in the first five years of registration, 1838–42, had been 3·88 per 1,000 of population; but it must be remembered that medical registration of cause of death did not become compulsory until 1874. Any wasting disease was apt to be called "consumption." In 1871–80 the death-rate from all forms of tuberculosis averaged 2·88, and it had become 1·43 in 1911–20 and 1·01 in 1921–30, and 0·76 in 1934.

In the Brussels report I pointed out that many factors were concerned in this decline, including diminished crowding in houses and their improved cleanliness, improved industrial conditions, and the educational influence of universal school education since 1870 on domestic and personal cleanliness, especially as regards intra-domestic expectoration, but I added that these "almost certainly are not the only factors concerned, and the means by which these factors have caused a reduction of tuberculosis has probably been in part misinterpreted." In writing this I referred to the attempts then already prevalent to belittle the importance of measures directed to controlling infection.

Some of the most important public health measures have directly diminished the opportunities for infection. Improvement in housing and the diminution of overcrowding undoubtedly have had this effect. The improved habits of the people have had the same effect to an even greater extent. Quite apart from the present crusade against spitting, there has been an immense improvement in national habits in this respect and in general domestic cleanliness, which must have had a material effect in diminishing opportunities for infection.

At the same time I deprecated neglect of the influence of crowded ill-lighted dwellings in favouring tuberculosis, adding "all who wish to effect the most good will endeavour to the utmost to control both sets of factors." Sir Hugh Beevor in 1899 had shown "a coincidence and a remarkable agreement between the fall in the phthisis rate, the number of paupers, and the rise in the average wage." He emphasised the importance of abundant food in the prevention of phthisis, and a diagram in my report at Brussels similarly showed a fairly consistent fall in the proportional price of wheat and the proportional mortality from phthisis.

In the same contribution, I quoted Robert Koch's statement in his startling London address, 1901, to the effect that

the only country that possesses a considerable number of special hospitals for tubercular persons is England, and there can be no doubt that the diminution of tuberculosis in England, which is much greater than in any other country, is greatly due to this circumstance.

I pointed out that Koch's statement as to special hospitals was not literally accurate, as the proportion of hospital beds in special hospitals to the total number of tubercular patients was very small; but that

if the total number of tubercular patients treated in general hospitals and still more those treated in workhouse infirmaries be included, there is good reason for attaching a high importance to the removal of these patients from their relatives and to the nursing of them under *conditions in which personal infection is greatly limited in amount*.

I illustrated this by the local experience of the infirmary of Brighton, in which during three years 211 phthisical patients were admitted to, and on an average each spent 316 days in the institution, either continuously or in successive periods. The above patients were equal to more than half the fatal cases of phthisis in Brighton in the same period.

Further investigations on the same subject led to my contribution to the Epidemiological Society (December 1905) on "The Relative Importance of the Constituent Factors involved in the control of Pulmonary Tubersulosis."[1] I pass over an earlier paper read at the Paris International Congress on Tuberculosis (October 1905), except to quote the conclusion at which, somewhat temerariously, I had already arrived.

The number of instances in which the point can at present be tested is relatively few, but so far as can be ascertained, the death-rate from tuberculosis has declined to the greatest extent in those countries in which the ratio of institutional to domestic treatment has been highest. This I regard as operating by segregating from the community the most potent foci of infection, while domiciliary treatment helps to retain such foci in the midst of the family.

The facts appear to justify the conclusion that the substitution of institutional for domiciliary relief of the consumptive poor has been historically a main factor in the reduction of the death-rate from tuberculosis.

This statement should be read with its context: otherwise it might appear to ignore the value of measures, including greater cleanliness and restriction of spitting and unscreened coughing, which diminish infection even when institutional segregation of open cases of phthisis is not provided to secure the same end with greater certainty.

I must refer the reader to the detailed statistics given in my paper published in the *Epidemiological Society's Transactions*. These figures were subsequently used by Robert Koch in 1910 in a paper entitled "Epidemiologie der Tuberkulose" (*Zeitschrift für Hygiene und Infektions Krankheiten*, Leipzig, 1910), and I reproduce here his diagram, rather than utilise my own, because of its historic interest.

[1] This paper is expanded in my *Prevention of Tuberculosis*, 1907.

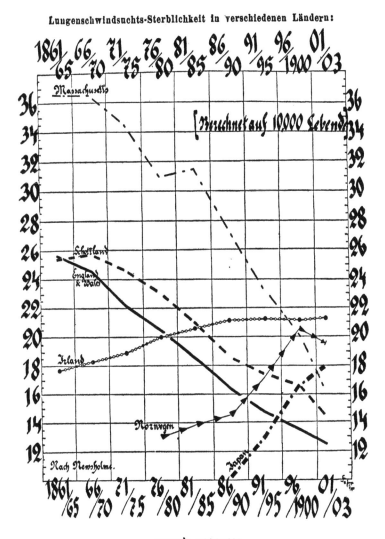

KOCH'S DIAGRAM

Death-rate from Pulmonary Tuberculosis in different countries

This diagram brings out clearly the difference in the course of experience of tuberculosis in Ireland and Norway on one hand and in Great Britain and Massachusetts on the other.

My own tables and diagrams showed the course in time of various measures of well-being compared with the course of the phthisis death-rate in a number of European countries, followed by a statement of the relative course of the best available (but necessarily imperfect) measures of institutional segregation of the sick and that of the phthisis death-rate.

I drew attention to the fact that, whilst the phthisis death-rate was then consistently higher in towns than in rural districts, nevertheless, although the proportion of the total population living in towns had steadily increased, the urban death-rate from phthisis had rapidly declined. And this had happened although, as shown by census figures, dwellings in towns in the aggregate were more crowded and room accommodation was smaller than in rural districts. Evidently some factor was at work counteracting the adverse influence of urbanisation. I added:

The main mischief of urbanisation consists in overcrowding and increased frequency of intimate contact both industrially and domestically; and consequently the influence which has been predominant not only in counteracting the effect of urbanisation, but also in obtaining great reductions in the phthisis death-rates, *must be one which tends to correct the effect of increased contact.*

Measured by logarithmic curves which exhibited the rate of change of factors, there was some imperfect concordance between evidences of improved nutrition (price of wheat, wages, or total cost of living) and the death-rate from phthisis in some countries, including England and Massachusetts, but in Ireland, France, and Prussia little or none; whereas when the death-rate from phthisis was compared with the amount of sickness treated in various hospitals, including workhouse infirmaries, there was a much closer correspondence. This was taken as a measure of segregation of the sick, and of avoidance of protracted continuous domestic infection. The good inverse relationship shown between phthisis death-rates and the extent of institutional treatment was confirmed by detailed local experience, showing that a large proportion of the total infectious life of consumptives in England and other countries is spent in institutions. The conclusion I drew from a general study of the evidence was that *institutional segregation, notably of advanced cases, is the most powerful single means available for controlling phthisis.*

And I drew satisfaction from this conclusion, inasmuch as the machinery to provide this segregation already existed, had been operating to a material extent for forty or fifty years, and could easily be vastly extended "at a far lower expense than would be incurred by the construction of a new machinery." In this sentence I implied my conviction that, from the public health standpoint, the institutional segregation of consumptives was immensely more important than the parallel attempt at cure of early cases by Sanatorium treatment. In other connections I had already emphasised my view that the chief benefit from Sanatorium treatment, in view of the frequency of belated diagnosis of cases, was through its training of patients to a hygienic life, beneficial to themselves, and reducing greatly the risk of the communication of protracted and therefore effective infection to the healthy.

Continuing my investigations, in October 1907, I gave an address on "Poverty and Disease, as illustrated by the course of Typhus Fever and Phthisis in Ireland," as the first President of the Epidemiological Section of the Royal Society of Medicine into which had been merged the separate Epidemiological Society. In it I made a careful study of the history of typhus fever in Ireland, especially during the nineteenth century, and compared it with the corresponding history of phthisis in that country. The comparison showed great decline of typhus and an absence of decline of phthisis. The story had been one of decimating epidemics of typhus among an impoverished people, among whom attempts at prevention of infection were almost entirely lacking. Alongside of this was the steady emigration, seasonal and permanent, of a large part of its population to the ports of England and Scotland and to New York and thence inland in these countries, typhus being inseminated by these migrants as they went. Typhus fever became more serious when potato crops failed in Ireland, and its people wandered in search of relief; and the potato famine of 1845–47 led to the culmination of typhus and then of emigration, Ireland losing the greater part of its people from disease and from mass-migration. Poor Law provision was made in Ireland in 1838, but years passed before hospital provision for typhus patients became available except on a small scale. When it was supplied and measures against vagrancy became effective,[1] typhus steadily decreased. The poor were willing to be treated for typhus in hospitals, but not for a protracted illness like phthisis; and after 1865 Ireland relaxed its institutional test for relief and gradually settled down to a vast dispensary system of home-relief for the sick, including phthisis.

A detailed study of typhus in Ireland shows the close association of this disease with infection, malnutrition, overcrowding, and vagrancy. These mostly occurred and varied together, and one cannot doubt that each of them is causally related to the disease. But although one cannot doubt that poverty and malnutrition favour the occurrence of typhus, no one would regard monetary aid on an adequate scale as the most immediate and powerful means of restraining an epidemic of this disease. So also with the abatement of overcrowding, unless this is associated with persistent effort on a large scale to separate the healthy from the infectious sick, reduction of typhus could only be partial. The reduction of vagrancy had a marked effect in reducing infection. Disease became immobilised in each parish and in institutions; and to this in large part must be ascribed the reduction of typhus in Ireland.

The course of Irish phthisis is different. Both typhus and phthisis occur especially in circumstances of privation and overcrowding. Both of these adverse conditions had greatly decreased in Ireland by 1906, when my address was prepared, but although typhus had declined, these ameliorations had "not sufficed to overcome other influences tending to increase the death-rate from phthisis." There had been much success in immobilising typhus, a disease of short duration, but little

---

[1] Through the localisation of poor-law relief.

or none against phthisis, a disease of protracted duration. I stated my main conclusion as follows:

The influence which had the predominant share in causing the decrease of phthisis in those countries in which decrease has occurred was the *immobilisation of infection*.

This, even when it was largely domestic, had succeeded for typhus (vagrancy had been almost stopped); but

immobilisation in a protracted infectious disease like phthisis, in order to be efficient, must be institutional, especially for advanced cases.

I may complete my review of contributions made in unofficial papers to elucidate "The Causes of the Past Decline in Tuberculosis and the Light thrown by History on Preventive Measures for the Immediate Future" by referring to a special lecture given by me under the above title at the International Congress on Tuberculosis, September 29, 1908, in Washington, D.C. This is published in the official transactions of the Congress, and received wide publicity in United States of America through its separate publication. I may be excused for giving here a statement made by Dr. Livingston Farrand, then executive secretary of the American Association for the Study and Prevention of Tuberculosis and now President of Cornell University. It is taken from an address given by Dr. Farrand at a national conference in 1910 presided over by Mr. Taft, then President of United States of America.

In a masterly paper presented at the International Congress on Tuberculosis, Dr. Newsholme of London showed from figures gathered from European sources that so far as inferences could be drawn from the data there was a direct proportion between the fall in the death-rate from tuberculosis and the amount of hospital provision for advanced cases. This simply means that as often as you take a case of tuberculosis and put it under such conditions that it no longer becomes an infecting centre you reduce the amount of tuberculosis in a community. This presents the situation in a nut-shell. If this be sound reasoning it would appear that in institutional care of consumptives there lies the principal means of preventing the disease.

If we can bring about, upon an adequate scale, provision for

E

tuberculous patients in all stages there can be little doubt of the ultimate result.

This view has been adopted as an essential part of the anti-tuberculosis fight throughout America. In a more recent discussion on prophylaxis in pulmonary tuberculosis (*Proc. Roy. Soc. Med.*, July 1935) Dr. D. A. Powell quoted a Canadian authority as affirming "the very foundation of all anti-tuberculosis measures is *beds*"; and he added:

Dr. Drolet (Statistician, New York Tuberculosis Association) has demonstrated that there is a striking correlation between tuberculosis hospitalisation and mortality in different countries, those with the lowest death-rate having the largest number of beds per hundred deaths, and vice versa. . . . The paramount importance of the segregation of open cases is apt to be lost sight of in these days—it has never been realised in some quarters.

I can regretfully endorse the last statement.

My Lecture to the International Congress at Washington concluded with the following summary:

The various elements of well-being do not in every community vary uniformly along with the phthisis death-rate which they are supposed to and undoubtedly do influence. Thus in actual history they have not had constantly predominant influence on the course of phthisis. Institutional segregation, on the other hand, while operating in the same group of adjuvant influences, has maintained its inverse relation with the course of phthisis. Each of the factors has been tested in the actual experience of many large communities over the same period of history under precisely the same opposing and adjuvant conditions. In the series of communities subjected to this test, institutional segregation has been the only factor the variation of which has been always associated with a variation in the prevalence of tuberculosis in a constant relative direction. It would not have been surprising had the influence of institutional segregation been masked by that of opposing factors, as has been seen to have occurred in many countries with the maleficent influence of urbanisation; or contrariwise if more than one influence had varied with the prevalence of tuberculosis in a constant relation. In either case the question as to which influence had predominated in affecting the prevalence of tuberculosis would have been left open. In fact, however, no influence except that of institutional segregation has appeared in actual experience in a constant relation to the amount of tuberculosis, and the evidence points to the conclusion that it has been the predominant influence in changing the incidence of this disease.

The institutional treatment which it is claimed has played a predominant part in the past reduction of phthisis has been in the main the institutional treatment of patients who were disabled by sickness, rather than of earlier and less severe cases. . . . There can, I think, be no doubt that advanced cases are more effectively infectious than earlier cases. But no responsible administrators having regard to the prevention of tuberculosis will content themselves with the treatment of advanced cases. They will treat early cases in the hope of securing recovery of the patient; and intermediate cases in the hope of restoring a modicum of health, as well as of educating the patient so that he will no longer be a source of infection to his family and his fellow-workmen. These points are evident; they can, so far as my experience indicates, be more completely ensured by institutional treatment than by the training which the patient receives at a dispensary or through a domiciliary visit. . . .

If we consider the closely aggregated conditions under which an enormous proportion of our city populations are housed, we shall be able to realise, what is I believe the fact, that had it not been for the steadily increasing extent of institutional treatment of the sick, and especially of the consumptive sick, which has characterised most of our great centres of population, we should have experienced not the decline of phthisis which has occurred, but an increase in its prevalence.

It is easy to deplore that statistics do not present themselves in that systematic form which permits wide conclusions from relatively limited experience. In this respect they differ from well-conceived laboratory experiments, in the deductive reasoning connected with which such form is rightly required. With equal truth and reason one might express regret that in pathology and medicine one is compelled to work backward from the investigation of the complex structure and functions of the human body rather than forwards from the simplicity of the microscope and the test-tube. The more cumbrous "clinical" methods of statistics might be dispensed with were we able to place the body under laboratory conditions. Social physiology and medicine are even more complex than the same sciences applied to the individual and statistics must be used to decipher their mysteries. As they are required, our plain duty is to use them with the same care to avoid fallacy and the same pains to control our results as are expected in deductive experiment. We are not engaged in academic labours, of which the prize goes to the winner, and each man may neglect his preparation if he choose.

The servant of public health is working on the lives of men, and should be laying the foundations of national prosperity and happiness. He belongs to an order of sanitary priests, and belies his vocation and betrays his trust, if he does not use the material at his disposal fully and faithfully. He is his brother's keeper; and as in these matters knowledge means added life and happiness and usefulness to the communities whose welfare is in his charge, he will reject no method of labour and spare no endeavour which offers the prospect of increased power over disease.

"The day is short, and the work is much, and the labourers are slothful, and the reward is great, and the master of the house presses."

I may finally quote Robert Koch's statement in 1910 ("Epidemiologie der Tuberkulose" in *Zeitschrift für Hygiene*), in the paper from which the diagram on page 125 is derived.

Newsholme seeks to draw the conclusion that in Norway also the tuberculosis mortality has increased because there is insufficiently extensive reception of the tuberculous in institutions. I may add that this lack has already been recognised in Norway, and pains taken to counteract it by the provision of special institutions for tuberculous patients. It would appear that following on this the death-rate has ceased to rise in the most recent years. Newsholme refers also to the notably high tuberculosis mortality in Paris, and connects this with the insufficient hospital accommodation, in consequence of which the stay in hospital is too short to be able to exercise any obvious influence on the prevention of infection.

I am fully in agreement with Newsholme in his view that *the most extensive and prolonged reception possible of the tuberculous in institutions for the sick is the most important measure for the prevention of infection by and spread of tuberculosis*.

A more complete discussion of the causes of decline of tuberculosis is embodied in my *Prevention of Tuberculosis*, pp. 429 *et seq.* (Methuen, 1908).

OBJECTIONS TO THE SEGREGATION HYPOTHESIS

The objections most commonly entertained are as follows:—

(1) This hypothesis assumes that the steady and increasingly

rapid decline in tuberculosis during the last fifty years has resulted from human efforts, whereas it may be that we are seeing a cyclical phase in the epidemicity of this disease, comparable to the partial disappearance of scarlet fever as a fatal disease.

(2) The hypothesis assumes that the prevention or diminution of massive infection from person to person is the chief factor concerned, whereas is it not more likely that increased resistance to infection produced by improved hygienic conditions and especially by the great national improvement in nutrition experienced in recent generations is responsible for the improvement?

(3) Is it not likely that habituation to minor doses of tuberculosis in successive generations explains our diminishing death-rate, and is not this illustrated in the experience of some native races?

(4) Has not the selective influence of heredity gradually eliminated the families most prone to tuberculosis?

A volume would be required to discuss these questions fully, and I can only give a few points here. In other writings of mine the reader will find these points more fully debated. But I must mention first the objections raised by Professor Karl Pearson, F.R.S., the distinguished biometrician, to my use of *correlation factors* in drawing conclusions from the degree of parallelism in time between reduction of phthisis and increase of institutional segregation of patients. By using factors of correlation, in accordance with Pearson's method, one was able to state as a fraction the total correspondence in time between the two factors concerned, for which otherwise elaborate diagrammatic curves or long tables of figures would be required. The correlation factor was a shorthand statement of these comparisons. I was and am as well aware as the father of biometrics, that such a correspondence in time fails to justify the conclusion that the two factors compared are causally connected. The concurrence may be accidental, or they may both—in this instance, death-rate and measures of segregation —be products of some independent cause. The correlations need to be and were, in fact, considered in the light of our scientific knowledge of tuberculosis, on the following among other points.

(1) This knowledge teaches us that the tubercle bacillus

is the essential cause of tuberculosis. "No tubercle bacilli, no tuberculosis" is an elementary fact; though the converse statement that the presence in the system of these bacilli means that the recipient develops the well-known wasting disease—phthisis—does not hold good directly and always, inasmuch as (*a*) some persons resist infection more than others; and the resistance of the same person varies from time to time; and (*b*) both in experimental animals and in man it is certain that disease is more certain to be started when the infection by bacilli is massive or frequently repeated.

In herds of cattle, tuberculosis can be and often is stamped out by measures directed solely to the elimination of infection. Cattle tuberculosis is a dramatic, but not the only, instance of success in annihilating a chronic infectious disease when complete systematic measures are adopted. Leprosy in Norway provides another striking example. (*The Prevention of Tuberculosis*, p. 263.) Unlike the rest of Europe in which leper asylums had been universal these were lacking in Norway, and leprosy still prevailed; but with their establishment and with action ensuring partial segregation, leprosy began to decline in that country towards almost complete disappearance.

(2) The international decline in tuberculosis has occurred chiefly in countries which have in practice adopted *measures reducing the dosage of infection*, among these being the treatment of open cases of tuberculosis during a large part of their infectious life-time in institutions. Hospital segregation is not the sole means to this end, though it is the most practical and efficient means.

These considerations give weight to the coincidences in time between segregation and reduced tuberculosis which I have shown to exist in this and other countries, and convert a coincidence into a probably causal relation.

(3) The institutional treatment of phthisis during its acute exacerbations and when the patient is bedridden is now universally accepted as extremely desirable, even more so than treatment of earlier cases in a sanatorium with a view to cure. It is being carried out in most civilised countries to an enormous extent.

And yet, strange as it appears, some still fail to study the past which points to the conclusion that prevention of persistent massive infection by segregation has been an important factor in causing the great reduction of phthisis which had already been experienced, before the fundamental importance in preventive medicine of Koch's discovery in 1881 of the tubercle bacillus became slowly appreciated.

Having stated the case for regarding institutional segregation of open cases of tuberculosis as not only an important public health measure in sanitary administration, but as having been historically a great factor in the reduction of tuberculosis already achieved, we can next touch on alternative explanations of this decline (p. 133).

Have there been great *variations in the virulence of tuberculosis* during cycles of time? There is no evidence from older clinical accounts of phthisis that this has occurred. In all countries in which tuberculosis is endemic, the clinical picture of the disease is fairly consistent. That it is especially fatal in races when they first come into contact with Western people is well known. I have never satisfied myself as to whether this excessive death-rate indicates with certainty special susceptibility to attack and to death among an "unsalted" people, or whether the alternative explanation holds good that these newly invaded people live densely crowded in their huts with utter disregard of precautions against excessively massive infection (see p. 216 of my *Prevention of Tuberculosis*).

That *susceptible strains of human beings* have been gradually eliminated in the course of time is even more unlikely as an explanation of experiences in the last fifty years. The fact that the amount of reduction of tuberculosis has varied greatly in countries in all of which this disease had been long endemic, points away from this conclusion. Hereditary susceptibility in exceptional families has never been proved, notwithstanding valiant efforts of the biometricians, for they have not been able to eliminate the infective factor from their elaborate estimations of the force of heredity. Susceptibility doubtless varies in any one individual from time to time, being increased by intercurrent disease, by depressing emotions, by alcoholism, by over-fatigue, and so on. But these almost certainly count but little in the scale when compared with the question, has the patient or has he not been exposed to persistent or massive infection from another patient, especially a member of the same family?

Does the great improvement in national well-being and the fact that the population is better fed than in the past account for the decrease of tuberculosis? This is a view widely held, and is the more difficult to exclude as largely responsible for diminished tuberculosis because undoubtedly improved nutrition has helped in decreasing deaths from tuberculosis. There was a somewhat close correlation in the course of events from 1877 to 1901 between the total cost of food and the phthisis death-rates in Great Britain, but the correlation was relatively poor in Germany and absent from Ireland. The fact that high nutrition in sanatorium treatment aids recovery has appeared to support the contention that it may also prevent the successful invasion of tuberculous infection.

Events in the Great War are widely believed to support the same view. In most countries the later stages of the war coincided with a great increase in the tuberculosis death-rate. This happened in America, more so in Great Britain; much less so in Ireland. In France and still more in Germany the increase in the phthisis death-rate was very marked. Doubtless this was a period of some scarcity of food for the civilian populations of the warring countries. Is not this convincing evidence?

By itself it is not. Other adverse factors were acting as well as malnutrition. There was a devastating pandemic of influenza in the later years of the war, and this disease—even when no variations in nutrition are involved—has always increased the registered death-rate from tuberculosis. Furthermore, in Great Britain, and presumably in other countries, sick and wounded soldiers occupied sanatorium and hospital beds which consumptives had vacated, returning often to unsatisfactory homes. Not only so, but there were enormous displacements of population, vast recruitment of women and of ex-patients from sanatoria into munition and other works to take the place of the fighting men. It is when such industrial and domestic overcrowding consists of *aggregations of healthy and unhealthy* all working at great strain that tuberculosis finds ready victims. Thus while not doubting the value of high nutrition, especially for the young, its share in lowering our national tuberculosis toll does not entitle it, in my view, to be placed in the first category. The facts given on page 230 must also be borne in mind. Nutrition is of primary importance for infants and children; and this was more than maintained during the War, as shown by the rapid improvement in their death-rates. On nutrition and phthisis, see also pages 140, 147 and 402.

CONCLUDING REMARKS ON THE PREVENTION OF TUBERCULOSIS

If the main gist of what I have written is accepted, I desire in a final paragraph to set out the wider view of prevention of tuberculosis. Neither orthopaedic hospitals for cripples nor sanatoria and hospitals for consumptives can be said to be our ultimate means for preventing crippling or tuberculosis. But until we have discovered how to prevent poliomyelitis (a chief cause of crippling) as we already know how to abolish bovine tuberculosis, another great cause of crippling, orthopaedic hospitals will continue to be needed for the curative treatment of cripples.

In regard to tuberculosis derived from human infection the position is not so simple; for sanatoria, colonies for the families of consumptives, and still more hospitals for advanced and bed-ridden cases are not merely indispensable means of treatment, sometimes of cure; they are also invaluable means of preventing a further crop of cases of tuberculosis. They can, therefore, never cease to be required until tuberculosis approaches—as it will—extinction. They will continue to hasten the pace at which this end is being approached; but as improved personal habits as to coughing and expectoration (both in recognised consumptives and in others) become more general, the need for the above provisions will diminish. Already in the administration of towns in which there is efficient anti-tuberculosis administration, there is slackening in the notification of new cases of tuberculosis. Soon "new crops" of tuberculosis will diminish and, eventually, almost disappear, and then each member of the population will possess his own domestic "sanatorium" maintained by his own intelligent co-operation in communal hygiene.

E*

CHAPTER XV

THE ADMINISTRATIVE CONTROL OF TUBERCULOSIS

My description of experience in the administrative control of tuberculosis must be partially a continuation of Chapters XXVIII–XXX, especially of Chapter XXX, in my *Fifty Years in Public Health*.

In those chapters I described the prolonged struggle to base preventive measures on knowledge not only of deaths from tuberculosis but also of cases notified by medical practitioners at an earlier stage of illness; and I especially emphasised the value of short stay in a sanatorium to secure the education of patients in a hygienic life.

I now continue the subject from the time of my becoming Principal Medical Officer of the Local Government Board; my annual reports during the following eleven years enable me to do this fairly completely. When attending the Washington Congress on Tuberculosis in September 1908, I had been authorised by Mr. Burns to announce at its opening meeting that he was about to issue an Order making all cases of pulmonary tuberculosis attended by poor-law medical officers compulsorily notifiable to the M.O.H. This Order came into force in January 1909, and the Order and my explanatory memorandum are printed in my Annual Report, 1908–9. The Order provided also for the notification of changes of address of patients. Subject to the condition that no action should be taken rendering the notified patient "liable to a disability affecting him or his means of livelihood," power was given to promote cleansing and disinfection, to provide sputum-flasks, etc., for the safe disposal of sputa, and to help the patient "in any way which will tend to prevent the spread of infection."

My explanatory memorandum included a detailed statement on tuberculosis and on known methods of its control. It urged educational work with the public, but more intensively with the patient and his family, especially as to coughing and spitting; it stressed the importance of early diagnosis, and of gratuitous pathological examination of sputum for the family doctor; set out the procedure recommended to be taken in official inquiries concerning notified cases; the action needed to control infection, including personal instruction and short-period training in a sanatorium; procedure in home training and supervision: the proper uses of the tuberculosis dispensary, and of sanatorium treatment; and in conclusion reiterated the supreme importance of institutional treatment for advanced cases of pulmonary tuberculosis. When this was impracticable, methods of home isolation were set out.

The tuberculosis dispensary was given its important place as a centre for diagnosis and for detection of further cases, and the need for domiciliary visitation and investigation was emphasised. The domiciliary work of the dispensary was recommended to be a sub-department of the M.O.H.'s work.

PROGRESS 1909–10

The first Notification Order had already led to great increase in notification of cases of phthisis in towns in which voluntary notification previously existed, and I recommended further extensions of notification. I noted that in a very considerable number of towns the initiative of Brighton in utilising empty wards of isolation hospitals for the treatment of phthisis had been followed, and in some other towns empty smallpox hospitals, as in Manchester, were being similarly employed. Exceptional voluntary activity in anti-tuberculosis work was noted, including a popular exhibition at Whitechapel, where Mr. Burns had given a stirring address.

PROGRESS 1910–11

In my annual report for this year more active progress was noted, and in a general review I pointed out that if the value of the annual loss of lives in England at ages 15–65, the working years of life, were reckoned at only £150 per death from phthisis, the annual money loss to the community amounted to over five millions sterling, though as compared with the average mortality experience in 1871–80 the death-rate in 1909 represented a saving in that year of nearly six millions sterling. I add here a statement in which I summarised the causes of this saving of life, and of national industrial capacity.

(a) There had been improved medical care, better housing, hygienically improved occupational conditions, more wholesome and more abundant food and clothing. While these have doubtless increased resistance to infection, they have "even more ensured diminished facilities for infection." Infection had also been decreased by

(b) Improvements in the habits of the people. The spittoon has disappeared from private houses; and there is greatly improved cleanliness in most homes.

(c) A much more completely separate treatment of the sick is now secured than has ever been practised in the past. Increased dissociation of the sick from the healthy has been one of the outstanding features of the last thirty years. I need not quote the figures bearing this out. But the following facts as to urban compared with rural life may be given. At the census of 1901 out of a given number of the total urban population ten times as many lived in one-roomed tenements compared with the corresponding rural population, and twice as many out of a given number lived in two-roomed tenements and overcrowding in each room was greatest in towns. And yet, notwithstanding the greater crowding in houses in towns, their phthisis death-rate has decreased to a remarkable extent. The town dweller can obtain better treatment for his illnesses in hospitals and infirmaries, . . . and has thus been able to overcome almost completely the relative handicap to health of town life.

(d) In the same report I discussed the influence of nutrition as follows:

The nutriment of the individual has much influence in increasing resistance . . . but among populations living under approximately equal conditions as regards nutrition the death-rate from tuberculosis is highest among those most exposed to protracted infection and to the effect of dusty occupations; and the greatest possibilities of fruitful action by sanitary authorities lie in the first instance in preventing protracted exposure to infection and dust . . .

I give first place to the adequate and satisfactory treatment of advanced cases of consumption, not only for the sake of the patient, but also as a supremely important means of preventing the receipt by others of massive doses of infection. In this respect history and pathology teach the same practical lesson. No other means for the prevention of tuberculosis compares, in prospect of early result in diminished prevalence of the disease, with the treatment under hygienic conditions of advanced cases of the disease.

(On nutrition in relation to the incidence of tuberculosis, see also pp. 136 and 230.)

In 1910–11, a further advance was made in the planned and deliberate extension of compulsion in notification of cases of phthisis. In May 1911 the duty of notification was extended to doctors attending on patients (in-patients or out-patients) at all hospitals for the sick.

PROGRESS 1911–12 AND 1912–13

Following on the two previous Orders of the Local Government Board, the obligation to notify cases of pulmonary tuberculosis to the M.O.H. was extended in November 1911 to cases of this disease occurring in private practice. I noted in my annual report that the information thus received was confidential, and that remarkably few instances had come to light of individual hardship resulting from notification to the extent it had hitherto been enforced. In February 1913, the Board's Orders on Notification of Tuberculosis were consolidated, and the duty of notification was extended to non-pulmonary forms of the disease.

In this year a new element was introduced enabling more complete measures for the control of tuberculosis to be initiated than had heretofore been possible.

THE SANATORIUM BENEFIT UNDER THE INSURANCE ACT

A Sanatorium Benefit was included in the National Insurance Act, 1911. It was among the most beneficent of the provisions of that Act, not only through the Benefit itself, but much more as the result of the associated arrangements for greatly increased national expenditure in administrative measures for the control of tuberculosis in the whole population, non-insured as well as insured. Section 16 of the Insurance Act required the Insurance Committees created under the Act to make arrangements for treating persons suffering from tuberculosis and a special sum was set aside from the insurance funds for this purpose. No right to special treatment in a sanatorium was created, but such treatment was given on a large scale and with inadequate discrimination for insured patients, and many of these, though unsuitable for sanatorium treatment, crowded the available institutions. For the United Kingdom a sum of 1½ millions sterling was contributed from the National Treasury for the building of additional sanatoria; and it was definitely laid down that the beds thus provided were not solely for insured persons, but were to be available for the entire population.

A great impetus was thus given to more complete schemes for the treatment of tuberculosis. In December 1911, even before this impetus was felt, sanitary authorities in England had already provided some 1,400 beds for phthisis, in addition to the 9,000 beds for this disease already available in poor-law institutions. There were also some 2,800 beds provided by voluntary bodies.

A Departmental Committee, Mr. (later Lord) Astor, Chairman), sat to advise on the provision of Tuberculosis Schemes, and very properly recommended that in them provision should be made for the whole community, and that their organisation should be undertaken by local health authorities.

To the Local Government Board and its medical department came the central organisation of this nation-wide movement, and in order that non-insured as well as insured persons should share in the new provisions, it was decided in the same year that

the Government were prepared annually to provide a sum of money equal to half the total estimated cost of treating non-insured persons, including dependents of insured persons, under any scheme approved by the Local Government Board.

Thus, so far as tuberculosis was concerned, treatment at the public expense (half Government and half local authority) was provided for non-insured, while it was assumed that the Sanatorium Benefit would give insured consumptives an equal or greater amount of institutional treatment.

In 1921 the Sanatorium Benefit ceased to be included among the medical benefits of the Insurance Act, 1911, the provision of institutional treatment of insured consumptives devolving upon the County and County Borough Councils as for other members of the community. This I regard as a first step towards removing also the Medical Benefit, for general domiciliary treatment of insured persons out of the Insurance Act, and its replacement by a national system of medical treatment for all wishing to join it (p. 117).

In the enormous central work connected with the preparation of schemes I had the invaluable help of Dr. J. F. H. Coutts, Assistant Medical Officer of the Board, Dr. Chapman, himself a tuberculosis expert, also giving active assistance. Further details are given on p. xli of my Annual Report, 1912–13. It is unnecessary to describe here the domiciliary treatment of insured consumptives.

Dispensaries, unhappily so called, were already at work in some areas, as centres for skilled diagnosis, for examination of contacts, and for deciding the best form of treatment needed for each consumptive. This form of institution in Britain had been first introduced by Dr. (later Sir) Robert Philip in Edinburgh, and the obvious need for a common centre in each area for the purposes indicated above and other collateral public health work soon led to this administrative and medical centre being generally provided. I do not propose to describe the relative work of voluntary and official dispensaries. The former did good work in showing the way, but frequently there was risk of the dispensary work not being satisfactorily linked up with the preventive work of the local authority. Of course they should be one and indivisible; but this was sometimes delayed by the inertia of individual medical officers of health, and sometimes by the dispensary officers limiting themselves to clinical work and not adequately furthering public health work for combating tuberculosis. Nor do I propose to enlarge on the question of Care Committees, essential in a complete tuberculosis scheme. I must refer the reader to the already quoted annual report for fuller particulars.

In my annual report for 1912–13 will be found not only details of the development and administration of Tuberculosis Schemes, but also a detailed study of the national statistics on tuberculosis. This included, *inter alia*, standardised death-rates from tuberculosis, supplied from the General Register Office. Thus one could eliminate any variation in these rates caused by differing age-constitution in the compared populations. This was the first occasion on which such corrected rates had been given. Each sex was dealt with separately.

In giving elaborate maps of the local incidence of tuberculosis, I discussed the influence of migration on these death-rates. Other maps showed that there were vast local differences in the age distribution of the phthisis death-rate in the male and female sex respectively, as for instance in contrasting Birmingham and Sheffield. It was shown that urban conditions of life do not imply the same excess of phthisis in women as in men.

PROGRESS 1913–14

During the preceding year there had been completed the policy of the Local Government Board gradually to make all forms of tuberculosis compulsorily notifiable. In that year also the Sanatorium Benefit had come into being for the insured third of the population, and as already indicated the large grant of the Treasury for erection of sanatoria for the general population had been made, and the important offer had been made by the Treasury that half the total expenditure incurred by local authorities with the approval of the central Board for non-insured persons would be defrayed from national taxation. In 1913–14 both the secretarial and medical staff of the Board were busily engaged in developing national tuberculosis work on the lines indicated by the three governing events just set out.

As recommended in the report of the Departmental Committee (p. 142) the M.O.H. of each county and county borough area was put in administrative charge of the local Tuberculosis Scheme, while one or more special tuberculosis officers were appointed to undertake the clinical work of diagnosis (acting as consultants to private doctors, or independently of these), of examination of contacts, and of advising as to the form of treatment appropriate for each patient. Sometimes the tuberculosis clinical officer also had charge of patients in residential institutions; more often these institutions had a distinct staff. In the metropolis arrangements were more complicated; public health work following notification of cases and dispensary work was under the Borough Councils, while residential institutions were provided by the London County Council. For a considerable period consolidation of the anti-tuberculosis work in metropolitan boroughs was imperfect; then voluntarily managed dispensaries became municipal. The change may here and there have involved some lowering of efficiency, where the M.O.H. was Laodicean, but the possibilities of efficient unification of administration had increased.

The co-ordination of dispensary work with that of local sanitary authorities was discussed fully in my 1913–14 report; among other problems the same report dealt with observation beds, the importance of early diagnosis, "following up," examination of contacts, domiciliary treatment, care and after-care, and the principles underlying treatment in residential institutions.

In the same report I returned to the subject of the *advantages of hospital provision for disease in general*, and I reproduce here by permission of H.M. Stationery Office the diagram on the next page.

I commented that

these figures represent an enormous change in the conditions under which disease is treated in this country: and in setting out the influences which have brought about the reduction in the death-rate from a large number of diseases, an important place must be given to the improved treatment of disease which is now secured in our medical institutions for a largely increased proportion of the total population.

For pulmonary tuberculosis some further figures were given. Thus in the year 1912, of the total deaths from this disease 56·5 per cent of male and 43·8 per cent of female deaths in London occurred in infirmaries and hospitals, while even in rural districts 11·4 per cent of male and 6·4 per cent of female deaths occurred in these institutions. I further commented as follows:

In London more than half the total deaths from tuberculosis occur in hospitals, under conditions in which greater comfort and help to the patients are secured than would be possible under the domestic circumstances of most of the patients. The relief of anxiety, the diminution of infection, the lessening of financial stress . . . must also be very great.

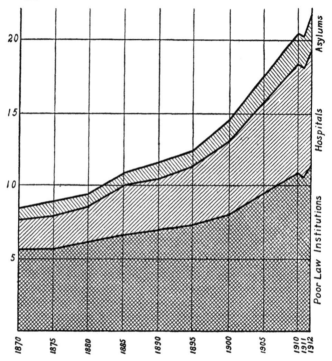

Per cent, of total deaths occurring in Institutions.

England and Wales 1870-1912.—*Proportion of Deaths from all causes occurring* (a) *in Poor-law Institutions,* (b) *in Hospitals,* (c) *in Lunatic Asylums.*

THE YEAR 1914-15

Prior to August 1914 six medical inspectors of the Medical Department of the Board had been employed in the development of tuberculosis work on behalf of the Central Government, but this number was necessarily curtailed under war conditions. Proposals for capital expenditure on sanatoria and other capital expenditure were temporarily held up. In some instances tuberculous patients in poor-law infirmaries were transferred to the isolation hospitals of public health authorities, so that the infirmaries might be used as military hospitals. But tuberculosis work was continued, although with difficulty, and much good work was accomplished.

THE YEAR 1915–16

Certain forms of anti-tuberculosis work, as for instance the systematic examination of home-contacts of patients, had to be abandoned, owing to lack of staff. Action had to be taken to prevent enthusiastic consumptives from enlisting as soldiers, and M.O.H's were required to supply the Army Council with a list of men aged 18 to 45 who had been notified as tuberculous during 1913–16.

THE YEAR 1916–17

I drew attention to the increased number of deaths from tuberculosis as compared with pre-War years. This was not confined to one sex, which meant that "conditions had arisen adversely affecting the health of persons of both sexes in these years." Naturally the impulse arose to ascribe the increase to the altered nutritional and other conditions of life during war-time, but a table given by me in my annual report and relating solely to the civilian population showed that inter-current circumstances not belonging necessarily to the War, had facilitated spread of infection. This table is reproduced in part below.

ENGLAND AND WALES: PROPORTIONAL MORTALITY (1913 = 100)

	1913	1915	1916
Pulmonary tuberculosis ..	100	112	112
Influenza	100	164	138
Pneumonia	100	130	101

This association of epidemic influenza with increased mortality from phthisis was not a new phenomenon; it was seen similarly in 1890–92 and in 1899–1900.

But apart from intercurrent influenza, war circumstances favoured the spread of phthisis. Some of these are noted on page 230. As I said on page XIX of my annual report for 1916–17:

A large number of unrecognised or partially recovered consumptives have entered the Army or have been employed at high wages in munition and other works. Often there has been overwork and excessive exposure to irritating dust, and owing to great migrations of military and civil population, there has been great overcrowding . . . notwithstanding great efforts of the Government to secure improved housing and conditions of work for munition workers.

In the report for this year I reviewed the general position as to the administrative control of tuberculosis somewhat fully. I concluded by "slaying" once more a persistent fallacy as follows:

Housing and institutional treatment for tuberculosis cannot properly be regarded as alternatives. They are necessary complements to each other, and there is needed increased expenditure on both. Housing is a problem in two divisions: for the healthy and for the sick. Special housing in institutions is needed for the sick when the care which their condition requires is not available in the home of the patient. This is so, whether the patient will be cured by institutional treatment or not.

THE YEAR 1917–18

I noted the continuance of war conditions. Referring to the excessive mortality from tuberculosis in women, I associated it with "their more extensive employment in munition and other industrial occupations, in conditions of exceptional stress and strain, associated with crowded lodging accommodation."

The problems of treating discharged soldiers and sailors suffering from tuberculosis were discussed, emphasis being laid on the "need to provide adequate useful occupation for the patient's mind and body," the lack of which was a common cause of sanatorium failure.

The above being my last annual report as Principal Medical Officer of the Local Government Board, subsequent progress in tuberculosis control can only be mentioned from an onlooker's standpoint. Administrative measures have been extended and consolidated, and there is now in operation a fairly complete and successful supervision and regulation of the life of consumptive patients.

I am convinced that had it not been for the somewhat lukewarm attitude of some local authorities and of their responsible officials concerned in anti-tuberculosis work, progress might have been more rapid. The M.O.H. or tuberculosis medical officer who attaches weight to the notion that we are in the grip of cosmic forces determining cycles of greater or less prevalence of tuberculosis; or who regards inherited resistance through natural selection as more important than anything he can do; or who regards the prevention of tuberculosis as being in the main a problem of high nutrition; or who has not cleared his mind by differentiating between housing for the sick and housing for the healthy, is unlikely to give enthusiastic and continuous impetus to the anti-tuberculosis work in the area for the health of which he is officially responsible. Under these and allied categories are the chief obstacles to much more rapid reduction of what is still a great national plague.

PERSONAL CONTRIBUTIONS

(For list of contributions on tuberculosis prior to 1909, see *Fifty Years in Public Health*, p. 266, and the two preceding chapters of this volume.)

The Present Position of the Tuberculosis Problem. A Lecture at the University of Chicago, May 10, 1926. (*Lancet*, 1926.)

Notification of Tuberculosis in Great Britain, A Historical Note. (*Brit. Med. Journal*, 1934, Vol. II, p. 75.)

Address on Private Medical Practice and Preventive Medicine to the Derby Medical Society. (*Lancet*, October 30, 1926.)

Retrospect and Outlook on the Tuberculosis Problem. (*S.C.A.A. News*, New York, February 1920.)

See the further references to personal contributions in the text of Chapters XII and XIII.

CHAPTER XVI

THE CONTROL OF VENEREAL DISEASES

DISEASE AND CHARACTER

The illnesses which man inflicts on himself, and in the control of which a high standard of conduct is necessitated, have had a special interest for me and, however inadequately, I have written much on this aspect of preventive medicine; for instance on "Considerations on the Relation between Government and Conduct" in Chapter x of my *Health Problems in Organised Society*,[1] and on "Medicine and Character" in Chapter xvii of *Medicine and the State*.[2]

Among these illnesses the foremost are the venereal diseases which a man voluntarily runs the risk of contracting; and the inevitable questions obtrude, shall we attempt to introduce such public health administrative machinery as will give "an artificial immunity to promiscuous fornication," or shall we trust to indirect social and moral measures, or is a middle course practicable and desirable? The history of changes of social outlook on these problems in my own lifetime goes far towards giving an answer to these questions.

Efforts in many countries to control the spread of venereal diseases by compulsory action against the female partner in illicit intercourse, have never extended in Great Britain beyond ports and towns where there were military stations.

Our Navy and Army consist chiefly of men living in almost compulsory celibacy; and during many decades venereal diseases were a chief cause of invalidity among them.

CONTAGIOUS DISEASES ACTS

Local Acts of Parliament followed, which gave powers in certain areas in which troops were stationed to subject prostitutes to periodical physical examination and to detain them while in a contagious condition. Hospitals were provided for

[1] P. S. King & Son, 1927.
[2] George Allen & Unwin, 1932.

the treatment of prostitutes found to be diseased; and these were regarded by the opponents of the Acts as being less concerned with treatment of the prostitute than with the task of making her "clean for hire." I must not follow the stages of the opposition to these local enactments, which steadily increased. The enactments probably were not entirely without effect in diminishing infection, and statistics were forthcoming which showed decrease of venereal disease in the localities concerned. I remember in the '80's studying statistics for and against this system; the results appeared contradictory. It was in fact the usual story: *non ceteris paribus*. More factors than the one—inspection and segregation of the infected—dealt with in the statistical tables of sickness, were in action. This has been shown by the course of events.

The Acts, which had been applied in eighteen military and naval stations, were suspended from operation in 1883 and repealed in 1886. The repeal was brought about, in part at least, because under the Acts power was given compulsorily to examine in the scheduled areas not only any prostitute, but also any one suspected of prostitution, as well as to detain in hospital any woman found to be suffering from a venereal disease. The fact that men escaped scot-free under this system aroused indignation; as did also the impression that a main object of the Acts was to render "promiscuous fornication" safe for men.

Among the factors producing the steady diminution of venereal diseases in the Army, which has occurred since the Contagious Diseases Acts were repealed, have been improved methods of treatment continued until the patient is cured, and, even more, educational measures and improved recreational resources for the soldiers. Temperance increased, and there was an improved moral tone amongst the men. Colonel Harrison, D.S.O., has stated that the incidence of venereal disease per 1,000 men in the British Army in the United Kingdom in 1905 was only one-sixth of that in 1885.

But although venereal diseases had diminished in the Army and Navy, the extent of the disease as seen both in hospitals and in private practice among civilians continued to cause much heart-searching.

INCREASED KNOWLEDGE FAVOURING CONTROL

Meanwhile scientific knowledge concerning these diseases had increased, rendering new and improved measures against them practicable.

In the year 1903 Metschnikoff and Roux transmitted syphilis from a human subject to monkeys by cutaneous inoculation, and they demonstrated that the application of strong calomel ointment at the site of inoculation prevented the transmission of disease.

In 1905 Schaudinn discovered in primary lesions of syphilis the protozoon to which syphilis is due; and Noguchi in 1911 succeeded in cultivating this artificially. Noguchi furthermore proved in 1913 that general paresis of the insane and locomotor ataxy are due to this protozoon, and actually found it in the brain and spinal cord of human patients suffering from these diseases.

In 1906 Wassermann and his co-workers discovered a serological test which enables a correct diagnosis of syphilis to be made when clinical evidence is dubious. It gives valuable evidence also as to whether anti-syphilitic treatment need be further continued after a course of treatment.

These discoveries rendered it possible to recognise syphilis when it might previously have been overlooked. Ehrlich's discovery of Salvarsan (606) opened out in 1910 a greatly increased prospect of cure of syphilitis; and what is perhaps even more important, rendered it possible promptly to free the patient from much of his power to infect others. This important new application of chemotherapy placed syphilis, from the public health standpoint, in a more favourable position than tuberculosis, in which efforts in this specific field have hitherto failed.

During this period a local form of gonorrhoea, one of the two chief venereal diseases, was being vigorously attacked by some local authorities. This was *ophthalmia neonatorum*, a purulent discharge from the eyes occurring in new-born babies, in most instances caused by gonorrhoeal contagion from the mother during the act of birth. In my report to the Local Government Board for 1910 I described the increasing extent to which local authorities were making this disease compulsorily notifiable, consent for its addition to the list of diseases notifiable under the Infectious Diseases (Notification) Act having been given in each instance by the Local Government Board. Into the activities against this disease, the President (Mr. John Burns) entered vigorously; and in 1935, only a few weeks before this paragraph was written, I received a gleeful message from him as to the number of children's institutions for the blind which had been closed. As the result of the prompt treatment of infantile ophthalmia which has rapidly become fairly general, many of these institutions are no longer needed. In February 1914 ophthalmia of the new-born was made universally notifiable, and preventive measures then became general.

These were among the factors which led the Local Government Board in March 1912 to arrange for an inquiry into the control over venereal diseases, with special reference to the adequacy and general character of the arrangements for institutional treatment of these diseases available in England and Wales.

DR. JOHNSTONE'S REPORT

Dr. Ralph Johnstone, a medical inspector of the Board, was nominated by me to undertake this inquiry; and his report on the subject (Cd. 7029), which was presented as a Parliamentary paper early in August 1913, gave an excellent account of our knowledge of the subject, and of the main lines of administrative action against venereal diseases which were immediately desirable and practicable. I reproduce here a small part of the remarks which I prefixed to this report, as it summarises the public health problems constituted by these diseases.

The inquiry was necessarily limited in extent, and of a "sampling" description; but the report, although thus limited, sufficed to enable certain broad conclusions to be drawn bearing on administrative action.

Extracts from my preface to Dr. Johnstone's report.

The venereal diseases requiring serious consideration are gonorrhoea and syphilis. The first-named is the less serious of the two, even though it is a frequent cause of chronic suffering and sterility in women, as well as the chief cause of blindness occurring as the result of ophthalmia of the new-born.

The serious extent to which syphilis affects the national health is not generally realised. It is an important cause of arterial degeneration and of heart disease, and the cause of locomotor ataxy and general paralysis of the insane, as well as of various forms of skin and bone diseases.

The virus of syphilis can be and commonly is transmitted from the parent to the foetus *in utero*. The immediate result often is abortion or miscarriage. . . . Apart from still-births, syphilis is a frequent cause of premature birth and of the "Marasmus" and "Atrophy" which bulk largely in the causes of mortality in the first month after birth. . . .

In his report, Dr. Johnstone has emphasised the practical point that syphilis is spread less by habitual or professional prostitutes than by women who are only occasional prostitutes and by men "who when infected have neglected to secure competent advice or to observe it when given." Hence it is impracticable to attempt to repress this disease by restrictive measures of the type of the former Contagious Diseases Acts. We must look to other means of control applicable with a fair degree of equality to all concerned, of both sexes. . . . It is of primary importance, in the public interest, that facilities for gratuitous Wassermann and allied tests should be made available throughout England and Wales.

Syphilis illustrates more forcibly even than tuberculosis the importance of *treatment as a means of preventing the spread of disease*. This was true in regard to the older methods of its treatment. If, as is now generally believed, the duration of active symptoms is greatly decreased and relapses are less frequent when salvarsan is administered, this truth becomes still more important. . . . Dr. Johnstone reports that for the vast majority of patients suffering from syphilis in its active earlier stages there is everywhere a great dearth of the best means of accurate diagnosis and of the best methods of treatment under acceptable conditions; and that in consequence a large amount of serious avoidable disease continues its ravages.

The essential remedies required to reduce this evil are set out in the following paragraph from Dr. Johnstone's Report:—

"It cannot be too strongly urged that the best method of controlling venereal diseases and protecting those free from infection would be the provision of means for early and accurate diagnosis, with skilled advice and adequate treatment, available for all infected persons. In short, the essence of the problem is how to get a willing patient at the earliest time to the doctor from whom or to the institution from which such advice and treatment is to be had."

ROYAL COMMISSION ON VENEREAL DISEASES

In November 1913 His Majesty the King appointed a Royal Commission,

to inquire into the prevalence of Venereal Diseases in the United Kingdom, their effects upon the health of the community, and the means by which those effects can be alleviated or prevented, it being understood that no return to the policy or provisions of the Contagious Diseases Acts of 1864, 1866, or 1869 is to be regarded as falling within the scope of the inquiry.

The appointment of this Commission was probably hastened by a letter urging it, which appeared a few months earlier in the *Morning Post*, signed by many distinguished doctors and others. The following were appointed to constitute the Commission: Baron Sydenham of Combe (Chairman), Sir David Brynmor Jones, Sir Kenelm Digby, Sir Almeric Fitzroy, Sir Malcolm Morris, Sir John Collie, Dr. Newsholme, Canon Horsley, Rev. Dr. Scott Lidgett, Dr. Mott, Dr. Mary Scharlieb, Mr. J. E. Lane, Mr. Snowden, M.P., Mrs. Creighton, and Mrs. Burgwin.

In my annual report for the next year, 1914, I stated that I had during the year prepared four memoranda for this Royal Commission on the following subjects:

1. *Ophthalmia neonatorum.*
2. The statistics of still-births.
3. The distribution of general hospital accommodation in England and Wales.
4. An administrative scheme for the control of venereal diseases.

I added that the enormous increase of military celibate life due to the World War had rendered the control of venereal diseases a matter of greater urgency than it had ever been in the past, and as the labours of the Royal Commission were drawing to a close, I hoped that soon it would be practicable to organise a scheme of national effort for securing improved diagnosis and adequate treatment of these diseases.

THE ROYAL COMMISSION'S REPORT

The main recommendations in the Royal Commission's Report (March 1916) were as follows:

1. Confidential registration of causes of death.

2. A uniform system of records of sickness in hospital and poor-law establishments should be organised by the Local Government Board.

3. Extended facilities should be made available for the diagnosis of venereal diseases by laboratory methods.

4. Measures should be taken to render the best modern treatment of venereal diseases readily available for the whole community, and the arrangements should be such that persons affected by these diseases will have no hesitation in taking advantage of the facilities for treatment which are afforded.

5. The organisation of these means of treatment should be in the hands of the councils of counties and county boroughs.

6. Institutional treatment should, so far as possible, be provided at general hospitals, by negotiation between them and local authorities.

7. This treatment should be free to all. There should be no refusal to treat a patient who is unwilling to go to his own doctor.

8. The treatment at any institution should not be restricted to persons resident in a particular area.

9. Subject to proper safeguards, local authorities should be empowered to supply salvarsan or its substitutes gratuitously.

10. The expenditure on laboratory diagnosis and on treatment by local authorities should be paid by the Local Government Board on the basis of 75 per cent from Imperial Funds and 25 per cent from local rates.

Of the above recommendations, 3, 4, 5, 6, 7, 8, 9, and 10 were promptly adopted by the Local Government Board, and Regulations, obligatory in character, were issued by the Board to local authorities in July of the same year. This promptitude was in part due to the urgency caused by war conditions; but to the late Mr. Walter (afterwards Lord) Long, then President of the Board, must be ascribed the chief credit for the prompt and effective action taken. I may be excused a personal reference. I was deeply impressed with the need for immediate action and was fearful that there might be official delay. On a given Friday when I knew Mr. Long was about to leave London for the week-end, he received an urgent personal letter from me addressed to him at the House of Commons. This letter set out the position and enclosed an article in a review on the subject in which I had contributed a summary of the evidence to and conclusions of the Royal Commission. In my letter to Mr. Long I stated that on the Monday he would receive my proposals for immediate action. On that morning I had a "chit" from him: "put forward your recommendations at once." The proposals recommended by the Royal Commission set out that 75 per cent of the cost of local treatment centres throughout the country should come from the National Treasury, leaving only 25 per cent to come out of local rates in counties and county boroughs. This I had urged on the Royal Commission, as I realised that without such liberal help local authorities might hesitate to act vigorously and some of them might refrain from action. Mr. Long minuted to the effect that the Treasury should pay the entire cost, but was persuaded to adhere to the 75 per cent. He walked over to the Treasury the same day, and came back with the Chancellor's sanction to the proposed expenditure. So it was at once a case of full steam ahead! I doubt whether this case could be paralleled in official experience.

Subsequent action is set out in my reports for 1916 and 1917. As already indicated the Royal Commission had recommended that treatment centres *should be* set up. The recommendation put forward from the Medical Department and accepted by the President was that the provisions for treatment and for diagnosis should be *mandatory*. Local authorities had the duty definitely imposed on them to provide these facilities.

Preference was expressed that the treatment centres should be at general hospitals, in order that no special attention would be drawn to the kind of illness. The Committees of a considerable number of voluntary hospitals objected to instituting special departments for venereal diseases, although the entire cost would be borne by the local authorities and the Exchequer. Some of these Committees held the older view that by so doing they would be condoning vice. More often objection was taken that it constituted a departure from the voluntary charitable work of the hospital, inasmuch as any patient applying was to receive treatment, *whatever his circumstances*, and whether or not he lived in the area ordinarily served by the hospital. This was a valid objection, though voluntary hospitals already were treating patients who were not very poor, and sometimes were exacting payment according to means.

There was the further objection that the medical staffs of these hospitals gave their services gratuitously, and this could not be expected for "State" patients. The Board agreed with this view, and as a rule a definite salary or a definite fee per attendance was given to the special venereal disease surgeon appointed by the hospital with the approval of the local authority. The majority of important voluntary hospitals, however, came into the scheme, the local authority paying for the costs of the clinic. No serious difficulty was encountered in meeting one condition of our scheme, that patients need not be inhabitants of the area of the given local authority. In the periodical returns made for financial adjustment it was found that the cost of outside patients could easily be relegated to the appropriate local authority.

An essential part of each scheme was the provision of laboratories to which medical practitioners could without any charge send specimens for Wassermann tests and for microscopic search for spirochoetes and gonococci. The cost was borne by the local authority and the Treasury. The method of provision varied. Large authorities added the new work to their already existent Public Health Laboratories. In other instances, independent arrangements were made, as for for instance with University Laboratories.

A condition of approval of a local authority's scheme was that the treatment should be confidential, and the patient's name and address should be known only to the surgeon in charge of the Centre. In order further to ensure secrecy, patients were authorised, if they wished, to attend Treatment Centres distant from their homes.

The regulations empowered local authorities to supply salvarsan free of cost to any medical practitioner asking for it for his private patients, subject only to his competence to give intravenous injections.

Local authorities were also urged to arrange for instruction of the public respecting these diseases. Much of this instructional work was done by the National Council for Combating Venereal Diseases, of which Lord Sydenham was the first president, and to it much credit attached in awakening the public to the danger of these diseases and the need for prompt treatment.

The control of venereal diseases is beset with difficult problems, some of which are discussed in this chapter.

GRATUITOUS TREATMENT OF ALL APPLICANTS

Although this was the first instance on a completely national scale of gratuitous provision of medical care at the expense of public taxation, it had been anticipated partially in certain directions. Public Health Authorities were already providing hospital treatment and pathological diagnosis for acute febrile diseases, mostly without charge; and similar provision was already being made, though incompletely, for tuberculosis. Poor Law Authorities were providing treatment, even though often unsatisfactory in character, for both venereal diseases and tuberculosis in workhouse infirmaries, but this was limited to the technically destitute. The new proposals as regards venereal diseases were a gigantic step forward in the provision of medical treatment for the entire community at the expense of national funds. Thanks are due to the British Medical Association, as representing the general practitioners of medicine throughout the country, for taking a statesmanlike view. Evidently there was risk of some interference with private medical practice, and the Association faced bravely the alternative of safeguarding private practice or of a great departure in policy demanded by the public interest. For, it will be noted, the State proposed to provide treatment to as many as asked for it, without any limit of income. True, there was no prohibition, and there was some aid, of private medical treatment of venereal diseases. Doctors wishing to treat syphilis could have a free supply of salvarsan, and could charge their patients for the medical care they gave. It is fair also to add that many private practitioners were unacquainted with the modern treatment of syphilis, and were glad to be relieved of its treatment; and so far as patients insured in the national system were concerned (a third of the total population), the national provision for venereal diseases lessened the practitioners' burden, while not affecting their remuneration.

The proposed Regulations of the Local Government Board were sent in advance to the British Medical Association for observations: and at their representative meeting, although at first there was some opposition to the proposal of gratuitous treatment *for all applicants*, the Association eventually adopted the official scheme by an overwhelming majority. This was done, although it was fully recognised that here was "a new departure of a most important kind." In doing this the Council of the Association were influenced by the consideration of

the exceptional nature of venereal diseases; the reluctance of patients affected by them to go to their own private medical attendant; the risk that they might, with disastrous results, go to unqualified persons for treatment; and the importance to the community that all sufferers should be induced to seek early and adequate treatment;

and for the above reasons the Council considered that the proposals of the Royal Commission, endorsed by the Local Government Board, should be accepted and approved by the Association.

In the third volume of my *International Studies*, etc., I have given rather full details on this subject, and in the *American Journal of Social Hygiene* I have adduced statistics showing the marked success attending the work of the Treatment Centres throughout the country. Similar figures have been given in the Registrar General's annual return. I may quote here some later figures given by Colonel Harrison, D.S.O., in the *Journal of Social Hygiene*, 1929. He concludes that in the civilian population of England and Wales the incidence of new infections of syphilis has decreased by five-sixteenths since 1918. I think this statement underestimates the total result.

Success was made more certain when resort to official

Treatment Centres was increased, by legal prohibition of treatment of venereal diseases by unqualified persons. In a memorandum prepared for the Royal Commission on Venereal Diseases (June 1914) I had suggested that

chemists and other unqualified practitioners ought to be *forbidden to treat any disease or disorder of the genito-urinary organs*, . . . *Such a prohibition should only apply in districts in which satisfactory gratuitous treatment for these diseases is available*. It would not, I think, be practicable to extend the inhibition to diseases such as skin diseases, sore throat, etc., which may be syphilitic; but the inhibition to the extent recommended above, if secured, would be most valuable.

The Commission in their report said:

We should have advocated legal provisions making the treatment of venereal disease by unqualified persons a penal offence, but we recognise the practical difficulties in securing the effective operation of such a law in present circumstances. The prohibition of advertisements is open to less objection on this ground, and we believe it would go far to remedy the great evils which have been emphasised by the evidence given before us. (Par. 195.)

In a memorandum to the President of the Local Government Board (Lord Rhondda) dated September 30, 1916, after quoting the above, I referred to conferences I had with Lord Sydenham and Sir Thomas Barlow of the National Council for Combating Venereal Diseases, urging the President to take steps.

to prohibit the treatment of venereal diseases by unqualified persons, and to prohibit any advertisement relating to these diseases.

Resolutions to the same effect were passed *inter alios* by the Royal College of Physicians, the General Medical Council, and the Municipal Corporations and the County Council Associations.

This was accomplished in 1917 when the Venereal Disease Act became law. This not only prohibited the advertisement of remedies for venereal diseases, but also made illegal the treatment of any person for venereal disease, or the giving of advice for treatment, except by a duly qualified medical practitioner;

F

but it was provided that these powers should not become operative within any area "until a scheme for the gratuitous treatment of persons in that area suffering from venereal disease has been approved by the Board and is already in operation." Ere long, owing to the general provision of gratuitous treatment, it became practicable to enforce the prohibition against unqualified practice for the treatment of venereal diseases universally.

It should be added that the success of the official measures is shown not only in the reduction of the prevalence of venereal diseases, but also in the diminution of such diseases as general paresis of the insane and degenerative diseases of the nervous system which are apt to result from neglected venereal disease.

The coexistence of other factors besides the general provision of treatment likely to reduce the incidence of venereal diseases makes it difficult to assess the relative importance of each factor. Thus the end of the War meant diminution of sexual promiscuity. The reduction of prostitution has been associated with an apparent increase of irregular unions of longer duration and therefore involving less risk of contagion. The increased use of mechanical provisions having a contraceptive intent may have also decreased contagion. Great social changes have occurred under each of these headings. But making full allowance for all these factors, there is no reasonable doubt that the national provision of universal free treatment of venereal diseases has been a chief factor in the reduction of these diseases experienced since 1918.

Pathological Facilities for diagnosis and control of treatment in a large number of diseases had been urged in my annual report for 1912–13, in which was set out a statement of the work already being done to this end by some large local authorities. This comprised in the main aids to the diagnosis of infectious diseases, but in a few instances suspected cancer material, etc., was being examined. The matter had gone so far as to make financial provision for the initiation of this more general pathological work through local authorities, in the financial estimates of the Government for 1913, but the Great War indefinitely postponed action.

PROGRESS IN 1916–17

The Board's Regulations on venereal diseases had been issued in July 1916, and during that year and 1917 a large portion of my time and that of Dr. Coutts, who had already given important aid in organising tuberculosis work, was occupied in active co-operation with secretarial colleagues in helping local authorities to initiate schemes for the diagnosis and treatment of venereal diseases. Formal conferences were held by the medical inspectors of the Board with local authorities and frequently with the Committees of local general hospitals. Among these inspectors was Dr. J. P. Candler, a pathologist who had worked some years with Sir Frederick Mott. Dr. Coutts and Dr. Candler gave special help in preparing the technical part of my memorandum, which was issued with the Board's Regulations. I addressed a number of conferences in important centres and many conferences were held at the Board's offices. This work of organisation, shared between the secretarial and medical staff, was an example of excellent co-operation than which no better could be found.

By the end of March 1917, 87 out of the 145 Councils which were charged with the execution of the Board's Regulations had submitted schemes for a population of 23½ millions, and nearly 140 voluntary hospitals in England and Wales had expressed their willingness to participate in the schemes of local authorities. In some districts, in which difficulty had been experienced in obtaining specially experienced medical officers for the Treatment Centres, the Army Council assisted by permitting Army Medical Officers to be appointed to this work. I would emphasise the fact that in the Army during the War venereal diseases were being successfully treated before civilian arrangements had been completed; and much of the diminution of mortality from venereal diseases in the post-bellum period shown in our national statistics is attributable to this.

In my report for 1916–17 will be found a statement of difficulties in detail, and the ways in which these were met.

PROGRESS IN 1917–18

During this year 127 out of the total 145 local authorities had schemes at work. There were fairly adequate arrangements for the more populous areas of the country, but difficulties in scattered areas still needed to be overcome. In some rural areas local authorities were authorised to pay travelling expenses to a town hospital for treatment. Already it was being found that to camouflage the treatment of venereal disease by arranging for it to be done at a general hospital for all diseases was not so essential as had been thought; for a few *ad hoc* clinics, opened where the Committees of general hospitals had refused to help, proved successful, patients coming to them readily. Although I do not particularise the good work done in subsidising Rescue Homes, in the treatment of sailors, of pregnant women for syphilis, and other special work, these developments had great importance. I must, however, comment on the subject of

THE COMPULSORY NOTIFICATION OF VENEREAL DISEASES

Appended to the Report of the Royal Commission (Cd. 8189) was a memorandum prepared by me for the Commission on the notification of infectious diseases in general, with particular reference to the question whether notification of venereal diseases would be of practical utility. I reported against notification, and the Royal Commission recommended that its consideration should be postponed.

In later papers I have suggested the desirability of applying compulsory notification to syphilitic diseases in childhood, e.g. interstitial keratitis, and that valuable action can be taken in discovering syphilis by pathological examination of tissues from cases of abortion and miscarriage. This is now often done, but only to a very partial extent. The essential difficulty is to secure that the private practitioner will feel free and be willing to act on the principle that he (like the M.O.H.) has a duty to the State as well as to his patient in detecting disease and preventing its spread. We often hear and read that we must think in terms of health not of disease. This is nonsense in so far as it suggests we are to put on blinkers when there is an opening to discover disease, and thereby pave the way for its treatment and for the organisation of measures to prevent its further extension.

Notification of every case of venereal disease would be valuable if, and only if, it led to the discovery of many sources of infection to counteract which effective action could be taken. This would imply attempts to trace a man's or men's disease to a particular woman, and to take coercive measures against her. Men would seldom be discovered as sources of female infection, and official activities would be almost completely unisexual. Attempts in this direction have occasionally been made in America, but I cannot be confident that they have had considerable success. Such attempts may, meanwhile, have inhibited many patients from coming for treatment for venereal disease to a doctor or centre from which notification is required. It is true that in Britain this risk is minimised by the prohibition of treatment of these diseases by unqualified persons; but, on the other hand, the fact that all cases must be treated by a doctor, whose duty it is to warn the patient as to infecting others, diminishes the importance of formal notification. Personally I revolt against coercive measures which must be chiefly directed against women. In a civilian population such measures would furthermore, I believe, have little effect in reducing infection. The lines of more complete control of these diseases consist in (a) attracting all who have venereal disease or suspect they have it to a Treatment Centre, where they receive instruction as to avoidance of transmission of their complaint, while benefiting by efficient treatment.

(b) The second line of practical control consists in utilising the information already possessed by private practitioners and by medical officers of health. There is much need for action on these lines. Thus more might be done to secure Wassermann and other tests after miscarriages, and when still-births occur, and to secure the examination of family contacts with patients under treatment.

I am aware of the difficulties in such circumstances as the above; but am certain that until information for action which is already within reach is fully utilised, little hope lies in action, which often would need to be coercive, against women who are believed to have infected several men venereally. Imagine such a case coming into Court, and the course of the cross-examination of the unwilling men-witnesses. Who will vouch for their chastity except in regard to the accused woman? Proposals for notification have been revived to secure the return to treatment of a venereal patient who has ceased to attend a Treatment Centre before he is freed from infection. Compulsion to accept a particular form of treatment is *ultra vires;* all that could be done if the doctor reported such a case, and the patient were recalcitrant, would be to remove him compulsorily to hospital, and those familiar with other instances of legislation to this end will appreciate how seldom it would be successful in regard to this disease. Even this would only be practicable under new legislation, and were this obtained, the procedure indicated is undesirable in public health work.

WAR EPISODES

A few jottings will illustrate some of our earlier difficulties. In 1916 I wrote to Sir Alfred Keogh, the Director-General of the Army Medical Department, who was always willing to co-operate in civilian work. I urged that the practice of refusing recruits suffering from venereal disease should cease, and that these should be placed under military medical treatment. This was done.

In 1918 when demobilisation was beginning, it was proposed to discharge venereal soldiers, sending a letter stating the man's address to the M.O.H. of the district where each patient lived. Sir Alfred, on my representation, at once agreed to regard information as to these soldiers as confidential, and decided to retain them temporarily in military hospitals, "until all signs of active disease had ceased."

New influences favouring the spread of venereal disease necessarily arose from war conditions. Vast numbers of men became compulsorily celibate, and temptations to promiscuity were everywhere prevalent. Perhaps even more serious than this was the displacement from their home surroundings of many thousands of young women, to some of whom it almost appeared that the giving of sexual favours to a soldier on leave was a species of patriotism. There is good evidence that in Britain venereal disease was spread less by prostitutes than by casual relationships.

One interview gave me a shock. A lady representing a group of social workers urged me to recommend the President of the Local Government Board to take action to secure the physical examination of all girls suspected of irregular relationships with recruits and soldiers. Nothing I could say in the way of reminding her of the proved futility of such attempts in the past, and of the gross insults likely to be inflicted on chaste women, could change her views, and she left me, regarding me doubtless as the most obstructive, stick-in-the-mud, wilfully blind official "as ever was!"

THE ETHICAL ASPECT OF VENEREAL DISEASES

It is impossible for me in this chapter to discuss this, the more important, side of the prevention of venereal diseases. In a lecture given for the British Social Hygiene Council (formerly the N.C.C.V.D.) and still published by the Council as a separate pamphlet, I have set out in full detail what I think is the teaching of morality and religion.

Perhaps I cannot better conclude this chapter than by quoting the last paragraphs of Chapter IX of my *Health Problems in Organised Society*.

I put aside the general teaching of chemical prophylaxis. It can only be effective in a fraction of cases; furthermore, non-personal and indiscriminate instruction of this kind will, in my view, increase the amount of promiscuity, which is the real enemy to be fought.

We must not lose our view of the final issues involved. To be successful, civilised life in communities necessitates a steady change and advance in the standards of morality. It necessarily involves partial suppression of our over-sexed instincts and a stricter adherence to the monogamy which civilised family life implies. . . . Partial failure in the past does not condemn to futility psychologically better directed and more intelligent efforts now within our reach. . . . This is the task of the pedagogue inspired by high ideals and by accurate knowledge of child psychology, and of parents who realise the extent of their responsibility and of their power to educate their children to resist venereal or any other form of moral infection.

Our knowledge of the processes by which habits of self-control can be initiated and fortified, and by which the social instinct can be made to restrain and in large measure to sublimate the sex-instinct—as well as of the possibilities of forming and directing public opinion towards higher ideals—goes far to confirm the conviction that further victory over venereal diseases will be gained chiefly on the ethical plane, and that on this plane we can achieve success. Although moral progress is slow, the rate of progress tends to become accelerated at each step, so that in the end vast masses of people accept a new truth in a short time.

These remarks have an important bearing on the relative value of education and compulsion. By education I do not mean merely intellectual instruction, but the systematisation, from the earliest age of each child, of efforts in the training of character and the development of self-control through example and teaching. Knowledge is necessary, but in practical life it is attitude more than knowledge that counts. The real failure in life consists in the shirking of the discipline of self-control. The exercise of compulsion runs some risk of atrophying self-control; but compulsion may be a means of training in self-control when it operates chiefly against those who cannot or will not exercise will-power. Indeed, the ideals of compulsion and of education of character are not irreconcilable in public health work. In the sequence of national life the policeman preceded the school teacher, but the success of the teacher renders the policeman less and less necessary if intelligent and conscientious parents enter into partnership in the task of education of character.

PERSONAL CONTRIBUTIONS

Public Health Education. (*The Hospital and Health Review*, 1921.)

The Relative Roles of Compulsion and Education in Public Health Work. (Address at Bournemouth meeting of the Royal Sanitary Institute, July 1922. Reprinted as Chapter IX in my *Health Problems in Organised Society* (P. S. King & Son, 1927).)

The Moral Aspects of Social Hygiene. (*American Journal of Social Hygiene*, December 1924, and a special pamphlet issued by the National Council of Social Hygiene.)

The Decline in the Registered Mortality from Syphilis in England. To what is it due? (*American Journal of Social Hygiene*, December 1926.)

CHAPTER XVII

THE EVOLUTION OF PREVENTIVE MEDICINE: ITS PHYSIOLOGICAL SIDE

THE headings of previous chapters show that these chapters have been chiefly concerned with the steady improvement of the treatment of sickness, and with the social and sanitary means for diminishing poverty, in the sense of deprivation of essential needs, and thereby lessening the sickness causing poverty and the poverty causing sickness. There are several reasons why the treatment of existent sickness has formed so large a part of total public health efforts (in which I include voluntary as well as official charitable work) up to the present day, and why for many decades treatment will continue to form a chief part of the work of Public Health Authorities.

(1) Our knowledge even now of the means for preventing a large proportion of the total sickness and mortality in the community is only partial. This is true of cancer, on the prevention of which we have hitherto but scant and incomplete light.

Cancer is in marked contrast with syphilis, a plague which vies with cancer in being a chief reason why men who have reached the end of their third decade of life fail to survive to old age; for syphilis, given abstinence from anti-social conduct, can be abolished entirely.

(2) More generally, even when knowledge exists which if applied would reduce avoidable illness, it has not become vitally realised by most of us, and many among us are completely ignorant concerning it. Many more are unwilling to live in accord with this knowledge, or are so circumstanced that their knowledge cannot be applied in their lives. I need not discuss here whether moral inability or intellectual ignorance are the greater destroyers of health. The answer as to the relative share of the two will depend in part on whether—as we ought—we include mental and moral as well as physical health in our review.

(3) Physicians, hygienists, and Public Health Authorities find themselves confronted by an embarrassing multitude of sick

F*

people needing immediate aid; and their primary duty obviously is *to give adequate and complete treatment of already existent sickness.* Ambulance work must precede work to prevent future accidents, though no ambulance work is fully satisfactory which does not include thorough investigation of the origin of the accident, and the full application of the conclusions from inquiry to the prevention of recurrent accidents. I do not imply that prevention of accidents—or of sickness—is being neglected. History teaches us all the time that the close investigation of each accident or case of illness has been the most fertile source of our present knowledge of Preventive Medicine. This has been so especially in regard to communicable diseases. In more recent years bacteriology has given us powerful additional means of preventing some of these diseases. But broadly speaking, attempts at separating the practice of curative and preventive medicine from each other have proved futile; and it is universally recognised that the practice of the two branches of medicine must always be intimately associated.

This being so, provision of satisfactory treatment of the sick must continue to be an important part of Public Health practice. So also the enforcement of sickness insurance, thus securing medical as well as financial benefits for many who are not technically poor, must be held to be, at least potentially, and in part actually, a means of improved health.

The work of these two organisations (Poor Law and Insurance) for preventing illness by treating it has been extended by various voluntary bodies, and even more so by the efforts during the last thirty years of Public Health and Education Authorities, as set out in preceding chapters.

On these two some supplementary remarks may be made at this point.

MEDICAL WORK OF PUBLIC HEALTH AUTHORITIES

Since Sanitary Authorities emerged into separate existence—at first as an offshoot of Poor Law Authorities—they have steadily increased their medical services. For some decades they were chiefly concerned with treatment as a means of preventing the spread of infectious diseases, including vaccination against smallpox. On the vast collateral effect of domestic and municipal sanitation in diminishing diarrhoeal and enteric diseases I have already written. (*Fifty Years in Public Health,* Chapters xxv and xxxviii.) Nothing written in this chapter casts into the shade the direct effect of elementary sanitation, of safe water supplies, and of better housing in reducing disease. But here I am concerned with treatment of sickness and with personal hygiene as means to the same end. Even aside from consideration of its possibilities of prevention of spread of infection, the hospital treatment of acute infectious diseases, especially of smallpox, scarlet fever, diphtheria, and enteric fever, has been continued and increased, and the social value of this treatment to the community, which pays for it through local taxation, has become universally appreciated. In recent decades the scope of hospital treatment by sanitary authorities has widely expanded, and such diseases as puerperal sepsis, erysipelas, ophthalmia of the new-born, measles, etc., are being treated. In recent years venereal diseases have been added to the list, special gratuitous treatment being given to all applicants at special clinics or in a hospital when needed; and some insight into the vast provision for the treatment of tuberculosis by Public Health Authorities is given in Chapter xv. Nor is this all; for Sanitary Authorities now provide homes and hospitals for many lying-in women, especially when home circumstances are unfavourable; for children who are crippled by tuberculosis or other causes; and for pre-school children, and sometimes for their mothers, especially for wasting conditions and for rickets.

In all these instances, prevention has been the keynote of the work of Public Health Authorities. This is conspicuous in their work for treating acute infectious diseases and even more so in their work for the prevention and treatment of the two great infectious diseases of protracted duration, tuberculosis and syphilis, in both of which they have secured conspicuous success in reducing the amount of sickness and thus elevating the general standard of health.

SCHOOL MEDICAL WORK

In Chapter xli of my *Fifty Years in Public Health,* I have set out the earlier stages of medical work for school children. Work for improving the health of scholars is not confined to what is done by school medical officers. Physical training, the cultivation by teachers of high ideals and good habits, and the general discipline of school life have an importance in their bearing on health which cannot easily be exaggerated. Perhaps the greatest direct benefit secured by the school medical service has come through the school nurses. The increased cleanliness and the vast diminution in verminous conditions among children must have been a large factor in improving the national health.

The treatment of special abnormalities in school children has been highly developed. Among these are squint and defects of refraction of eyes, adenoids and allied conditions, rheumatism in scholars, and various deformities, for all of which a vast organisation has gradually developed. Some of this work—a decreasing amount—has been done by voluntary hospitals, very little under the Poor Law.

Here is a second flourishing branch of municipal and State medicine, which has not seriously encroached on the work of private practitioners of medicine. Most of it had never previously been undertaken by them for the masses of the people.

As the Local Education Authority is now a constituent Committee of the County Council or the County Borough Council, school medicine functions side by side with the work of the Public Health Committee and its sub-Committees, and is therefore closely related to an extensive system of medical and hygienic aid for mothers and their children of pre-school age.

This association of the medical work of local authorities for pre-school and for school children and for their parents, has opened up possibilities, previously impracticable, for the complete hygienic guidance and help for mothers and their children.

That school medical work has hitherto been concerned mainly with the detection and remedying of the end products of sickness and neglect cannot be denied. But such work possesses high value, though it would be even more valuable could departure from health be more often anticipated, or treated at an early stage. This is now being rendered practicable by close co-operation and indeed identification in local administration of the medical and hygienic work for school children with that for infants and pre-school children.

A generalisation on possibilities may be permitted at this point. The defects found in school medical inspection, somewhat in the order of frequency, are carious teeth, diseased tonsils and adenoids, enlarged glands, rickets, discharging ears, etc.; and broadly these conditions are the effects of prolonged malnutrition, or other domestic evils, or are the end products of earlier catarrhal and specific febrile infections. Malnutrition often occurs apart from necessitous parental circumstances, and then it can be prevented in both the mother and her infant by a better balanced dietary which will help in increasing resistance to infections. How is this to be done? An official service alone will not suffice, though at child welfare centres and through the work of health visitors vast good can and is being accomplished to this end. Most of all it will depend on the infiltration into the minds and consciences of mothers and future mothers of accurate teaching of hygiene, not only in child welfare centres but also in the course of elementary and secondary education. There is great need to enlist every general medical practitioner in this work.

THE MEDICAL SIDE OF CHILD WELFARE WORK

The evolution of the physiological side of Preventive Medicine is seen best in the child welfare work of the last thirty or forty years. This work throughout has had a clinical background. In my Annual Report, 1913–14, I showed that over 21 per cent of the total deaths in infancy and nearly 33 per cent of the total deaths in the first five years of life are due to various infective diseases; and if we add bronchitis and pneumonia to this group, as is justifiable, then more than half of the total deaths 0–5 are due to infective agents. We can agree that the antecedent health of each child will have played a part in determining death or recovery when attacked. A lowering of the death-rate at ages 1–5, immediately following infancy, was occurring many years before specialised child welfare work began (see p. 327, *Fifty Years in Public Health*). The importance of clinical medicine in child welfare work is still further

evidenced by the success now being attained in the reduction of measles and of diphtheria by specific immunisation. In producing these modern developments laboratory
research has been directly or indirectly responsible; but for
some important improvements in child hygiene it is to clinical
research that we are chiefly indebted. Physiological investigations have brought important help to medicine, while the study
of disease in children has led to great advances in physiology.

CARE OF INFANTS

The interaction of the two is especially seen in the improved
care of infants. Perhaps the greatest outstanding accomplishment in Preventive Medicine is that Summer Diarrhoea has
ceased to be the annual scourge to infancy which it was in the
last century. Greater municipal cleanliness, including the reduction of horse manure, cleanliness in the preparation of infants'
artificial foods, the practice of domestic asepsis by the mother
and nurse, the more efficient selection of appropriate foods and
allied measures have brought this about; and in securing it the
credit must be given to trained health visitors, to infant consultation centres, which have led to improved infant hygiene,
not only for the parents directly influenced, but also by diffusion
of knowledge and example for the whole community.

RICKETS

Last century children and adults with deformed limbs,
resulting from this disease, were common. Now they have
almost disappeared. Rickets in its more severe forms is seldom
seen. (See Chapter XXVII of my *The Story of Modern Preventive
Medicine*, 1929.) For long it has been known that cod-liver oil
was an admirable remedy for this disease, and its specific
value as a remedy for it was proved experimentally in 1919 by
E. Mellanby. The work of many investigators on both sides
of the Atlantic has shown that deficiency of vitamin D is the
chief factor determining the occurrence of rickets, as well as
of defectively formed teeth. This vitamin can now be obtained
in isolation, and the therapeutics of rickets is thus facilitated.
The value of ergosterol and irradiation in the prevention
of rickets I need only mention. Rickets can be completely

avoided when expectant mothers have an ample well-balanced diet, including milk and green vegetables, and live during part of each day in the open air, and when their infants are similarly treated and are given an additional daily dose of cod-liver oil. It is only necessary to mention scurvy and beri-beri, in which the knowledge given by medical observation has been fortified and extended by experimental work, as further illustrations of the importance of the physiological side of medicine.

NUTRITION

The importance of Nutrition in ensuring a high standard of health has been fully established by field observations and experiments. Especially noteworthy have been the scientifically conducted mass observations on children in residential schools, proving that the addition of a daily pint of cow's milk to their already satisfactory diet resulted in better growth, increased weight, with improvement in mental alertness, when these children were contrasted with other children living under the same conditions, except as to the additional milk.

GENERAL REMARKS ON NUTRITION

The many investigations showing the importance of varied and adequate food which have been made in recent years, have resulted in a marked advance in Preventive Medicine. This is not only because of our rapidly increasing knowledge of vitamins initiated in 1906 by Gowland Hopkins; the importance of these investigations is now fully appreciated. They enable us, as McCollum has put it, to appreciate more fully "the sensitiveness of the animal body to an improperly adjusted inorganic content" of food, and the necessity for "protective foods," especially milk and leafy edible vegetables. They have also brought into relief the teaching as expressed by Hess that

the harmful effects of food deficiencies should not be associated in our minds . . . chiefly with specific diseases such as scurvy or rickets, but rather as disorders of nutrition, producing slight and manifold disturbances of function.

The subject of Nutrition in relation to susceptibility to infection, as Mellanby reminds us (*Nutrition and Disease*, 1934), is only in its infancy, and as yet "we know too little to lay down specific rules as to what criteria" (of malnutrition) "should be used according to recent knowledge" (*op. cit.*, p. 75).

It is clear, however, that experimental animals become more liable to some infections when fed on food deficient in fat-soluble vitamins. Dr. G. Mellanby's observations showed that in two experimental groups of pregnant women, the group treated by vitamin A therapy suffered less from puerperal sepsis than the corresponding group not thus treated. This evidently is a tentative result, having only dubious significance. Were it confirmed in more general experience, a great advance in preventive therapy would have been made, worthy to be placed side by side with the therapy by which we can ensure the total abolition of rickets.

NUTRITION IN TUBERCULOSIS

Preceding remarks bear on what I have already written (pp. 136 and 140) in this volume and more fully elsewhere on the part played by improved nutrition in the general reduced incidence of tuberculosis; as also on its increased incidence during the Great War (p. 230). The influence of improved nutrition in reducing tuberculosis, in my view, has been exaggerated by writers who have failed satisfactorily to assemble all the factors contributing to this result, and have not also weighed each factor in accordance with the lessons derivable from comparative experience. To arrive at a satisfactory conclusion in this complex problem, there is needed con-temporaneous study of various communities, and historical study of the course of events in each single community. When this has been done, I do not doubt that, while attaching weight to all contributory factors, the overwhelming importance of avoiding protracted or massive exposure to infection will not remain in doubt. But the wonders done by special diets in rickets, beri-beri, scurvy, and some other diseases excite even fantastic hope that eventually there may be discovered some specific food or medicament which will have real power to inhibit the development of the seeds of tuberculosis, although these have been already implanted. It may be that this dis-covery—if ever—will be made before tuberculosis has so far declined, as the result of present public health activities, that it has little more than academic value. (See also page 402.)

CHAPTER XVIII

OFFICIAL INQUIRIES AND REPORTS ON INFANT AND CHILD MORTALITY

IN my *Fifty Years in Public Health* I described the earlier efforts made to save infant lives by various health organisations and authorities, four chapters being devoted to this subject. In those chapters I endeavoured to disentangle the various factors in improved infant hygiene, and discussed the extent to which the lowering of the infant death-rate has been due to the special work of M.O.H.s, of health visitors, and of child welfare centres—specific child welfare work—and to what extent to more general causes of physical improvement, domestic sanitation, a higher standard of general and specific cleanliness, more general temperance as regards alcoholic indulgence, a higher standard of comfort, and so on. Of the importance of specific child welfare work I have no doubt and, as is shown in the next chapters, the importance of this specific work has increased as the years have passed.

In taking part in the forward movement for Maternal and Child Welfare I prepared in the earlier years of my work at the Local Government Board four special reports, which were national studies of the whole subject. In this chapter the outstanding points of these reports are indicated.

FIRST REPORT ON CHILD MORTALITY

The first of these reports, entitled "Report by the Medical Officer of the Local Government Board on Infant and Child Mortality" (Cd. 5263, pages 142), was issued in 1910. In a preliminary letter to the President of the Board (Mr. John Burns) I said:

To the subject of this report more work has been devoted by the Board and by sanitary authorities during the last four years than at any previous period. There has been a widespread awakening to the national importance of child mortality, and a concentration on efforts to diminish it such as has never previously occurred.

In bringing about this change, public addresses by Mr.
Burns had a large share. I have already mentioned the address
given by him in June 1906 (p. 27). It is reprinted in full in
The Early History of the Infant Welfare Movement, by Dr.
George McCleary, 1933, and I may quote the following from
among Mr. Burns's aphorisms in the same address:

> We must concentrate on the mother. . . . The stream is no purer
> than its source. Let us glorify, dignify, and purify motherhood by
> every means in our power. . . . Nourish the mother, you feed the
> child.

The object of my report as set out in the preface addressed
to Mr. Burns was threefold: (a) to determine on the basis of
our national statistics, whether reduction of infant mortality
implies any untoward influence on the health of survivors to
later years; (b) to point out the communities which are characterised by a continuing high rate of infant mortality and to
warn them of the need for reform; and (c) to assess, so far as is
possible, the relative weight of the different factors of excessive
infant mortality.

The first problem (a) is considered in Chapter XXI.

Dealing now with (b) I quoted from my first annual report to
the Board, in which I had summarised the experience of the
infants born during 1908 in 217 larger provincial towns and
in 29 metropolitan boroughs. Among these

6·2 per cent of the total infants born had an infant mortality
under 90 per 1,000 births,

and in an ascending series, which need not be quoted in full,

> in 15·5 per cent the infant mortality was 130–140
> in 20·3 per cent the infant mortality was 140–150
> in 15·9 per cent the infant mortality was over 150.

My special report (1910) on Infant Mortality was concerned
with an analysis of infant mortality and of mortality at ages
1–5 in the year 1908. There was no difficulty in demonstrating
the immense inequalities in the distribution of infant mortality
throughout England and Wales. The following illustrations
refer to four counties, two chiefly industrial, two chiefly rural.

In the following table I have picked out infant mortality under one month, and at ages of 6 to 12 months.

DEATH-RATE PER 1,000 BIRTHS

	Under 1 month	6–12 months
Durham	52	42
Glamorgan	46	43
Hereford	31	16
Oxford	31	15

The comparison here given refutes the very persistent error that mortality in the first month after birth is fairly uniform and not capable of reduction, for in the example given above it was nearly 70 per cent higher in Durham than in Oxfordshire. I extended the comparison to variations in individual causes of death; and without entering into detail, such extreme instances as the following may be cited:

Development and wasting diseases, Durham 57, Berkshire 34; *Diarrhoeal diseases*, Glamorgan 27, Hereford 6.

SECOND REPORT ON CHILD MORTALITY

In this report (Cd. 6909) an analysis was made of the infant and child mortality in 241 urban areas of England and Wales in the year 1911. The prefatory statement to Mr. Burns indicated that

for the first time the sanitary authorities and medical officers of health of these 241 urban areas will be able to ascertain the exact relative position of the areas for whose public health welfare they are responsible, not only in respect of total mortality at ages 0–1 and 1–5, but also in respect of mortality in the different parts of infancy and from the chief causes of death.

In view of the experience of 1911 it could be claimed with a high degree of probability that the great saving of child life which had been effected in the last few years was

the result of improved sanitary and housing conditions, of more efficient municipal and domestic cleanliness, of education in hygiene, of increased sobriety of the population, and of the widespread awakening to the national importance of child mortality, with concentration on efforts of child welfare work such as had never previously occurred.

The report had a definite practical object:

Although the exact causes of excessive infant mortality are complex and vary in different towns, comparison between towns of low and those of high mortality brings out the irresistible conclusion that a high proportion of the excess of mortality in the less favoured towns can be removed, if the appropriate social and sanitary improvements which are within reach are adopted.

The report proved that the highest infant mortality occurred in the chief centres of industry, in large tracts of the Midlands, of the north of England, and in South Wales. Even within the same county and under similar climatic conditions, extreme variations in infant mortality were experienced. There was no difficulty in concluding that

geographical position and climatic circumstances have, within the area of England and Wales, only a minor influence on infant mortality; and that particular local conditions special to certain limited areas or in certain social classes are responsible to a high degree for the variations which occur in the infant mortality rates.

Already in this second report I deprecated the assumption that the rate of mortality in the first weeks after birth had not declined (see also p. 198). Comparing national experience in 1911 with that of the preceding six years:

A decline of nearly 4 per cent occurred in the first week after birth, of 13 per cent in the next three weeks, and of 20 per cent at ages 1–3 months.

Comment was made on the amount of decline in the death-rate secured in infancy and in the next four years of life. Thus comparing the average experience of 1871–75 with that of 1908–10 the infantile death-rate had declined 34 per cent, and in the next four years of life 41, 50, 53, and 50 per cent respectively; furthermore "the decline in infant mortality began much more recently than that in the next four years of life." This would not be surprising, "even on the hypothesis that avoidable infant mortality is a product solely of environment"; for "at both ends of life the balance between health and disease is more sensitively held than at other ages."

The general conclusion was drawn that high rates of infant

mortality depend very largely upon certain social conditions differing locally in degree or in kind from those prevailing in districts with a low infant death-rate.

An analysis of these special conditions was made in detail; but much of what I should otherwise write here is stated in the chapters on "The Safeguarding of Development and Growth" in my earlier volume (pp. 321–380).

The following paragraphs, summarised from my Annual Report for 1909–10, written soon after I went to the Local Government Board, although they give in substance what is more fully stated in Chapter XL of my earlier volume, are given here because the problem is stated from a somewhat different angle.

A GENERAL REVIEW OF INFANT MORTALITY

My first two special reports were intended to give a bird's-eye view of the incidence of mortality during childhood in the different areas of sanitary administration of the country, and to determine in which of these areas further administrative control over the causes of infant mortality was most urgently needed.

The three main branches of the subject necessarily over-lapped and interlaced; for infant mortality varied with the personal character and knowledge, the social well-being, and the sanitary well-being of parents.

In my first report I set out in particular the serious responsi-bility of sanitary authorities in relation to excessive mortality. Evidently this did not cover all the ground. Thus infant mortality formed a partial measure of vice. The records of deaths due to inherited syphilis are very imperfect; but the evidence available shows that if to the deaths of children born alive with this terrible heritage be added the total aggregate of premature and still-births due to the same cause, syphilis would rank as a serious cause of infant mortality.

Along with syphilis must be placed alcoholism as a serious cause of infant mortality. Parental neglect is a common result of alcoholic habits, and this implies a high rate of mortality among the children affected by the neglect. The same habits obviously tend to poverty, and to a direct lowering in the standard of life.

Alcoholism can, however, scarcely be placed in its proper relation to other causes of excessive child mortality, unless it is regarded as part of a vicious circle, of which ignorance and carelessness, poverty—in the sense of privation of some of the necessaries of life—and insanitary houses, yards, and streets, form other important portions.

No fact is better established than that the death-rate, and especially the death-rate among children, is high in inverse proportion to the social status of the population concerned. Not only are poverty and a high death-rate always closely related, but a high death-rate implies also a high rate of sickness and of inefficiency among those who survive.

Evidently poverty is a complex, comprising many constituent elements, having varying weight in the production of excessive child mortality. Economic problems are involved; but the most promising course in immediate practical administration consists in removing those elements of poverty and of excessive mortality which can be attacked separately. Among these stand out prominently neglect of means for the prevention and the treatment of disease.

Failure to recognise conditions of life favouring disease, and difficulty of access to prompt and efficient medical treatment form important causes of excessive child mortality; and action helping to secure recognition and early treatment of illness will do much to equalise the possibilities of healthy child life in the different social strata. The national system of medical inspection of school children reveals among school children defects and disease which are difficult to eradicate or to cure, but many of which might easily have been prevented or cured in early childhood. For most children a healthy youth and adult life cannot be secured if the circumstances of the first few years of life are unsatisfactory in character.

THIRD REPORT ON CHILD MORTALITY

My third report dealing with Infant Mortality in Lancashire (Cd. 7511) was published in July 1914. In this report were contributions by Dr. Copeman giving the results of an investigation of infant mortality in Burnley, Colne, and Nelson; by Dr. Farrar (Wigan and Stretford); and by Dr. Manby (Widnes and Farnworth), prefaced by an introductory study of their data by me. Dr. Janet Lane-Claypon added an account of child welfare work in Lancashire.

In the above-mentioned seven towns total infant mortality in 1913 varied from 91 (Nelson) to 215 per 1,000 births (Farnworth).

FOURTH AND FIFTH REPORTS

Two further reports were issued, which had been long in preparation. In October 1915 my "Report on Maternal Mortality in connection with Childbearing and its relation to Infant Mortality" (Cd. 8085) was published, and will be summarised in Chapter XXIII; and in March 1917 was published my "Report on Child Mortality at Ages 0–5 in England and Wales," which completed my studies and review of the whole range of maternal and child mortality from the points of view of investigation and of administration. The chief points in this report may be indicated here.

The hope with which it had been prepared had been "to secure a bird's-eye view of the extent of unnecessary child mortality still occurring, of the places in which the need for combating this is most urgent, and of the appropriate means for combating it."

As I set out in my prefatory statement to Lord Rhondda, then President of the Local Government Board,

the one outstanding fact is that the centres of excessive child mortality are those in which the chief industries of the country are carried on. That this association is not inevitable is shown by the great reductions in child mortality already secured in these centres, and by the great variations in present child mortality in towns having the same or closely allied industries.

I added that

in every area a very high proportion of the total present mortality can be obviated; and it is well within the range of administrative action to reduce child mortality within the next few years to one-half of its present amount.

This report dealt with the experience of 575,078 children who died in England and Wales in the years 1911–14 at ages under five. These formed 28·2 per cent of the total deaths at all ages during these years. In this report I dealt with the relative mortality in each of the first five years after birth (see Fig. 9 in my earlier volume), and discussed the fact that

the reduction in the first year after birth is less in amount and began at a later period than the reduction in the first four years of life.

In this as in preceding reports each district and town, sometimes also each ward of a town, was classified in accordance with its favourable or invidious position in respect of death-rate in each of the first five years of life. I devoted a special chapter to two industrial towns, Middlesbrough and St. Helens, in which the death-rates at ages under five per 1,000 births were terribly high, 251 and 242 respectively. In these towns the same rule held good as elsewhere: thus in certain wards of Middlesbrough the child death-rate was 2½ times as high as in some other wards of the same town. A similar analysis showed that the excessive mortality from pneumonia experienced in Middlesbrough was not fully explained by the sulphurous and other fumes incidental to its main industries; for it was experienced by children as well as adults, and its amount varied greatly in different wards of the town. Having described the lamentable housing conditions and the low standard of domestic cleanliness which then prevailed in the inner wards of the town, I gave my final opinion that

if the public-houses in the town and within a few miles of it could be closed for six months, the population now living under housing conditions inimical to health and to self-respect would secure an immense improvement in health and efficiency even in their present houses . . .

With regard to St. Helens I stated

as in Middlesbrough, much continuous work in improving housing, in clearing out crowded areas, and in enforcing municipal and domestic cleanliness is needed if work directed to promote temperance, and to secure improved personal hygiene, is to have a rapid prospect of success. The two classes of work are dependent on each other for their joint success.

To this period belongs my Lady Priestley Memorial Lecture

on "The Enemies of Child Life," which I gave on November 21, 1917. It was published in the *Nineteenth Century and After*, January 1918.

At such a time, when the World War had been sacrificing our national capital, of men and money, to an unexampled extent I stated

it was being realised that the restitution of national prosperity after the War will come early or late in accordance with the number of young and capable workers who will be available for the nation's work. . . .

The wanton destruction of life in war has led to a general appreciation of the value of child life: and it is not surprising, therefore, that while national economy has been urged in other directions, the Local Government Board has urged the continuance and extension of social work for the welfare of mothers and their infants . . . and that this work has been greatly extended throughout the country, notwithstanding the war-time difficulty in securing social workers. . . . Now that we appreciate more fully that the mother is the maker of the home, the link between the past and the future, the transmitter of life and civilisation, and that each child may not irreverently be named a Holy Child, the protection of mother and child will become to an extent not hitherto attained an all-important part of future work to secure the welfare of our nation and of civilisation.

DO INFANTS START FAIR?

In this address I adduced evidence showing that experience does not support the statement often made that infants are born in a fairly equal state of health. The incidence of syphilis, for instance, varies very greatly; and the proportion of still-births (and doubtless correspondingly of infants born alive with inferior health) also varies within wide limits. The variations in mortality of mothers in childbirth—from 3 per 1,000 live births in London to from 6 to 8 in some textile towns—are

associated with a lamentable amount of sickness and weakness of mothers who survive—and this must mean a corresponding excess of sickness and deaths of infants both before and after birth.

Varying vitality in the first month after birth as measured by the death-rate during this first month of extra-uterine life is shown in the experience of some groups of population, the rate being seven times as high in some as compared with other groups.

Various other problems were discussed in the same lecture; but I will only mention here my remarks on the *Advantages of Urbanisation*, which partially counterbalance its inimical influence on health.

Urban life has rendered available auxiliaries to family life, which can be made to go far to counterbalance its evils. Among these the school and the hospital stand pre-eminent, though many other municipal and voluntary agencies are valuable aids to home life. The home is the basis of family life; the city is the larger home, and the institutions of the city are good and useful in so far as they conduce to the health, efficiency, happiness, and character of its constituent families.

PERSONAL CONTRIBUTIONS

Report by the Medical Officer of the Local Government Board on Mortality during the First Five Years of Life, dealing with the Statistics of Sanitary Areas (grouped) and of Administrative Counties of England and Wales. (Cd. 5263.)

Report by the Medical Officer of the Local Government Board on Mortality during the First Five Years of Life, dealing with the Statistics of 212 Towns and 29 Metropolitan Boroughs during the Four Years 1907–10 (grouped) and in 1911. (Cd. 6909.)

Report on Infant Mortality in Lancashire, with special reference to Seven Towns within the County by the Medical Officer of the Local Government Board, and by Drs. Copeman, Manby, Farrar, and Lane-Claypon. (Cd. 7511.)

Report by the Medical Officer of the Local Government Board on Maternal Mortality in connection with Childbearing and its relation to Infant Mortality, with contributions by Dr. Janet Lane-Claypon and Dr. Isabella Cameron. (Cd. 8085.)

Report by the Medical Officer of the Local Government Board on Child Mortality at Ages 0–5. (Cd. 8496.)

1910. The National Importance of Child Mortality. Lecture to the Congress of the Royal Sanitary Institute at Brighton. (*Journal* of the Institute, Vol. xxxi, No. 9.)

1916. Local Government Board, Circulars and Memoranda on Maternity and Child Welfare.

1918. The Enemies of Child Life (Lady Priestley Memorial Lecture). (*Nineteenth Century and After*, January 1918.)

1920. Address on Neo-Natal Mortality. The F. A. Packard Lecture of the Philadelphia Pediatric Society. (*Lancet*, May 22, 1920.)

1922. Mortality in the 1st Month after Birth and Possibilities of its Reduction. (*National Health*, 1922.)

1923. Midwifery Work and Social Welfare. (*Maternity and Child Welfare*, June 1923.)

CHAPTER XIX

PUBLIC ADMINISTRATION AND CHILD HEALTH

IT will have been plain, especially to those who have read the four chapters in which I discussed Infant Mortality in my *Fifty Years in Public Health*, that voluntary workers have taken a great part in initiating specialised work for the welfare of children. If in this chapter it should seem that voluntary effort has not received sufficient consideration, I ask the reader to bear in mind that I am engaged chiefly in reviewing official work. It is, however, satisfactory to record that while voluntary work for child welfare persists and is to be seen in all well-governed sanitary areas, it is in large measure voluntary work "in a municipal setting."

THE BEGINNINGS OF OFFICIAL CHILD WELFARE WORK

I have already set out (*op. cit.*, p. 335 *et seq.*) some of the earlier work of Public Health Authorities. Huddersfield was the first town to secure a Local Act making it obligatory to notify to the M.O.H. each birth within thirty-six hours of its occurrence. This example was rapidly followed by other towns, and the Act of 1907 gave the same powers to every local authority, with the consent of the Local Government Board.

In 1915 the Notification of Births Act came into force over the whole of England and Wales. It had already been widely adopted in towns throughout the country. By its means much valuable work has been done. It has enabled prompt visits to be made to advise the mother as to the hygiene of infancy, and it has led to consultation centres being started at which mothers attend with their infants and receive individual counsel based often on a medical overhaul of the infant.

HEALTH VISITORS

Already local effort, sometimes voluntary, sometimes official, had secured many suitable women visitors to the mothers. This earlier history is described on p. 26 *et seq.* of McCleary's *The Maternity and Child Welfare Movement* (P. S. King, 1935).

At first some difficulty was experienced. There was no statutory power to appoint visitors who were not also sanitary inspectors. For several years local authorities appointed female sanitary inspectors, with instructions to give personal counsel as to infant feeding, etc., whilst arranging for the putting-right of domestic sanitary defects. In 1908 the London County Council obtained special power from Parliament enabling metropolitan borough councils to appoint "health visitors"

for the purpose of giving to persons advice as to the proper nurture, care, and management of young children and the promotion of cleanliness

in addition to any other duties that might be assigned to them; and the Bill also provided that the Local Government Board might regulate the qualifications, mode of appointment, duties, etc., of all such health visitors. The first of these regulations was issued in September 1909. Ere long health visitors were appointed throughout the country; and their number has rapidly increased.

PREVENTIVE WORK BASED ON EARLY NOTIFICATION OF BIRTHS

In my Second Special Report on Infant and Child Mortality (Cd. 6909) published in 1913, after indicating the indispensable connecting link between improved general sanitation and the work of child welfare, I emphasised ignorance as an impediment to reform.

The object of child welfare work is to ensure that each parent has within reach accurate counsel as to the hygiene of childhood, and as to the general and domestic conditions necessary for ensuring its maintenance. On the medical side this implies such advice as will conduce to the prevention of minor ailments, to their prompt discovery, and to that early treatment which is essential for the prevention of more serious disease.

In the fulfilment of this ideal, I outlined the main lines of work, as follows:

1. The question of infantile hygiene antedates the birth of the infant. The need for further study and further action was illustrated by the great variations in infant mortality in the first week and the first month of extra-uterine life.

2. There was needed the co-operation of better trained midwives for improvement of both the ante-natal and the post-natal condition of the infant. Much work in this direction was already being done; but

to achieve the desired end the administrative machinery for working the Midwives Act will need to be brought into more intimate relationship with that of the Notification of Births Act.

3. Home visits to mothers and definite personal instruction in general hygiene and in methods of feeding were called for and—

The experience of many counties shows that the maximum efficiency of this visiting is reached when the children are referred to an Infant Consultation Centre.

4. The Infant Consultation

should be a department for practical instruction in infant hygiene, presided over by a medical officer possessing special knowledge of the diseases and minor ailments of infants and young children. The mother thus has the advantage of personal instruction and also of the collective influence of the other mothers who have previously received correct instruction.

The importance of these Consultations was stressed, not only for instruction of mothers, but also for medical students, midwives, and health visitors. "The establishment of an Infant Consultation at each Medical School in the country would have an immense influence for good. They could easily be built up in connection with the Maternity Departments of Medical Schools."

5. This skilled supervision needed to be continued, until it bridged over the interval between infancy and school life. This would reduce the total amount of neglected illness found when children began their school life.

HEALTH VISITING AND CONSULTATIONS

In my Annual Report for 1913 I summarised the history of the work of voluntary and official agents in promoting health visiting. There was already evidence that great good had been effected, but I deprecated excessive trust in comparative statistics between districts which had and those which had not adopted this Act.

The case for child welfare work cannot be based on statistics, in which it is difficult to compare homogeneous populations, under conditions which are equal, apart from notification of births. It is reasonable to act on the assumption that the hygienic advice secured by the visits following notification must have valuable influence in improving health in childhood.

Already there was striking evidence of increase in the number of Infant Consultation Centres.

I stated that "much of the success so far achieved in improving the health conditions of infancy and childhood has been secured by co-operation between voluntary and official workers."

In achieving this result the conferences on Infant Mortality already mentioned (p. 178) had greatly helped, as had also the National Association for the Prevention of Infant Mortality which organised these conferences. I may specially mention resolutions signed by Sir Thomas Barlow, late President of the Royal College of Physicians, on behalf of this Association, urging that degree and license-conferring bodies should require each medical student to have attended a course of clinical instruction on infant hygiene, management of infants, and the diseases of infancy; that this course should include instruction in the relation of the medical practitioner to the work of health authorities, of the midwife, and of health visitors; and that the certificate to be given after the required course of instruction should include instruction in ante-natal hygiene, and in the management of mothers and their infants during labour and the period of lactation.

SPECIAL EFFORTS re DIARRHOEA

In 1911 a step was taken to assist in securing more exact information as to deaths from diarrhoea and enteritis. After negotiation with the General Register Office it was arranged that all deaths from diarrhoea and enteritis under the age of two years should be classed together, as this gave perhaps the most satisfactory measure of the incidence of epidemic diarrhoea. This arrangement had the additional advantage that it facilitated international comparisons of deaths from diarrhoea. Although by many local authorities this was already done, the Board in 1911 sent a circular letter to all local authorities in which *inter alia* was urged the giving of exact advice as to the feeding and management of children. The point was emphasised that although printed leaflets were useful, "even more important are personal visits and the offer of practical advice to the mothers of babies born within the last twelve months. Exact and simple instructions are most likely to be followed if given during a period of special danger."

It was urged also that special and more frequent visits should be made in quarters of a town where past experience had shown excess of diarrhoeal sickness; and prompt efforts made to control diarrhoea in districts in which this disease had been made compulsorily notifiable. Emphasis was laid also on hospital treatment of such cases, and of the marasmus of children (often fatal) left after a severe attack of diarrhoea. During the same year three special investigations were started under the small scientific grant of the Board, with the hope of further elucidating the pathology of epidemic diarrhoea; and an inquiry as to flies as carriers of infective matter was started, Dr. Copeman being entrusted with this. Two further reports issued from the Medical Department of the Board during this year had bearing on the prevention of diarrhoea. Dr. Janet Lane-Claypon contributed a report on the value of boiled milk (not including milk boiled for prolonged periods) for infants. (*Loc. Gov. Board Reports*, N.S. 63.)

Dr. Coutts's report on Condensed Milks (N.S. 56) also bore on this subject. It led the way to regulations controlling the sale of condensed milks insufficiently or inaccurately described on the labels, and to the prohibition of machine-skimmed condensed milk for the feeding of infants. In the same year regulations were made prohibiting the use of preservatives in milk and insisting on the adequate declaration of their presence when contained in preserved cream.

CHILD WELFARE WORK IN WAR TIME

In my Annual Report 1914–15 I noted that child welfare work was being vigorously pursued notwithstanding the altered social circumstances produced by the Great War; and the next report for 1915–16 showed that the number of health visitors appointed by local authorities had increased to 1,000 as compared with 600 in March 1914. The Board in a circular letter about this time urged that, notwithstanding the War, child welfare work was nationally important.

At a time like the present there is urgent need for taking all possible steps to secure the health of all mothers and children and to diminish ante-natal and post-natal mortality.

The Board's circular also emphasised that

steps should be taken in the directions indicated, even at the present time, when strict economy is required in the expenditure both of public bodies and private individuals.

This counsel was in accordance with public opinion, which was fully roused as to the urgency of all measures for promoting maternal and child welfare. More general action had been facilitated by making the Notification of Births Act applicable in every sanitary area from September 1915, and by giving to County Councils the powers of a Sanitary Authority for the purpose of the care of expectant and nursing mothers and young children.

During the year 1916 the infant mortality rate for England and Wales as a whole fell to 91 per 1,000 births, the lowest recorded rate up to that year.

In my last Annual Report for 1918 I reviewed the whole subject of child mortality, but must refer the reader to that report for details.

I may, however, quote a sentence from its conclusion, as follows:

The history of 1917 and of preceding years shows that we can anticipate a reduction of the national rate of infant mortality to 50 per 1,000 births,

a rate which had already been experienced in some parts of England and in New Zealand as a whole. In 1933 the infant death-rate in New Zealand was 32 and in Australia 40.

Writing in 1936 it is evident that, following on the rapid strides made in child welfare work during post-War years, an even lower figure will be attained in infant mortality rates than is named above. But the preceding forecast and my suggested forecast for future years (in words italicised in my report of 1918) *can only be secured by improving the welfare of every mother.*

This aspect of child welfare work is discussed in Chapters xx and xxii.

The formation of the Ministry of Health in 1919 happily put an end to the wastefulness of duplicated and divided efforts in official child welfare work, on the past history of which more is written in Chapter xx.

In future developments of medical practice the family practitioner will, I anticipate, do much, but not all of the work now carried out in Child Welfare Centres. As stated on page 293 of my *Medicine and the State* (George Allen & Unwin, 1932):

The official procedures for the medical care of childhood and youth have two characteristics which differentiate them from private practice as ordinarily conducted. In the first place there is undertaken a searching out of minor departures from the normal and the application of remedial measures; and, secondly, counsel is given and action is taken to increase psycho-physical fitness, and thus raise an additional obstacle to the onset of illness, whether physical or extra-physical.

The infant consultations conducted by special medical officers do work, chiefly hygienic, which for the vast majority of infants would otherwise be neglected.

But this position need not persist.

CHAPTER XX

RIVALRY BETWEEN GOVERNMENT DEPARTMENTS

MY account of the rapid growth of official Maternity and Child Welfare Work if it is to be complete must include remarks on the duplicated activities during the years 1908-18 of the Local Government Board and of the Board of Education in the promotion of infantile and child hygiene. This duplication had advantages compensating in part for the difficulties and friction involved in the persistent and partially successful efforts of the Board of Education to undertake work which—as I see it—was the work of the Local Government Board, the central authority concerned in initiating and organising local public health work.

It would not, of course, be completely accurate to state that the Local Government Board was the only Central Health Authority, for Parliament had recently imposed on the Board of Education (p. 197) powers which implied responsibility for detecting, and in some instances treating, illness or defects found in children in attendance at elementary schools. This fact must have inclined the Board of Education to "take a hand" in giving grants to local organisations to help them in undertaking the hygienic and medical care of children under school age. The control of elementary education in this country is highly centralised owing to local educational finance being largely aided by grants from the Central Government.

The giving of grants by the Board of Education facilitated the opening of a few schools for mothers by voluntary bodies, and of some nursery schools, at which children less than five years old—the age at which school attendance becomes compulsory—attended and received such training and personal care as is appropriate to their tender years. There is further discussion of this early schooling on page 389 of my *Fifty Years of Public Health*.

I referred in a previous paragraph to the advantage resulting from the rival zeal of the Board of Education in hygienic matters concerning children not in attendance at an elementary school. Writing as one whose steady endeavour was to stimulate the Local Government Board to proceed further and more quickly in the prevention of child mortality and the improvement of child health than appeared feasible in the complex conditions of official life, I can testify that the intrusive efforts of the Board of Education to occupy part of this field were a useful stimulus to increased efforts in child welfare on the part of the Local Government Board.

It is unnecessary to recall in full the stages of the almost competitive efforts of the two Boards in this initial period of official child welfare work. I can summarise most of what needs to be written from memoranda written by me in the early months of 1914, when Mr. Herbert Samuel had become President of the Local Government Board. The prospect of extended official child welfare work owed much to the stand he took in defence of the position that this work formed a part of public health administration. The memoranda in question recalled the efforts of the Local Government Board during six years and more to promote infant and child hygiene, and showed how this aim could not be completely fulfilled, unless we secured improved maternity work and ante-natal work. At that very time the Board of Education had put forward proposals for an Education Bill, one clause of which, had it been adopted, would have empowered Education Authorities to provide consultation centres, to make home visits, or otherwise to give medical assistance to mothers with regard to the care of their children from birth onwards. Writing many years afterwards, it is almost unbelievable that such preposterous proposals should have been advanced. At the same time propaganda were rife to the effect that no good thing could come out of Nazareth, as represented by the Local Government Board.

In memoranda I set out the points in which the two Central Boards of Local Government and Education were in agreement. Each of them alike was concerned that every child, so far as practicable, shall be enabled to become an efficient citizen.

I added that Education Authorities had been concerned hitherto chiefly with mental and moral fitness for citizenship; relatively little had been done to train children attending schools for physical fitness. In 1907 additional powers had been conferred on them by Parliament, namely to make arrangements . . . for attending to the health and physical condition of the children educated in public elementary schools.

Prior to this, much health visiting had been carried out by many Public Health Authorities; and when in 1907 the above-stated power was given to the Board of Education and Local Education Authorities it was clearly stated in correspondence between the two Boards that "any developments in this direction would be such as would fit in with the general public health administration of each area."

It was also formally agreed that the additional work of the Board of Education should be so organised, that it might be easily transferred to the Local Government Board should this be deemed desirable.

The tendency up to this time had been to make the Local Government Board the chief centre of imperial and international health organisation. The Foreign Office and the Colonial Office co-operated in this functional assimilation. The action of the Board of Education as regards medical inspection was separatist; and one regrets the inertia and timidity of the Local Government Board which made it possible.

Writing in 1914, I stated that notwithstanding the good work already done, medical inspection of scholars was inadequate, because at too long intervals; that the health work of Education Authorities still left much physical disability without diagnosis and prompt treatment; furthermore, that earlier attention to children's health, i.e. attention before school attendance begins, would be needed if the sickness and defects now found by school doctors were to be greatly diminished. The problem was, who should give this attention?

It was now (in 1914) being urged in support of the view that the Board of Education centrally and Education Committees locally should undertake this work, that the problem of poor health in childhood was one which could be met only by a reformed system of education, based upon physical health and upbringing. On this basis the question, it was alleged, was one of education and not one for Health Authorities.

I pointed out that this contention, placing personal and

environmental hygiene in two categories, was a false antithesis. For

the habits, training, and health of the parent, both during the intra-uterine life and after the birth of her infant, are as much a part of the infant's environment as the house occupied by both mother and infant.

Furthermore, no practical line of demarcation could be drawn between the dangers to child health due to ignorance or carelessness of the mother, and those due to conditions over which she was entirely without control. Even though it may involve some repetition, I repeat what I wrote in 1914 on this point.

Poverty, and what it implies, is commonly a more potent influence than ignorance. A dirty house and unsatisfactory methods of storage and preparation of infants' food may result from lack of training of the mother; but they are also commonly caused by the fact that her life is lived under adverse conditions, for which she is not responsible, and which can only be improved by public health measures, improved domestic sanitation, separate water supply for each tenement, etc., etc., and by more adequate aid in the relief and prevention of poverty.

The officers of the Health Authority, including health visitors, were, I maintained, prepared for special work in both these directions. In the same memorandum I traced the increasingly successful work done by Public Health Authorities and voluntary organisations in both these directions, though much was as yet left undone, because adequate staffs had not everywhere been appointed.

I then adduced the excessive mortality in the first three months after birth, in some districts as compared with others, as showing that evil ante-natal conditions, poverty, and insanitation were concerned even more largely than ignorance. This was still more so in the first month after birth. To bring, as was proposed by the Board of Education,

another Authority on the ground already occupied, implies not only the wastefulness of overlapping effort, but the neglect which is commonly experienced when two bodies are both partially concerned in identical work.

I pointed out that one-fifth of the total deaths in infancy occur in the first week after birth, one-third in the first month, and more than half in the first three months after birth. I added that

one might say that approximately at least a quarter and probably a third of the total infant mortality now occurring in the first year of life and a still larger proportion of the impaired health in survivors beyond the first year, are due to unfavourable circumstances of parturition and to ill health and disease in the expectant mothers.

I pointed out the significant fact that deaths of infants during intra-uterine life were probably as many as total deaths during the twelve months following birth, and added

it is suggested that "infant welfare work does not include maternity work"; *but it is in fact impossible to dissociate successful maternity and child welfare work.*

The machinery for discovering and preventing these conditions at birth and in the years before school-life began, was possessed by medical officers of health, being provided by the Notification of Births Act. There was in fact no justification for the contention on behalf of the Board of Education that the administration of ante-natal hygiene, midwifery, the postpartum period . . . must be kept, as far as administration goes, separate and distinct from questions of infant care.

I had no difficulty in concluding that "there is no valid reason for a *policy of discontinuity,* by which an artificial division is made at birth or a few months after it;" for infant consultations were being carried on, some voluntary, and many by Public Health Authorities, and it was already clear that women and their infants, born and unborn, can be brought into touch with such Centres to an extent which is *impracticable with any organisation working back from* school life, and thus only able to reach a minority of cases.

THE DUTIES *QUA* PERSONAL HEALTH OF PUBLIC
    HEALTH AUTHORITIES

On the side of the Board of Education it had been contended that the difference between the Sanitary Service and the

Educational Service in each area is a difference between the environmental factor and the personal factor. Even if this misleading nomenclature and classification were accepted, this contention was unjustified historically.

For:

(1) Under the Public Health Act, 1875, Public Health Authorities had been empowered to provide temporary medical treatment for the poorer inhabitants of the district, and hospital treatment when required.

(2) A specific duty of M.O.H.s was to "ascertain the causes and distribution of diseases within their district."

(3) Public Health Authorities were supplying antitoxin for the home treatment of diphtheria, and occasionally nurses for the home treatment of infectious cases.

(4) Many of them were the supervising authorities for midwives, and had already some control over bad midwifery arrangements, puerperal sepsis, and ophthalmia of the new-born, and could aid in the training of midwives.

(5) Already many health visitors had been appointed by Public Health Authorities, these nurse visitors being engaged in giving appropriate hygienic counsel to mothers and their infants, as well as helping to remove domestic and other conditions militating against the child's or the mother's welfare.

In addition already a considerable number of Infant Consultations had been started under the control or the supervision of the Public Health Authority. This personal hygienic work did not stand alone; similar work was being done for the prevention of tuberculosis and diarrhoeal and other diseases.

In the year 1936 it may seem superfluous to state these and other equally obvious points; but they form a necessary part of the story of the stages of development of official work on child hygiene, and the obstacles which this work met.

The statement summarised above indicates the then relative attitude of two Government Departments both of which were concerned with child welfare.

GRANTS FOR SCHOOLS FOR MOTHERS

The Board of Education had one great advantage over the Local Government Board, in that they had already subsidised the expenses of voluntary associations working for child welfare at "schools for mothers." These grants were limited by the Board's Regulations for Technical Schools and could be given only in respect of organised class-teaching. They were thus, as Dr. McCleary has put it (*The Maternity and Child Welfare Movement*, P. S. King, 1935), "subject to conditions that were unsuitable for instruction in mothercraft, which, to be successful, must be based on individual attention." The first of these schools for mothers was started by Dr. J. F. J. Sykes, M.O.H. of St. Pancras, London, and his colleagues in 1905–6. The "school" was very successful in its aggregate activities: baby weighings, dinners for nursing mothers, infant consultations, a provident club, classes on cookery, and on making of babies' clothes, etc. There were similar activities in Glasgow, St. Marylebone, and elsewhere.

Naturally existing centres for teaching health and for medical consultations for infants and pre-school children laid stress on the class-teaching side of their work, although it formed but a small part of their total activities, as thus they were enabled to obtain grants from the Board of Education in aid of their expenses. In the memoranda already abstracted, I emphasised the difficulties of connected and consecutive teaching, and emphasised the central truth that what is most needed is personal, medical, and hygienic advice, supplementing the advice given by health visitors at their home visits.

The position at that time, in short, was that Public Health Authorities could do, and were doing, much child welfare work without fresh legislation, while the Board of Education was doing extremely little of such work and could do no more without fresh legislation.

DISCONTINUITY OF MEDICAL ADVICE

Further, on a point previously mentioned, I concluded in the memoranda already summarised that there is no justification for discontinuity of medical and hygienic work which is natal and ante-natal from that which is post-natal: and in principle discontinuity of medical work before and during school life cannot be defended.

G*

The second discontinuity, however, already existed and still in 1936 continues in part: but, as I urged in the interest of future success of fully organised public health work, the area of discontinuity should not be allowed to be extended.

It followed naturally that I urged the Local Government Board to secure power to give Grants in Aid to the large Public Health Authorities for extension of medical work and of work in personal hygiene, including maternity centres, infant consultations, and the work of health visitors.

At the same time the extension of the work of the Board of Education was welcomed so far as it encouraged technical instruction in housewifery and child welfare to present and future mothers, definite class instruction to mothers in schools for mothers, and still more so far as it secured a better educated class of midwives.

The time was ripe for settlement of the disputed sphere of work of the two Boards. The problem was submitted to a high legal arbitrator. He gave his award early in July 1914. It sanctioned the continuance of the dual work of the two Departments of State, and the decisions of the award were incorporated in subsequent circulars sent out to local authorities. An immediate practical effect of the award was that the Treasury, actuated by Mr. Herbert Samuel, at once enabled the Local Government Board to give grants to local authorities to the extent of fifty per cent of their approved expenditure, coming within the spacious four corners of the following schedule appended to the circular letter issued by the Local Government Board to Public Health Authorities on July 30, 1914. When these public health grants became available, the difficulty of the "rivalry" between the two governmental Boards became insignificant.

MATERNITY AND CHILD WELFARE

A complete scheme would comprise the following elements, each of which will, in this connection, be organised in its direct bearing on infantile health. The following statement of these elements, prepared by me, was embodied in the Board's letter sent to local authorities, in July 1914.

1. Arrangements for the local supervision of midwives.

2. Arrangements for—

   ANTE-NATAL

   (1) An ante-natal clinic for expectant mothers.
   (2) The home visiting of expectant mothers.
   (3) A maternity hospital or beds at a hospital in which complicated cases of pregnancy can receive treatment.

3. Arrangements for—

   NATAL

   (1) Such assistance as may be needed to ensure the mother having skilled and prompt attendance during confinement at home.
   (2) The confinement of sick women, including women having contracted pelvis or suffering from any other condition involving danger to the mother or infant, at a hospital.

4. Arrangements for—

   POST-NATAL

   (1) The treatment in a hospital of complications arising after parturition, whether in the mother or in the infant.
   (2) The provision of systematic advice and treatment for infants at a baby clinic or infant dispensary.
   (3) The continuance of these clinics and dispensaries, so as to be available for children up to the age when they are entered on a school register, i.e. the register of a public elementary school, nursery school, crèche, day nursery, school for mothers, or other school.
   (4) The systematic home visitation of infants and of children not on a school register as above defined.

LOCAL GOVERNMENT BOARD, WHITEHALL, S.W.

July 1914

CHAPTER XXI

NATURAL SELECTION AND INFANT MORTALITY
INVESTIGATIONS IN EUGENICS

THE most debatable part of my first Report on Infant Mortality (published in 1910) was the comparison made between high and low death-rates respectively in infancy and in the successive four years of life. Let me first state the facts. They are summarised for counties in the diagram on page 205, reproduced by permission of H.M. Stationery Office from the report itself.

The figures indicated in the diagram are relative, i.e. the infant death-rate in England and Wales, 1908, which was 120 per 1,000 births, has been taken as 100 and all the infant death-rates in counties are stated in proportion to it. The diagram shows correspondence in magnitude between the infant death-rate in a county and that in the same county in the age-period 1–5. A similar correlation was visible when aggregate county boroughs and rural and urban districts were taken. The conclusion I drew was that

a high infant death-rate in a given community implies in general a high death-rate in the next four years of life, while low death-rates at both age periods are similarly associated.

The comparison was extended to ages up to twenty; and although the rule stated above did not hold good to the full extent, there was evidence of continuation of a similar experience.

In my Annual Report to the Local Government Board for 1909–10 I had approached the same problem from a different angle. Use was made of two Life Tables in the decennial supplement to the Registrar General's annual reports, showing the life-table experience in 1891–1900 of England and Wales and of selected healthy districts.[1]

[1] These life-tables both related to the same decade, and were constructed by the same method. Their data were therefore not incomparable, as were those mentioned on page 208.

ADMINISTRATIVE COUNTIES.

RELATIVE MORTALITY FIGURES, 1908.

AT AGES 0-1 AND 1-5.

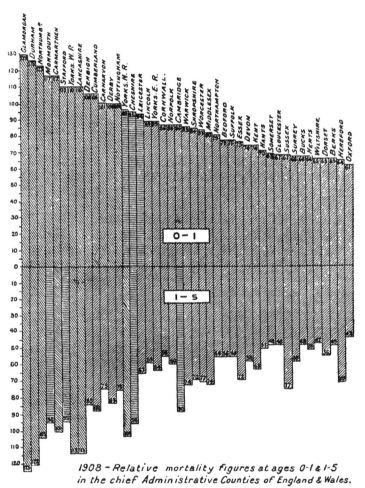

1908 – Relative mortality figures at ages 0-1 & 1-5
in the chief Administrative Counties of England & Wales.

The general result is shown in the diagram on page 207, reproduced from my report by permission of H.M. Stationery Office.

In healthy districts fewer deaths in earlier ages were followed by an excess of survivors at all higher ages, as compared with the whole country.

These were the facts. What could one conclude? Did it enable me to answer the first of the three questions on p. 178? I deprecated any conclusion going beyond the facts.

No attempt has been made in the preceding pages to settle the moot point as to whether a heavy infant mortality has any selective influence on the population surviving beyond infancy. The matter cannot be put to the test of actual experiment. To do this it would be necessary to transfer a large sample of the infant population of, say, the county of Durham, who had survived the excessive dangers of the first year of life in that county, to a county like Oxford, transferring an equal number of survivors from Oxford to Durham.

I added:

If natural selection during infancy in the county of Durham has left a juvenile population less prone to disease, the effect of this selection is most effectively and completely concealed by the evil environment in that county, which causes the hypothetically stronger survivors to suffer from excessive mortality, so long as they can be traced through life.

Mr. G. Udny Yule, F.R.S., a distinguished biometrician, subsequently President of the Royal Statistical Society, contributed to my report a valuable study of its statistical data, as to possible selective influence on the children surviving beyond the first year of life, and concluded that

there is little definite evidence of such selection beyond the second year of life, and after the third year the environmental influences even of infancy alone appear to preponderate over any possible selective influence.

My moderate statement, as quoted above, excited the indignation of Professor Karl Pearson, F.R.S., who was convinced that "a too busy official" could not be trusted to discuss such a biological subject, but I resumed its discussion in my "Second Report on Infant and Child Mortality," 1913 (Cd. 6909).

	Mean Population, 1891–1900.	Mean Infant Mortality per 1,000 Births.
England and Wales	30,643,479	... 157
Selected Healthy Districts ...	4,477,485	... 109

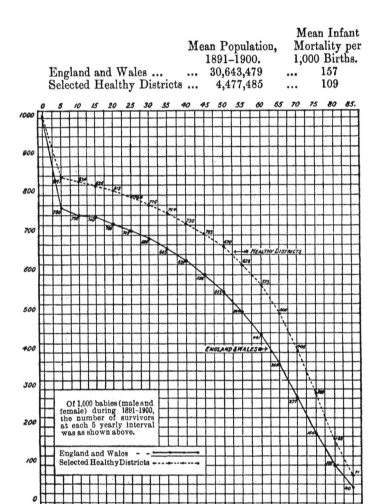

Of 1,000 babies (male and female) during 1891-1900, the number of survivors at each 5 yearly interval was as shown above.

England and Wales
Selected Healthy Districts

This table is to be read as shewn in the following examples :—At age 20 the number of survivors was 812 in healthy districts, 726 in the country as a whole ; at age 60 was 573 in healthy districts, 441 in the country as a whole ; and so on.

In this report I repeated that my statement did not settle whether efforts to save infant life meant preventing the "weeding out" of the unfit; and I took the opportunity to correct Professor Pearson's statements (*Proc. Roy. Soc.*, B, Vol. 85, 1912) to the effect that infant mortality had been "steadily rising since the restriction of families," and that "it is certain that the improved environment of the last thirty or forty years has not effected any improvement in the infantile death-rate." This statistical error had arisen from his comparing life-table death-rates, calculated by methods which were not comparable. The actual facts were in the opposite direction.

On the main point as to selection, several efforts have been made to trace children at successive ages, but no concordant results have been secured, the methods adopted having failed to give weight to the epidemiological history of the years under investigation. Meanwhile I am contented to rest satisfied with my statement in 1923 (in *The Elements of Vital Statistics in their Bearing on Social and Public Health Problems*, by A. Newsholme).

The conclusion arrived at in my official report stands. Environment has a preponderant influence in determining the magnitude of infant and child mortality in a community; and the increasing efforts of hygienists to improve environment (this includes the mother) need not be embarrassed by suggestions that such efforts may exert an inimical influence on the quality of mankind.

INVESTIGATIONS IN EUGENICS

This opportunity is convenient for mentioning other biometrical investigations which appear, until they are critically examined, to throw doubt on the value of many public health activities. The usefulness of not a few medical officers of health has been dulled by these doubts; and this diminution of enthusiasm for their life-work has been increased by their inability to check the statistical measures employed by biometricians, and by their too ready belief that pontifical statements based on (to them) incomprehensible statistics must be accepted implicitly. But in fact these biometrical, like other, statistical investigations are often vitiated by two chief errors:

the data may be untrustworthy, especially by being heterogeneous and therefore unsuitable for statistical use; or the methods employed in using them may be fallacious.

Let me deal first with this second point, as it is the error into which I was regarded by Professor Pearson as having fallen, in my inquiry into the influence of segregation on the phthisis death-rate (p. 133) and in my inquiry into the relation between death-rates at ages 0–1 and 1–5 (p. 206).

I have already expressed my appreciation, which has never failed, of the elementary consideration that no satisfactory cor.clusion can be drawn from the fact that two variables exhibit close correlation, when these change with time, and have always realised that the close correlation in a series of years of a declining death-rate from phthisis with increasing segregation of cases of this disease, needs to be considered alongside of the biological facts on tuberculosis and in the light of collateral facts (p. 133). Thus considered, the relation between segregation of infectious cases and reduction of disease can be, and by me has been, profitably investigated and conclusions of much practical importance have been reached.

So likewise in regard to child mortality. To establish the operation of natural selection, the same children should be followed throughout the entire five years under consideration, which could not be done with the national statistics used by me (p. 204). But the conclusion I stated as regards the total aggregate effect of possible natural selection and of the certainly existent important environmental influences holds good. Later investigators—Brownlee, Snow, and Falk—have attempted the more difficult task of assessing the separate influence of selection. Of these Dr. Falk has confirmed my results by studying a group of children traced from 0–1 to 1–5, while Dr. Snow has arrived at an opposite conclusion; and Dr. Brownlee has expressed doubt as to whether any method proposed to measure the influence of the death-rate as a selective agent can be trusted.

Underlying all Professor Pearson's biometrical work appears to be his conviction that hereditary are much more important than environmental factors in life, while the methods of social workers and of legislators imply the assumption that "better environment means race progress." I share the belief in the importance of heredity, but am equally convinced of the importance of environment, including infection and parental habits of life, in health problems.

PHTHISIS AND HEREDITY

In 1907 Pearson concluded that in the causation of tuberculosis in the artisan class heredity has many times the influence of environment. Evidence has been advanced similarly to show that only rarely is a wife or husband infected by the consumptive partner. Statistical evidence on the last point is shaky, and cannot allow for dosage of infection and for protracted latency of infection; and as to heredity one cannot in experience separate the hereditary factor from the coexistent opportunities of infection.

Pearson considered that firstborn children were more likely to be tubercular than their brothers and sisters, but Greenwood and Yule have shown the statistical fallacies latent in this conclusion.

Iu *Biometrika* in 1918–19, Pearson wrote on the check in the fall in the phthisis death-rate beginning about 1895. The death-rate somewhat later was increased by influenza and war conditions, but it was considered by Pearson when writing on pre-War experience that "the general trend of our graphs" (as indicated before the War) "is that somewhere about 1915 the fall in the phthisis death-rate which had been less rapid since 1895 would cease altogether and probably be followed by a rise." For a demonstration of the fact that broadly speaking there has been, on the other hand, an accelerating rate of decline of the tuberculosis death-rate, I must refer the reader to the Registrar General's Statistical Review, 1921, p. 52, and to the fuller discussion and diagrams on this point given on p. 587 of my *Elements of Vital Statistics*.

I must similarly refer the reader to Chapters XLIII to XLV of the 1923 edition of my *Elements of Vital Statistics* for other illustrations of the fact that accurate mathematical calculations made on the basis of dubious data, cannot be allowed to carry influence in social investigations. In the above instances the mathematical methods of investigation were, I doubt not, admirable, but the data were unworthy of use or were wrongly used. This appears to have been the case in the famous bio-metrical inquiry in Edinburgh into the relation between alco-holic habits and the weight, general health, and intelligence of the children of the alcoholics. The statistics appeared to show that the children of these alcoholics were somewhat superior to other children. Such a highly improbable conclusion naturally led to criticism, one point of which was that it had not been made clear whether the alcoholic habits of the parents preceded or followed the conception of their offspring (see p. 548 of *Vital Statistics*).

Similarly in testing intelligence in school children, publica-tions from the Galton Laboratory have arrived at the conclusion that heredity counts for much more than environment, but dispassionate examination shows that complete separation of the two main factors, heredity and environment, has not been effected, and probably in the instances given is impossible.

We cannot doubt that the newer investigations on genetic lines will give us results freer from fallacy than the biometrical school hitherto has obtained. As Hogben has put it (*in Nature and Nurture*):

The application of statistical technique in the study of human inheritance is beset with pitfalls. . . . There is the danger of con-cealing assumptions which have no factual basis behind an impres-sive façade of flawless algebra.

Hogben quotes the following from Wilhelm Ostwald, which aptly summarises the subject of this chapter:

Among not a few scientific articles . . . the logic and mathe-matics are faultless . . . but are worthless, "because the assumptions and hypotheses upon which the faultless logic and mathematics rest do not correspond to actuality."

CHAPTER XXII

MOTHERHOOD

IN preceding chapters I have repeatedly emphasised the principle that the health of the infant and of the young child depends on the health of the expectant mother and of the mother in the early years of the child's life. This has always been recognised; although, as so often happens, administrative effort by central authorities did not pursue the natural sequence, the health of the school child being the subject of financial aid from the Board of Education before the Local Government Board was empowered to give financial aid to Public Health Authorities for specific work for the care of infancy and of motherhood. This remark as to sequence of work does not apply to Public Health Authorities, for as early as 1892 the Bucks County Council had appointed health visitors, and similar action by other local authorities in the later years of the twentieth century have already been noted. In 1872 the Obstetrical Society of London had started an Examination Board for midwives, giving a certificate to competent women; but it was not until 1902 that the Midwives Act became law, prohibitng future practice of midwifery (after a few years' interval) by unregistered women. Before this enactment was secured many years of strenuous advocacy were needed on the part of Dr. C. J. Cullingworth of St. Thomas's Hospital and his co-workers. Opposition to this Act was based on various grounds. It was anticipated that mothers, especially in country districts, would be deprived of the services of the handy women who usually helped them in their time of need. It was further contended by medical practitioners, some of whom opposed action for training midwives, that not only would their own medical practice suffer, but that the State recognition of midwives would also create the impression that they were qualified to practise medicine. Many doctors contended that in the public interest the practice of midwifery should be chiefly by qualified medical practitioners.

The Act of 1902 created a Central Midwives Board, to keep

a roll of certified midwives, and regulate the conditions of their certification and practice; and entrusted to Local Supervising Authorities, who were the Councils of Counties and County Boroughs, the local supervision of midwives within their area. The Central Midwives Board worked nominally under the Privy Council and not under the Local Government Board, the Central Health Authority. Parliament, and perhaps this Board also, had not yet realised that the care of the mother as affecting the health of both mother and child was essentially a public health problem.

I need not enter into details of the difficulties of the new work. The provisions of the Act came only slowly into operation.

The midwife was required to advise the patient's relatives to send for a doctor when abnormal conditions were discovered by her, but no provision was at first made to pay the doctor's fee. The Local Government Board, looking at the difficulty from a chiefly Poor Law point of view, did not at first favour giving these fees except under Poor Law conditions. Some local authorities made independent arrangements, but it was not until the Midwives Act of 1918 was enacted that it became the duty of the midwife to call in a doctor herself when, in accordance with the rules of the Central Midwives Board, this was required. The same Act made it the duty of the local supervising authority to pay the doctor's fee, in accordance with an authorised scale. The midwife unfortunately may call in any registered medical practitioner in emergencies. This practitioner may be inexperienced in midwifery work, often his skill is not adequate for the serious emergencies which arise, and it is earnestly to be hoped that the movement now increasing to secure that the practitioner called in by the midwife shall be a skilled obstetrician will ere long become actual practice. This may necessitate the employment of consultants in each administrative area.

I may now narrate some activities with which I was personally or indirectly concerned.

As already seen the intimate relation between maternal and infantile health had been appreciated from the beginning, but the movement in infant welfare work was well advanced before, in 1914, these two aspects of complete work were firmly united by the giving of Government grants in aid of both maternity work and child welfare work (p. 202).

In my Annual Report as Medical Officer of the Local Government Board, which dealt with my first year's work at the Board, I recalled the evidence I had recently given before the Departmental Committee on the working of the Midwives Act, 1902 (Cd. 4822, 1909, p. 25). This Committee had sat for some time, and its report suggested valuable reforms in the administration of the Act.

In a memorandum prepared for this Committee I made the following among other suggestions:

(1) I forecasted the investigation by the Local Government Board which is summarised on page 216 on the great variations in the death-rates from puerperal sepsis in the different counties of England and Wales, and on the need to attempt to correlate these differences with the number of still-births notified by midwives and with the midwifery arrangements in the same counties.

(2) I pointed out that, under present conditions, midwives and health visitors, except in county boroughs and a few counties, may work under several different authorities; and active co-operation between these authorities was needed. I suggested that in scattered county districts it might sometimes be advantageous to combine in one person the duties of health visitor and of village midwife.

The desirability of combining in some instances the duties of midwife and of district nurse, or these with the duties of school nurse, was also considered, as also the practicability of combining administrative work under the Notification of Births Act with that under the Midwives Act.

(3) The desirability of systematic county investigation of infant mortality was pointed out. By analysing the returns under the Notification of Births Act, the county medical officer of health could learn whether there had been an excessive number of still-births in the practice of any midwife.

PUERPERAL MORTALITY

I embodied in my next Annual Report (1910–11) a study of puerperal mortality. The total registered puerperal mortality was decreasing. But although decreasing, it remained true that among all women aged 15–45 puerperal sepsis and accidents of childbirth caused 3,341 deaths in one year, while in the same year among men of the same age general accidents and negligence were responsible for 3,938 deaths.

Childbearing therefore demands a toll on the lives of women which, stated in proportion to total deaths at these ages (8·2 per cent), is nearly equal to the corresponding toll paid by men in connection with accidental causes (8·8 per cent).

The local differences emphasised in my evidence to the Department Committee are shown graphically in the diagram on p. 216 (reproduced by permission of H.M. Stationery Office) taken from my annual report for 1910. In general, London and the Home Counties showed the lowest rates under both of the above headings; while

the highest "sepsis" rates were experienced in South and North Wales, Lancashire, Monmouth, and Cheshire, and the highest "accident" rates in Westmorland, North and South Wales, Cumberland, and Monmouth.

I need not summarise this report further, except to draw attention to my preliminary conclusion, which was confirmed in my later report (p. 218).

The lower mortality in London and the Home Counties from "accidents of childbirth" in comparison with Wales and outlying parts of England is probably due in part to the fact that the latter comprise districts which are sparsely populated or difficult of access, and where consequently emergency treatment is difficult to obtain; and partly to the greater facilities for obtaining institutional treatment or the assistance of consultants in London and its neighbourhood.

The facts given in preceding pages showed that although rates of infant mortality showed remarkable decline, the "concentration on the mother and the child" urged by Mr. Burns had so far been effective chiefly for the child, and that there was needed further action to secure safe childbirth, and through this additional safety for the child.

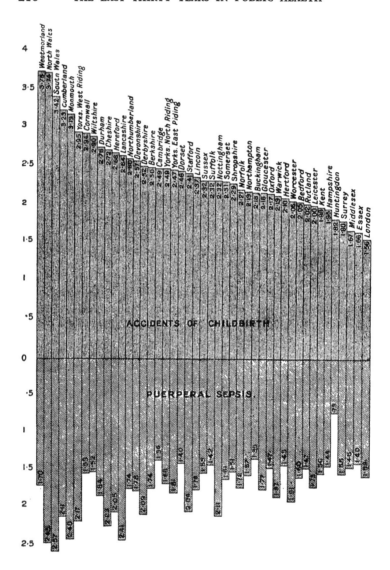

3   1897-1908. DEATH-RATES, PER 1000 BIRTHS, FROM
ACCIDENTS OF CHILDBIRTH AND PUERPERAL SEPSIS
IN REGISTRATION COUNTIES.

I added that

the attainment of these ends is important as much in the interest of the child as of its mother. That the welfare of the child is wrapped up in that of the mother was fully recognised in the Board's circular letter of July 31, 1914 (p. 202), and the schedule appended to that letter; and each year it is becoming more fully realised that, in order to secure healthy infancy and childhood, it is necessary that, both during pregnancy and at and after the birth of the infant, increased maternal care and guidance and medical assistance should be provided.

My complete report to the Board on "Maternal Mortality in connection with Childbearing and its Relation to Infant Mortality" (Cd. 8085), owing to the stress of work before and during the War, was not completed and published until 1915. It gave an elaborate analysis of puerperal mortality in each county and its constituent towns, and included special contributions by Dr. Janet Lane-Claypon and Dr. Isabella Cameron, members of the Medical Department's staff. In my prefatory statement to Mr. Walter (later Lord) Long, then President of the Local Government Board, I said that

childbearing is still associated in some parts of the country with very excessive mortality, and in every part of the country with much avoidable sickness and mortality.

The present report is intended to draw attention to this unnecessary mortality from childbearing, to stimulate further local inquiry on the subject, and to encourage measures which make illness and disability due to childbearing much rarer than at present.

This report showed a fairly uniform experience throughout England and Wales in respect of puerperal fever, while from other conditions affecting childbearing adversely, London's experience was more favourable than that of the provinces. A saving of 1,100 lives of mothers would be effected in England and Wales by the elimination of sepsis, which had already been almost accomplished in the experience of many Lying-in Hospitals. Welsh counties had the highest mortality from childbearing, Westmorland, Lancashire, and Cheshire the next highest, and in great towns there were even more striking differences. The incidence of puerperal mortality showed that "special local factors, other than topographical, were chiefly concerned in causing local excesses of mortality from child-bearing." Intensive inquiries in each county and in each of the towns showing vast differences in their sinister experience was needed, more fully to disclose the significance of these. Meanwhile an interim conclusion could be drawn:

General experience, apart from statistical evidence, appears to point to the conclusion that *the differences are caused in the main by differences in availability of skilled assistance when needed in pregnancy, and at and after childbirth.*

The special report on Maternal Mortality in connection with Childbearing included valuable reports by medical members of the Board's staff, one by Dr. Janet Lane-Claypon on the Economic Aspect of Midwifery and on the conditions under which medical help is sent for; and one by Dr. Isabella Cameron on Maternity Hospital Experience of Maternal and Infant Mortality. No further direct reference is made to these reports, but they should be read as throwing valuable light on the position in 1914–15.

My main conclusions, based on these reports and on my analysis of national statistics, were that:

(1) in order to take official action for reducing maternal mortality and suffering, we must ascertain what cases need help:

by providing skilled help at Maternity Centres;
to some extent through the notification of births;
by more effective notification of puerperal sepsis;
by the collection of the statistics of hospital experience;
and by the provision of pathological aids to diagnosis.

(2) Ante-natal work at consultations and clinics together with home-visiting should be organised.

(3) A better distribution of midwives and a stricter super-vision of their work are needed.

In my Annual Report 1915–16, I wrote that—

the urgent call of the Army for all available medical practitioners has interfered with the rapid development of maternity and child welfare centres under medical supervision, to the extent which the Board consider imperative to secure the full measure of success:

though nevertheless good work was being done.

In my next report (1916–17) I reported progress in the provision of Maternity Schemes, including hospital provision for complicated cases of confinement, or for complications arising after confinement either in mother or infant, and for infants found to need in-patient treatment.

During this year Dr. Janet Lane-Claypon reported on the Midwifery Service in London (N.S.111). This report showed that there appeared to be adequate hospital provision for in-patient maternity cases, but considerable inequality in its distribution. Her report confirmed the conclusion given on page 215, that the low mortality from non-septic causes of mortality in childbirth shown in London is due to the ample provision made for attendance on its midwifery cases when complicated.

In my Annual Report to the Local Government Board, 1917–18, I drew attention to the fact that already midwives attended nearly three-fourths of the total births in England and Wales, and that they were required to notify to the local supervising authority all births, including abortions and still-births without any limitation as to the period of pregnancy, which opened up important lines of public health investigation. My fuller remarks on this subject are given on p. xxvi of that report.

CHAPTER XXIII

MATERNAL MORTALITY

IN reviewing my already quoted remarks on the mortality of mothers associated with pregnancy and childbirth I am struck with their hopefulness, and with my persistent unwillingness to abandon this attitude. The course of events appears, in part at least, to have falsified my forecast; for in recent years we are constantly being reminded of the stationary or even increasing mortality from childbirth in Great Britain. Indeed the failure to secure improvement in this toll on the life of mothers—so strikingly in contrast with the spectacular decline in the rate of infant mortality—has made it a subject of Parliamentary questions, of resolutions at social conferences, and of a crop of official and non-official reports.

But are these statements as to non-success of the many and increasing efforts already being made to reduce puerperal sickness and mortality correct? Or have changes occurred in the factors contributing to maternal mortality, which make national returns of thirty years ago not strictly comparable with those of to-day?

If we use the classification of causes of death in use by the Registrar General before 1911, total puerperal mortality in 1911–15 was 5·02 and in 1931 was 5·55, while if the classification revised in 1911 be used throughout, total puerperal mortality has increased from 4·03 to 4·11 in 1931.

The comparison between 1911–15, after a revised classification of puerperal deaths was introduced into the Registrar General's reports, and the three years 1931–33, is as below:

ENGLAND AND WALES
Death-rate per 1,000 live births from

Year	Puerperal Sepsis	Other Puerperal Causes
1911–15	1·42	2·61
1916–20	1·51	2·61
1921–25	1·40	2·50
1926–30	1·73	2·54
1931–33	1·70	2·58

There has been some increase during recent years in the registered death-rate from sepsis, while the incidence of other causes of death in connection with pregnancy and parturition has remained stationary.

But are the figures, although comparable as regards allotment of certification of causes of death, strictly comparable throughout in other respects? And even if so, may not additional dangers in recent years have cancelled the saving of mothers' lives during parturition which would otherwise have emerged from the greater and better care now given to childbearing women?

There is a strong *a priori* probability that the recorded *rates* of mortality do not accurately represent the course of events. This grave doubt is reasonable for several reasons.

Sepsis in parturition ought now to be less prevalent than in more remote years when antisepsis and asepsis had not become the definite aim in all departments of medical practice. Listerism now is assumed to be the common practice alike of nurses and doctors, even though sometimes neglected. And yet the registered death-rate from puerperal sepsis has increased. If Listerism is more generally practised in midwifery than in the past, are we not driven (assuming that the figures are comparable) to search for some additional provocative of sepsis, or an old provocative acting on a much larger scale?

The declining birth-rate gives us the clue as to such a likely provocative. (1) The practice of contraception is not always successful, and when pregnancy in such cases occurs, there often arises the desire to secure its speedy termination. Statistical evidence of the annual amount of intentionally produced abortion in Britain is unobtainable; but obstetricians appear to be satisfied that it has increased, and the proportion of total puerperal sepsis ascribable to this cause has been placed as high as 20 per cent. If this be so, and if—as is highly probable—abortion is more frequently attempted now than in the past, a large share of the present death-rate from sepsis is thus explained. There may be, and almost certainly has been, increased care of the mother in childbirth; but a very serious cause of sepsis apart from childbirth at term has emerged. The Registrar General's figures give the annual number of deaths attributed to abortion during recent years, and these show no definite evidence of increase. But it is likely that these figures do not display the whole truth.

(2) Our national mortality statistics depend for their accuracy on the individual certificates of cause of death given by doctors throughout the country. There has always been unwillingness to associate death with childbirth, which should be a normal function of life; but accuracy of medical certification has increased and it may reasonably be assumed that this increased accuracy has increased the number of maternal deaths recorded.

(3) Maternal deaths associated with parturition—including deaths after abortion—have, in the Registrar General's annual summaries, been compared with each other in their ratio to the number of live births. Evidently it would be desirable to compare these deaths with total pregnancies, but this is impracticable. Now that the number of deaths due to abortion are given in our national returns, we shall be able to estimate separately the share of abortion (whether accidental or intentional) in producing the total puerperal death-rate, though we shall continue to be unable to state the death-rate from abortion in terms of total abortions.

(4) The greatly lowered birth-rate means on the average much smaller families, and therefore a higher proportion of first to subsequent births than in the past. It is most unfortunate that in English birth-registration a statement of the order of the birth is not required, and therefore, although we know that maternal mortality is higher for first births than for the next three or four in sequence, we cannot state exactly the influence of this factor on the registered puerperal mortality. That it has to some extent increased puerperal mortality as registered is certain, other things being equal, but only indirect evidence is available as to how much.

Matthews Duncan, dealing with deaths in Edinburgh in the year 1855, showed the result set out below: with these are compared Coghlan's figures for New South Wales relating to the eight years ending in 1900. Both sets of figures show the excess mortality (in relative figures) in the first pregnancy.

For consecutive pregnancies the figures up to and including the sixth pregnancy are as follows:

RELATIVE MORTALITY

(*1st pregnancy* = 100)

	1	*2*	*3*	*4*	*5*	*6*
Scotland	100	62	73	48	63	43
New South Wales ..	100	53	66	57	74	75[1]

The effect on total puerperal mortality of the greater risk in first pregnancies would be very considerable; in the absence of more complete statistics it has been placed tentatively as high as 15 to 20 per cent and as low as 4 per cent. I think the last-named figure will prove to be much too low.

Thus certain factors have been tending to increase the figures of puerperal mortality, as registered, to a considerable though not measurable extent, namely altered certification, smaller families, and probably increased abortions, which have counteracted to that extent the tendency of puerperal mortality, as registered, to decline. The statistics do not justify us in concluding that the quality of the aid rendered by doctors or midwives has become less efficient.

I have not added to these the psychological effect of the extravagant statements so often publicly made as to excessive puerperal mortality. These statements must have increased the fear of childbearing and the desire to avoid it, and their share in making childbirth more dangerous is not negligible.

The preceding considerations should reduce the amount of semi-hysterical writing on the subject, which if it continues may still further increase the modern fears of what should be a normal event.

But these considerations do not justify complacency in regard to the excessive mortality associated with pregnancy and childbirth. The facts are serious; and much more so are the differences experienced in various communities.

A Departmental Committee of the Ministry of Health has concluded that "at least one half of the maternal deaths occurring in this country are preventable," and some Glasgow investigations put this proportion as high as three-fourths.

[1] See McCleary's *The Maternity and Child Welfare Movement* and the recent Report on Maternal Mortality in Scotland, by Drs. C. A. Douglas and P. L. McKinlay (1935, pp. 35–37, 215).

There is now much hope that administrative measures making childbirth safer and freer from suffering will become general. In bringing this about it is clear that midwives who already attend about three-fourths of total births will need greater aid to render their services more efficient. In some districts subsidies in aid of their salaries will be required. They will need to receive a better training than they have hitherto had; and this educational need applies even more strongly to the training given to medical accoucheurs, if they are to retain any midwifery work, beyond ante- and post-natal medical care. An early reform called for is that in every administrative area there should be an obstetric consultant or a small panel of doctors with special obstetric experience, and that the midwife, when faced with abnormalities requiring medical aid, should only be permitted to send for those doctors on the official list of experienced obstetricians.

CHAPTER XXIV

THE GREAT WAR

GARRISON quotes Sudermann's description of the War as "the most gigantic imbecility since the Crusades." This is true. Unrestricted nationalism and inter-national misunderstanding, disputes, and greediness found their climax in war of almost world-wide extent. Happily this was not the only side of War; for it elicited self-denial and sacrifice on an almost unbelievable scale, not only in active belligerents, but in the masses of the peoples contending with each other.

From a medico-hygienic point of view the War had momentous results. It hastened research and shortened the protracted incubation between discovery and practical action on it which is the usual experience. In the prevention and treatment of sickness and in the treatment of wounds, there was almost immediate application of every available investigation. While many communicable diseases were spread with unexampled rapidity, due to war movements, and their virulence was increased, other diseases also communicable were almost entirely prevented by the unexampled application of preventive medicine. It is difficult to garner into one chapter the lessons of the War in its medico-hygienic aspects. I propose to consider it chiefly from the point of view of my work at the central health offices in the Local Government Board.

Although our medical staff was much depleted by detachment of men for special war work, we were able from the first to organise active co-operation between the local health authorities and the military officers of the camps established throughout England, for the protection of the food of recruits and the provision of satisfactory water supplies and drainage for each camp and in billets. From August 4, 1914, the work of the Medical Department centred almost entirely around the military position. In particular the importance of the following points was stressed:

(1) Each medical officer of health was asked to give information and assistance to military sanitary officers as to—

Water supplies,
Disposal of refuse,
Drainage and conservancy arrangement,
Control of infectious diseases, etc.

(2) The importance of the co-operation of the sanitary inspector was indicated.

(3) A system of inter-notification of infectious diseases, both by military and civil sanitary inspectors, was arranged.

(4) Attention was drawn to the value of anti-typhoid inoculation.

(5) The probable need for increased hospital accommodation for smallpox and enteric fever was indicated.

(6) The services of the medical staff of the Board were offered to medical officers of health for consultation; and local visits by medical inspectors of the Board were arranged.

By co-operation with the Medical Department of the War Office, corresponding military instructions were given to all commanding officers. The assistance given by the civilian health service throughout the country was handsomely acknowledged by the Army Council, who stated that the civilian co-operation in the unexampled circumstances of the first eight months of the War was "invaluable in safeguarding the health of the forces and in preventing the spread of infectious diseases." Until separate military arrangements for disinfection and disinfestation had been organised, sanitary authorities undertook this. The work of Dr. MacFadden and his staff of the Food Division of the Medical Department of the Board in safeguarding food supplies was especially appreciated.

Many special problems arose in which co-operation was needed between civilian and military health authorities and some notes may be added on these.

Unlimited vaccine lymph against small pox was supplied from the Board's stores and no considerable outbreak of smallpox occurred throughout the War. *Typhus fever* was almost completely absent either in Britain or in the British forces on the Western front and the amount of *typhoid* and *paratyphoid fever* was lower, in proportion to numbers of combatants, than in any past experience. The credit for this, especially abroad where sanitary conditions were imperfectly controllable, belongs chiefly to anti-typhoid inoculation, but our civilian experience during the War showed that protection against this communicable disease may be secured apart from artificial immunisation, when good sanitation, safe water, absence of contaminated shell-fish, and isolation of those already sick can be secured. I must recall that the insistence on chlorinated drinking water played a part in the diminution of military typhoid fever.

Soon after the War began, *cerebro-spinal fever* was occurring both in the troops and among civilians, and in January 1915 Surgeon-Colonel R. J. Reece, C.B., of my Department was seconded for the oversight of both military and civilian cases of this disease. The Canadian recruits who flocked to the Flag were heavily hit. It was thought that some of them had brought over with them a more virulent type of meningococcic infection, and visits made by me with other members of the Army Sanitary Committee to the Canadian camps on Salisbury Plain appeared to confirm this view. Many soldiers who had been in contact with cases of cerebro-spinal fever were found to be "carriers" of meningococci in their throats, and for some months efforts were made to curtail the quarantine imposed on these by spraying their throats with a solution of sulphate of zinc. Little if any good was effected by this means. Investigations made in the pathological laboratory of the Local Government Board brought out the important fact that when systematic examinations were made of throats of out-patients of general hospitals and others who had not, so far as could be ascertained, been near clinical cases of cerebro-spinal fever meningococci in numbers not very dissimilar from the number found among the contacts of a clinical case were found.

If my memory is correct, this gave the quietus to the attempt to clear throats of harboured meningococci. The amount of cerebro-spinal fever was in fact a partial index of the sanitary condition of the troops, and the practical remedy was widespread spacing of soldiers in barracks, free perflation of air, and the splitting up of infected units of men into smaller groups.

Encephalitis lethargica like trench-fever was a newcomer among diseases during the War, or was at least then first recognised in England. It made its appearance in London and in

a number of provincial towns in the early part of 1918. My
attention was first drawn to it by a request that I would see
some anomalous cases of illness in a general hospital in London.
The patients showed stupor, associated with other cerebral
symptoms, sometimes partial paralysis. The first suspicion was
that the cases were botulism, but this suspicion soon disappeared. There was little or no evidence of infection from patient
to patient. Careful investigations were undertaken by the
Medical Research Committee and by members of my staff. On
looking into medical literature, similar cases were found to have
occurred in Vienna and Paris, and Von Economico had given
the disease the name standing at the beginning of this paragraph. I recommended that the disease should be made compulsorily notifiable under this name and this was done. In the
light of subsequent cases of the disease, one can say that
encephalitis lethargica is one of a group of diseases, comprising also acute poliomyelitis and cerebro-spinal fever, in which
many more persons may harbour the contagium than suffer
from clinical symptoms. The infectivity of each of these
diseases is low and beyond what has already been indicated
one cannot give directions which afford satisfactory protection.

In the later years of the War *Dysentery* was found in troops
sent home from Eastern war countries. Shortly excellent
military arrangements were made for its control. Patients from
the East were sent only to a limited number of hospitals in
Britain and patients were only discharged after rigid bacteriological tests. Dysentery was made notifiable in civilians, but
although a few outbreaks of Flexner's dysentery occurred these
did not spread widely.

The Army Medical Service made important investigations
on dysentery, as did also the Medical Research Committee,
and Drs. Candler and Wilkinson of the Board's staff visited
some fifty camps and hospitals in co-operation with the military
medical officers.

The occurrence of *Anthrax* derived from shaving brushes
was noted in my earlier volume (p. 234). At first it was suspected
to be due to infected shaving brushes of German origin, but
soon it was found to be caused by Japanese shaving brushes

which had replaced the no longer obtainable brushes of German origin.

Malaria, like dysentery, was introduced from Salonika and other Eastern war centres. During 1918 some 30,000 carriers of malarial infection were evacuated to England and many in earlier years and later. In the summer of 1917 a few soldiers in certain camps, who had never left England, were attacked by malaria and there were also some "indigenous" cases of malaria in the civilian population and in some naval stations. It is known that the freedom of England from malaria is not due to the absence in warm seasons of anopheline mosquitoes, but to the absence of human links to continue the carriage by mosquitoes of the human contagion. Convalescent malarial soldiers from abroad provided these links, though happily not in adequate numbers to make malaria a serious public health problem in England. After consultation with the Army Medical Department, malaria was made a notifiable disease and the Local Government Board undertook the examination of all suspected blood films. Areas involved were visited by Colonels James and Wilkinson of the Board's staff, who had former experience of malaria in Army service in India.

Although practically no *Typhus* occurred on the Western front, this disease was terribly fatal in Russia and in Serbia. Its louse-borne causation is now well known. British, like other troops on the Western front, as well as recruits before they crossed to France, were much infested with lice in the earlier years of the War, and this condition was only improved when "de-lousing" stations were set up and systematically utilised. And yet no typhus occurred, and one must infer that the special infection of this disease failed to gain a footing on a considerable scale among the troops infested with lice.

But although typhus fever failed to appear, a new (or newly recognised) disease, *Trench Fever*, was recognised which was also spread by body lice. This disease was identified in Flanders in 1915. It was seldom fatal, but it caused serious illness and during the War it became a major cause of disability. So serious was it, that from one-fifth to one-third of the total illness of the British Armies in France and Flanders has been attributed to it. I cannot describe here the steps by which British military investigations showed that the disease was transmitted by the excreta of lice scratched into the skin. An American Commission, with Colonel R. P. Strong at its head, completed the elucidation of the life history of this disease.

It is strange, but true, that "fighting the cootie" was one of the chief sanitary problems of the War, taxing the ingenuity and administrative capacity of all concerned.

It is scarcely necessary for me to add to what is written in Chapter XVI concerning *Venereal Diseases* during the war, but I desire to emphasise the debt the civilian population owes to the venereal specialists of the Army Medical Service, who organised the efficient treatment of these diseases in the services, before the Local Government Board had secured adequate power to deal with the problem among the civilian population.

I have briefly discussed in Chapter XIV and XV the increase of mortality from *Tuberculosis* which was observed during the War in all the combatant countries and only mention it here also because this increase was a result of prolonged warfare and of its associated social misery. The close association of this increase with the pandemic of influenza, which scourged the world in the last year of the war, is undoubted (p. 147). Historically it has repeatedly happened that influenza increases the fatality of other diseases and especially of tuberculosis. Quite apart from this terrifically increased risk to the chronic tuberculous part of the population, there were the new risks involved in displacements of civilians, and overcrowding on an unexampled scale in modern life, and in the fact that many consumptives were impelled by patriotism and high wages to engage in munition and other works. What additional share deficient nutrition took in promoting the increased death-rate from tuberculosis is doubtful, but in Britain, this part, in my view, was relatively small (see pages 136 and 230).

But apart from the fatalities of war itself, the most devastating event of the latter part of the war period was the occurrence of

PANDEMIC INFLUENZA

It is no exaggeration to state that this pestilence which swept through the entire known world killed more people than were killed in the Great War, and alas! it is still an enemy against which mankind is almost completely unarmed.

These pandemics occur at irregular intervals. The last great one prior to 1918 was in 1889–1893, a previous outbreak having occurred some forty-three years earlier.

The provocatives of a particular tidal wave of this disease are unknown, though we know that during the wave it is spread from person to person by personal infection. During the War the whole world was in movement and human interchanges occurred on an almost unparalleled scale. The influenzal wave leaped over all possible obstacles, and the disease spread and multiplied with a rapidity which gave some excuse for the erroneous view that it was miasmatic in origin and spread irrespective of human contacts. America suffered even worse than England and earlier in the War. A personal incident of this period may be recalled. I received a cablegram from a friend in San Francisco, stating that face-masks had been insisted on for everyone suffering from catarrh, and suggesting that in London, which had then begun to suffer badly, this apparently useful method should be adopted. I did not adopt the friendly recommendation, and it soon transpired that in other American towns which had not adopted masks, a decline parallel to that in San Francisco had occurred. The key to this was found in the fact that masks or any other promising methods of inhibiting infection will appear to succeed if they are introduced when the natural down-trend of an epidemic curve has started! I do not of course minimise the value at all stages of an epidemic of individual precautions to avoid spread of infection and especially for young children and the aged, for whom disease is especially dangerous; and in support of this may quote the following paragraphs from a memorandum prepared by me, which was published and circulated in October 1918.

The occurrence of epidemic catarrhs would be greatly decreased by continuous flushing with air of each occupied bedroom and living-room. This implies the need for adequate warm clothing, and especially for persons engaged in sedentary occupations and for children and old people.

Overcrowding in dwellings or in unventilated assembly rooms and places of entertainment, should be avoided.

The aggregation of large numbers of persons in one room, especially for sleeping, is dangerous when catarrhs are prevalent, even though the floor space for each person may appear to be adequate. The smaller the unit of aggregation of persons, the less is the risk of infection.

Dirtiness, whether personal or of living or working rooms, and dusty conditions favour infection. The wet cleansing of all invaded places is important.

Indiscriminate expectoration is always a source of risk of infection; and is especially dangerous during the prevalence of influenza.

Persons with septic conditions of the mouth, teeth, or nasopharynx are especially prone to catarrhal attacks. The treatment of these conditions is important.

Prolonged mental strain or over-fatigue, and still more alcoholism favour infection; and complication by pneumonia is especially fatal among immoderate drinkers.

It is particularly important that sick persons and old people should be protected against exposure to influenza.

If every person who is suffering from influenza or catarrh recognised that he is a likely source of infection to others, that some of the persons infected by him may die as the result of this infection and took all possible precautions, the present disability and mortality from catarrhal epidemics would be materially reduced.

Influenza should be regarded as a member of a group of catarrhal infectious diseases which in the aggregate are perhaps the chief enemies of human health.

The only safe rule is to regard all catarrhal attacks and every illness associated with rise of temperature during the prevalence of influenza as infectious and to adopt appropriate precautionary measures.

OTHER WAR EPISODES

As one writes, many War incidents come to mind. I recall one remarkable series of coincidences which enabled me to give timely advice to a naval officer coming home on leave. I had been visiting hospitals in France and about 9 p.m. went on board ship which was crossing that night from Havre to Southampton. Being tired I went at once to my cabin, where I found that the second berth was engaged for Sir St. Clair

Thomson, a distinguished throat surgeon, who has had remarkable success in operations for cancer of the larynx. I rose at daybreak and went on deck and talked with a naval officer who had been without leave for a prolonged period. He was extremely hoarse, and in answer to questions said he had been hoarse for many months, but "had had no time to see to that sort of thing." In view of the chronicity of the condition and the officer's age, the likelihood of possible cancer forced itself upon me and I urged him as soon as he had reported at the Admiralty to see the best throat specialist surgeon in London. Then I recalled that this surgeon was on board, and later in the morning brought doctor and patient into touch. A few days later I heard from Sir St. Clair that the patient had at once been admitted to a nursing home for operation; and not many weeks later I had a grateful letter from the naval officer and his wife. It may interest the reader to add up the number of "coincidences" involved in this intervention on my part. I may add that whenever I have met Sir St. Clair in recent years, I still learn that "our patient" keeps well.

It would unduly lengthen this chapter were I to recall Sir Robert Jones's important orthopedic work (on this see p. 364 of my earlier volume), or my contacts with Dr. W. H. Rivers, who did much to throw light on the real nature of "Shell Shock" in soldiers. The valuable work of Dr. (Sir Frederick) Mott in this connection is well known. I do not attempt to describe the changes in the treatment of wounds during the War. The conquest of wound infections was one of the great achievements of the War. Anti-tetanic inoculation saved many lives, and so also did the prevention of gas gangrene caused by invasion by the bacillus Welchii. I merely allude to the use of Wright's hypertonic solution, then of the Carrel Dakin physico-chemical irrigation and finally the method of excision of devitalised tissues from the wound followed by primary suture. The use of Roentgen rays on a grand scale was another great diagnostic life-saving agent.

To sum up, the War, notwithstanding the notable advances in medicine and surgery incited by it, was the greatest calamity in the history of civilised life. Although I do not discuss the "changed morality" in sex matters which was so pronounced

H*

in the War, it had and must still have grave effect on family life. Whether or not the too prevalent result that "sinners (were) purged of conscience and made happy in their sinning" (Mencken) will gradually diminish or not, all who regard monogamous family life as the highest ideal for the community must mourn over even temporary lapse in regard to it.

I have indicated that in my view the intensification and hastening of scientific investigation and its application was one of the most hopeful sides of war experience. I will mention two other beneficial bye-products of the War.

An immense impetus was given to direct work on behalf of mothers and their infants (on this see p. 192); and, as I have indicated on page 159, it may be doubted whether the Local Government Board would have succeeded in carrying its scheme for the universal gratuitous offer of treatment for venereal diseases, had it not been for the special stress of war. It is seldom appreciated that this is the one extreme instance of complete treatment provided by the State, without any expenditure on the part of the recipient, whoever he may be, except what he has in the past paid in the shape of rates and taxes.

PART II

RECOLLECTIONS OF AMERICAN PUBLIC HEALTH AND SOCIAL WORK

CHAPTER XXV

THE RED CROSS IN PEACE TIME

I DO not pretend to have more than outside knowledge of the extremely valuable work done by National Red Cross organisations, both before and since the Great War, but I saw something of their work during that War.

The value of that work is universally recognised and especially so in America; and it is not surprising that on the initiative of Mr. Henry Davison, who had led the great work of the American Red Cross, an effort was made to retain and maintain for the years of peace the immense army of nurses and other social and public health workers who had been mobilised under the impetus of war.

With this end in view an international Conference was called in 1919 at Cannes by the Americans, to discuss how best the beneficent health activities created or phenomenally developed during the War could be utilised in post-bellum circumstances. In this I had the good fortune to participate. My own recollection of that Conference is re-enforced by the fact that it was at Cannes that I received from Dr. W. H. Welch the invitation to the School of Hygiene at Johns Hopkins University which determined my course for the next two years.

Mr. Davison, a greatly respected American banker, member of the firm of J. P. Morgan & Co., arranged the Cannes meeting; and prior to this meeting American experts had prepared preliminary plans for continued international co-operation of Red Cross Societies. These were submitted to the Conference. Dr. Emile Roux was elected President of the Conference and Dr. W. H. Welch, the doyen of the American medical profession, led the American section of the Conference, which comprised distinguished men and women from all the allied countries.

At its opening meeting Dr. Welch stated that Mr. Davison had conceived the idea that the resources and energies brought into action by the Red Cross during the War should continue for the benefit of mankind, and he forecasted that the League of Health, which it was proposed to found, would signify as much to mankind as the Peace League of Nations, then under consideration in Paris.

The main conception for the proposed organisation was that in the maintenance of health on a national scale there was scope in each country for devoted Red Cross work and support, which would be not less valuable than work to reduce physical suffering during war.

This general outlook evidently embodied the value attached, in America even more than elsewhere, to voluntary organisations, in helping forward the work of the official agencies in public health administration. With this central idea there could be no quarrel. As will be seen in subsequent chapters, a very important—often a preponderant—share of the burden of promoting the public health in America has been borne by unofficial organisations; and if in some other countries, including Great Britain, "voluntary" efforts in public health have been partially displaced by "official" work, the difference is not so great as is usually supposed; for in a democratic country in which popularly elected representatives have the final word in both local and central governmental work, voluntary workers "in a municipal setting" still maintain their power, to the extent to which they choose to use it.

To me a chief interest of the Conference was meeting, with time for friendly talks, many American and foreign epidemiologists and hygienists. I particularly recall talks with Dr. Emile Roux, the head of the Pasteur Institute, with Sir Ronald Ross, with nearly all the American delegates (including Dr. Welch, Hermann Biggs, E. R. Baldwin, Livingston Farrand, S. McC. Hamill, Emmett Holt, W. F. Snow, and others) and with Dr. (later Sir) Truby King of New Zealand.

The main proposal of the Conference was the establishment of an International Health Bureau, which would focus information and give guidance respecting various branches of public health administration in each country. The organisation was to be supported by subscriptions from national societies; but in the issue the needed support languished and the Bureau was kept alive for a few years chiefly by American funds. It did useful work in the interchange of information, and prepared the way for the Health Section of the League of Nations as now organised. This, so far, has been more efficient in promoting international hygiene than the parent body in ensuring international peace. But it is premature to judge. The Rockefeller Foundation has supported handsomely the yearly expenses incurred by the Health Section of the League of Nations in collecting and circulating epidemiological and other information.

I have already indicated that the chief personal episode of the Conference was the invitation to lecture (on public health administration) at the new School of Hygiene, Baltimore.

This I discussed with Dr. Livingston Farrand, then the Director of the American Red Cross, and now President of Cornell University, and with other American delegates, and accepted before the Conference closed.

It was at this Conference that I heard Dr. Farrand enunciate what I have always regarded as the fundamentally sound view of social work by voluntary workers: "The final object of every voluntary public health agency is to render itself superfluous." This is profoundly true: and yet it is also true that voluntary work, both within and without the official fold, will persist and even increase, for new avenues are always opening out, and voluntary workers have greater freedom in experimental social efforts than can often be accorded to officials. But in public health administration the greatest experiments have been official, as witness the earlier efforts of Chadwick and Simon and of their successors and of many medical officers of health both in America and in Britain.

As illustrating the extensive work in Europe undertaken by the American Red Cross during and in the earlier post-bellum years, I add a note here on a subsequent Conference of American Red Cross workers in many European countries which I was asked to attend in Paris in February 1922. It was proposed that I should review this work, now about to be brought to an end.

Dr. J. H. Mason Knox, Jr., of Baltimore, was the medical director of this European work, and to him I owed the invitation. There were present medical directors, nearly all American doctors, of Field Operations representing work in the following countries: Baltic States, Czechoslovakia, Austria, Poland, Hungary, Montenegro, and in Serbia, Albania, and Greece. Associated with Dr. Knox in this admirable work was Dr. A. C. Burnham, an indefatigable co-worker, whose death in middle life a little later is deplored. My task, after hearing the national reports, was to attempt an "evaluation of the work."

The work had begun during the War. It was directed chiefly towards help for mothers and their young children; and in the acute distress of war conditions in the countries enumerated above it is not surprising that at first the relief of suffering preponderated, though throughout an attempt was made to organise health centres in congested areas and to conduct these on the lines of such centres in America and England. Social work and nursing were organised, stress being laid on the public health aspect of nursing.

American dollars—several millions—were spent on relief through these countries; and, although these millions could not compass the entire work of relief which was needed, the American organisation was so conducted that the generous but still limited funds available would go far in helping the children. Most valuable work was achieved by these American workers, as may be seen by reference to the report of this Conference printed in 1922, by the Medical Department of the American Red Cross. Permanent maternity and child welfare work was begun in backward countries, and has since made great advances.

In Vol. II of my *International Studies*, etc., I have particularised the important work done by the American organisation known as the Serbian Child Welfare Association of America. Many health zadrugas have been opened in what is now Yugoslavia. The work done by Mr. Kingsbury and Mr. Homer Folks in this part of Europe cannot be described here, but a fascinating account is given in Folks' *The Human Costs of the War* (Harper Brothers, 1920).

It should be added that the efforts in America to incorporate direct health work under the ægis of the American Red Cross were gradually dropped, and a few years later their direct health programme almost entirely ceased (see also p. 292).

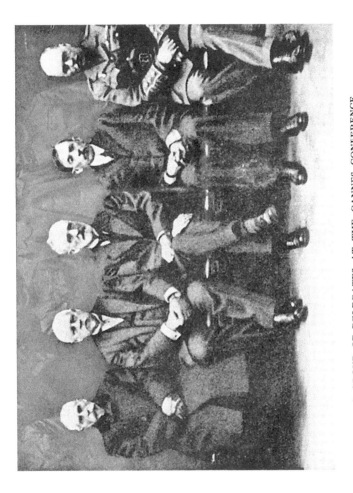

A GROUP OF DELEGATES AT THE CANNES CONFERENCE

Left to Right.—DR. EMILE ROUX (President of the Conference), DR. WILLIAM H. WELCH, SIR A. NEWSHOLME, DR. HERMANN H. BRIGGS, SIR RONALD ROSS

CHAPTER XXVI

ITINERARIES

THIS chapter is devoted mainly to personal items, which, although they are unimportant and sometimes may appear frivolous, throw some light on other chapters in this volume.

1919

At the end of the International Red Cross Conference in Cannes, my wife and I sailed for America, to fulfil the engagement already made with the Children's Bureau of Washington, and after that to undertake the new work at Johns Hopkins University to which I had committed myself while in Cannes.

We left Cannes on April 11, 1919, and on the 16th took the official berths reserved for us on the *Leviathan*, the ex-German *Vaterland*. This was at Brest, and on the 18th we sailed with about a dozen passengers, several of whom, including Dr, René Sand, were engaged on the same mission as ourselves. The crew, we were told, numbered some 2,000, and there were on board some 14,000 American soldiers on the way home, including many who were mentally or physically sick or disabled. It was a wonderful trip. The American doctors and soldiers were most friendly. We were entertained nightly with a cinema or a variety show. There was a daily newspaper, and one morning we learnt that on the previous day nine tons of turkey had been consumed for dinner! For us two, accustomed to war-time margarine, the greatest treat was the unlimited supply of good butter.

On April 25th we arrived in New York harbour, and although snow was falling, the soldiers had a wonderful reception. At Washington our quarters had been taken at the Wardman Park Hotel, and we met for the first time Miss Julia Lathrop, head of the Government's Children's Bureau, and Dr. Anna Rude its medical adviser. The latter travelled with us to California and back, and ensured our comfort and happiness. Miss Lathrop was a great social worker, a friend of Jane Addams, in whose settlement she had worked. Both have now "passed on"; both of them have been responsible for invaluable social work, and their influence lives on. Julia Lathrop and Grace Abbott, her successor at Washington, have done marvellously good work in promoting child health, especially on its industrial side. Miss Lathrop succeeded in obtaining Federal legislation, under which grants could be given to each of the forty-eight States of the Union for specific child welfare work. A few, including Massachusetts, declined this Federal Aid, as seeming to detract from their status as Sovereign States.

We stayed in Washington until May 9th. I attended and took part in meetings, and came into fruitful contact with many social workers.

The Washington Conference did much to inform the foreign delegates of American activities and American workers of what had been done in Europe during the Great War to safeguard the children; and the interchange of experience and aspirations in each successive city and State visited by us must have helped to promote further advance.

During my stay in Washington I gave an address at the central offices of the American Red Cross on "Red Cross Organisation in relation to the Preventive Medicine of the Future." Its chief object was to emphasise the great opening in work as public health visitors for those women who had been doing Red Cross work.

On May 9th I addressed a child welfare Conference in New York; and on the 15th, after an intermediate visit to Knoxville on a like errand, was in Boston where I met President Lowell, and among public health workers, Dr. Kelly, Commissioner of Health for Massachusetts, and Professors Rosenau and Edsall. On Sunday, May 18th at 8 a.m., we had reached Chicago, a city of profound interest, in which the worst and some of the best features of American life can be studied; for it has a great University, and a variety of social agencies doing admirable work. There followed two of the most strenuous days of my life. I was drawn into giving four addresses in one day, including an after-lunch address. My wife was similarly engaged at Ladies' Clubs. We visited Hull House, and the meetings at the Congress, including my lantern-illustrated lecture, were attended by over a thousand people.

On the 21st we had reached Minneapolis, and between public meetings had time to see and appreciate the work at the University of Minnesota for insuring the health and care in sickness of its students. Later, I saw an even better example of similar work under Dr. Sundwall, at Ann Arbor University. I was impressed in most of the cities visited by the fact that advanced social and hygienic work was much more manifest outside than in the official work of the municipality.

On the 24th of May we reached San Francisco. We had crossed the Salt Lake on a railway embankment thirty miles long. It was very hot; we passed over vast patches of dried salt. The desert of Sierra Nevada was also distressingly hot, but as we began to wind up the mountains of Sierra Nevada —reaching eventually 8,000 feet high, and passing through great banks of snow—we realised what a country of contrasts America is.

I addressed meetings at San Francisco and a large group of men and women students at the University of California at Berkeley, and made interesting contacts with Californian doctors. I cannot define in what respects the western differs from the eastern American mentality; but climate, social conditions, and perhaps greater remoteness from Europe have produced a distinctive type.

The fascinating journey north to Seattle confirmed this impression. Tropical rice fields of vast extent were succeeded in Oregon by upland country of apple and peach orchards. It is not surprising that some Western people appear more interested in Japanese and Mexican workmen than in European problems. Seattle had a bustling active life, not limited to its great port which is rivalling San Francisco. The workers in Seattle live in wooden houses widely scattered in its woodlands, which in England would rank as "middle-class villas." I was impressed by a Seattle school clinic visited by me. Every scholar is overhauled three times annually by a "graduated nurse," who has had "special training in diagnosis." Dental hygienists, in addition to qualified dentists, are employed, and women nurses are specially trained—as also in eastern America—in the administration of anaesthetics.

From Seattle we returned to Chicago, thence to Atlantic

City, which was reached on June 6th. Here I became engaged in what may almost be described as an orgy of public conferences more or less bearing on my subjects.

From Atlantic City I visited Baltimore to meet the staff of the new School of Hygiene and to discuss my proposed curriculum. The meeting was presided over by Dr. Goodnow, then the very wise legal President of the Johns Hopkins University.

From Atlantic City, to which I returned, I travelled to Toronto. My engagements with the Federal Children's Bureau were now ended; but I had been invited to address the Academy of Medicine at Toronto, and did so on June 20th on "Some Problems of Preventive Medicine of the Immediate Future."[1]

This with two exceptions was my last public engagement until I began my work at Baltimore in the following October. In Toronto I met most interesting public health and University men, and was guest at a public dinner, where I was impressed by the evidence of loyalty to the British Crown, surpassing in fervour what would have been shown in a corresponding function in England.

We now had two to three months to spare, and began with a memorable trip down the St. Lawrence, changing boats at Prescott for the exciting passage of the rapids. After a stay in Quebec we went down stream to Murray Bay and settled at Chamard's Hotel. I must not linger to tell of the scenery, or of the interesting people in the province of Quebec, mixed French, British, Highlanders and others. Nor of my visit to Mr. Taft, formerly President of the United States, who had a summer villa at Murray Bay, and discussed with me at length the health problems of the Philippine Islands, where he had been Governor. I must mention the hotel library, partly because it was the best I have seen, partly because the volunteer librarians were three Misses Fenimore Cooper, granddaughters of the author of *The Last of the Mohicans*, *The Spy*, and other novels, my favourite books as a boy. Year by year they were guests at the hotel, and added to the pleasure of all other guests by this labour of love.

While at Cannes I had promised Dr. Baldwin, Trudeau's

[1] Published in *Public Health and Insurance: American Addresses* (Johns Hopkins Press, 1920).

successor at the famous Saranac Sanatorium, to give two addresses to the summer school of tuberculosis which annually assembled at Saranac. To meet this engagement we travelled on July 21st to Montreal, to visit child welfare institutions as guests of a lady who had been with us at Chamard's Hotel. From Montreal the same lady drove us in her car to Lake Placid, some 150 miles distant. Here, at a bungalow in the grounds of a large country club, we stayed until September 5th, and enjoyed the varied life of the Club, and the forest and lake scenery of the Adirondacks. Saranac was only twelve miles distant from Lake Placid, and there we met many tuberculosis doctors, and saw the valuable work initiated by Trudeau in Saranac, and now greatly extended under Dr. Baldwin's leadership. Trudeau began the Sanatorium movement in the States, and some of the best tuberculosis work is still being done at Saranac, which has become a great colony for consumptives and their families.

I must mention though I cannot enlarge on two fascinating visits to American summer camps, one to the summer home of the late Dr. Emmett Holt, at Panther Point Camp, Upper Saranac Lake, and the other to Keen Valley to the summer home of Dr. Hatfield of Philadelphia, who for years has been a mainstay of anti-tuberculosis work in the States.

A bye-product of my medical contacts at Saranac was that I was persuaded to learn to drive an automobile, and travel in it by easy stages over 800 miles to Baltimore. For this purpose a two-seater Ford coupé was obtained, and after what I confess was inadequately assimilated instruction, we started on this adventurous journey. Looking back I do not know which was more remarkable—my wife's courage in entrusting herself to my driving, or my unlearned audacity in undertaking it.

Our first destination was Boston. We took a course due east, crossing Lake Champlain by ferry, then through the White Mountains to Portland, Maine; then by the coast road to Lawrence and Methuen, where a niece of mine lived; and thence on to Boston.

Were I to attempt to describe our adventures in this journey and in the further journey to New York and Baltimore, the reader's appreciation of my wife's courage would be enhanced.

But although I knew next to nothing of the working of "Henrietta," the name we gave the car, every American we encountered knew, or thought he knew, everything about it, and help was always forthcoming. Henrietta had no self-starting gear, and "cranking" was a horror. I only failed once to obtain help, and then only partially. It was in New Hampshire, and Henrietta stalled in going up-hill. The village blacksmith also failed to start the engine, but he suggested a method which proved successful. We pushed the car to the brow of the hill. It started down hill under the influence of gravity, and movement soon roused the engine into activity!

OTHER ADVENTURES OF HENRIETTA

I am tempted to expand the story of this motoring trip. Remember it was undertaken in 1919, when self-starters had not been perfected, and when, furthermore, only a few main roads were as good as most roads now are.

While these main roads were under repair, we were repeatedly invited to undertake a détour, and often it was many miles before we reached the smooth main road again. The side roads were "dirt roads," and often the car wheels were partially buried in thick dust. This was not all, for these side roads were also very bumpy. We were amused on one occasion by a notice some wag had posted up at the junction with the mainroad: "Now you can talk again." At one danger point we were informed, "Our cemetery is not yet full," and we heard of this in the expanded form: "Put your foot on the gas! Our cemetery is only half full." Among the interesting notices to motorists, perhaps the best we saw was "Say it with brakes and save flowers," which I have at various times utilised as an illustration of preventive medicine; but I have added that the wise chauffeur is not easily taken by surprise, and preventive medicine goes further back than the use of brakes.

When, after leaving Boston, we came to the northern outskirts of New York, I confess I was nervous. I inquired the route of a man who stood on the side-walk. Our destination was the Ferry some twelve miles distant, near the Pennsylvania railway station. The man—he appeared to be a Pole—was going there and he would drive us through New York City.

What a relief! Although somewhat cramped for space, we drove the length of New York in comfortable irresponsibility. I managed to drive the car on to the enormous ferry-boat, and ere long we were on the New Jersey side. I refrain from narrating our many other difficulties. They did not prevent the drive from being on the whole most enjoyable; and on September 20th we arrived in Baltimore.

But I have omitted the most exciting incident of this trip. I had promised to give an address in Boston on the occasion of the Fiftieth Anniversary of the Massachusetts State Board of Health. We arrived on the day in September preceding my address, the subject of which was "Public Health Progress in England during the last Fifty Years."[1]

I had noticed an absence of traffic control in the streets, and on arrival at our hotel, near the State House, the hotel manager informed me that owing to the police strike he could not undertake charge of Henrietta, now left unprotected in the street. I telephoned to Dr. Kelly, the Commissioner of Health.

In a few minutes he arrived and informed me that for several days he had been trying to communicate with me, that Governor Coolidge had instructed that the celebrations must be abandoned, and Dr. Kelly advised us to leave the city immediately; so we hastily repacked our baggage and Dr. Kelly guided us to the outskirts of the city, heading towards New York. *En route* we examined our accumulated correspondence, and found it included an invitation from Dr. and Mrs. Lyman, asking us to spend a few days with them at Gayford Farm Sanatorium, near Wallingford in Connecticut, and this was at once arranged by telegram. It was a delightful and instructive break in our travelling. Dr. Lyman is a leader in tuberculosis work in the States; and the friendly relationship has since then been renewed in Newhaven, Conn., and in an English motoring tour.

I may add here one more to the stories of my mismanagement of Henrietta. On our way to Wallingford we found ourselves in a cemetery into which I had inadvertently turned. The road

---

[1] This address was subsequently published by the State Board of Health, and it is printed as Chapter I of my *American Addresses on Public Health and Insurance*, 1920.

narrowed as we went forward, and it became impossible to turn. Were I to give an estimate of the distance travelled before an exit was discovered, I should be suspected of exaggeration.

My recollection of these travellings has been aided by my wife's diaries. I wish I could give more of her "human" descriptions. But I will quote one sentence, which was written before we reached Baltimore, and would have been even more deeply appreciative had it been written later:

We have found the American people idealists at heart, with a reverence for the old country and for old-fashioned virtues, and an admiration for those who make good. They are a people of good common sense, most hospitable and full of loving kindness.

It is convenient to give in this chapter a summary of our itineraries in subsequent years, as I can thus allude to various points of medical interest not mentioned in other chapters.

OCTOBER 1919

On October 24th, soon after the beginning of my work at the School of Hygiene, I was under an engagement to address the American Public Health Association, of which that year Dr. Frankel of New York was the president. The visit meant travel by train for two whole days, and we had a panorama of the harvesting of cotton, sugar beet, and tobacco leaves for drying, and of maple-trees being tapped for sugar. At New Orleans I met many public health friends. We visited parts of the city showing evidence of the former French and Spanish ownership. I had already read Cable's novels, dealing with life in New Orleans (see also p. 329). On our return journey we had Dr. and Mrs. Charles Chapin as our travelling companions.

DECEMBER 1919

We spent Christmas in New York, and through the kindness of Miss Ellen Babbitt, shown in this and in many other ways, stayed as guests at the National Arts Club, Gramercy Park. The club has an atmosphere not unlike that of an old London square. This was our New York home in many subsequent visits.

On the 29th I attended a Conference in Boston, which is

further described on p. 274. During the same visit we supped with Miss Lilian Wald at the Henry Street settlement, and were able to visualise her valuable work in combined district nursing and health visiting.

1920.—January 21st. Lecture to the students of Professor E. A. Winslow at Yale University, Newhaven, Conn.

February 9th. Packard Lecture in Philadelphia on Maternal Mortality.

1920

My first year's work at the School of Hygiene was completed in April 1920, and we came to England for the summer, returning to America in September, with an English maid. We had taken a flat or "apartment" in Baltimore, and now had some months of interesting American housekeeping. We had a negress as daily cook. She arrived in her own Ford car, wore silk stockings, and was most efficient as well as expensive. The negro lift-man was much better dressed than I was. Those were the days of very high wages. Our American housekeeping enabled us to have weekly groups of students to dinner, and I hope they enjoyed these evenings as much as we did.

One instance of American kindness I give here. Commemoration day, November 1920, was a general holiday. It is a day kept almost as religiously as Christmas Day. A friend, who is a well known pediatrician, arrived at our flat: were we engaged anywhere? Then we must come and spend the day with his family. I could mention many like instances. No wonder my wife wrote in her diary at the end of this winter:

To me the American people have a peculiar charm. They are outspoken and enthusiastic, many-sided, and wishful to give their views and to hear yours, and always ready to help you.

During this second winter, we made two interesting visits.

I was asked by Dr. E. Williams, the Health Commissioner of Virginia, to address a Health Conference in Kingston, Virginia, and thus had the opportunity to learn something of Southern people and their work. Here for the first time we saw a lady wearing a live chameleon attached to her brooch. The colour changes were startling.

We were also guests at Hampton on Chesapeake Bay, where is the famous residential school for coloured boys and girls aged 16 to 20 years. It is a fine example of co-education, and the training given is such as to fit these young people to be leaders among their own people. We arrived on the Anniversary of Emancipation Day, when Lincoln made his famous announcement, and it was celebrated by a great assembly of old and present pupils. Over a thousand were present in the Great Hall, where we were introduced from the platform; and one can never forget the wonderful singing of old plantation songs and hymns which followed.

We had several opportunities of hearing the Jubilee Singers and their successors, and of admiring the wonderful gift of vocal music which is the possession of the negro.

I do not propose to detail our subsequent experiences in the United States during several revisits.

In 1926 I visited a number of Universities, and gave addresses on public health and social subjects. My visits in connection with the Demonstrations for the Milbank Fund are mentioned in Chapter XXXIII. One of these "Milbank" visits was made on our return from California, where, for health reasons, we spent the winter of 1927–28.

VISIT TO CALIFORNIA

We sailed from England in October 1927, and crossed the Continent by the Santa Fé Railway to Los Angeles. This route was chosen to enable us to visit the Grand Canyon, but we found it completely enveloped in fog. Determined to see it, we took the same route back eastward, and were well rewarded by the views then obtained.

We spent six months at an hotel in Montecito, a few miles from Santa Barbara. The hotel consisted of a number of bungalows grouped round a central dining-room, each bungalow having its separate porch and living-rooms. The climate and surroundings were perfect, and were it not for the distance from intimate friends, the temptation to remain there might have been irresistible. Two kind friends in the same hotel took us for daily drives in their car. Sometimes, however, one had recourse to the district omnibus, and I recall while waiting for it being invited to drive into Santa Barbara by the owner-driver of a passing automobile. I gladly assented, and he amused me by this story.

"It is not very safe now-a-days to give people a lift. A friend of mine did so, and soon after they had started he noticed his watch was missing. Skilfully extracting his revolver from his hip pocket, he pushed it into the passenger's ribs, with the demand 'Give me that watch.' The watch was handed over. Then the passenger was told to 'git.' He 'got,' and eventually the owner-driver reached home. There he was accosted by his wife: 'Do you know that you left your watch on the dressing-table this morning?' "

Motor buses go everywhere in California; and more than once we travelled thus to Los Angeles, that wonderful collection of widely spread millions in a vast city area. Here I gave a public health address, renewed my friendship with Dr. Anna Rude, and formed one with Dr. Pomeroy, who was doing fine public health work in the county of Los Angeles. From Los Angeles, on April 17th, we drove inland across the desert, which was just beginning to blossom, and we caught the wonderful colour patches of desert flowers characteristic of the desert at this season. We saw much of the life of the retired wealthy Americans while at Santa Barbara, and received delightful hospitality. I also saw something of medical practice in this paradise for doctors. There was, I thought, too much concentration on "keeping down one's blood-pressure." It was but natural that in a district devoted to fruit growing, cure by large quantities of orange-juice should be rampant. One of the most brilliant doctors of St. Barbara was a namesake; but in America the spelling had become phonetic (Nuzum).

On the whole, I think it is a mistake for retired people to collect almost exclusively in one area. They are more likely to do good and remain in good health when they live in a natural environment where many social strata are found in normal proportions.

1924.—Our West Indian itinerary is given in Chapter xxxvii.

1928.—During this year I made my second survey of the Demonstration Work of the Milbank Fund.

In July I attended the International Congress on Social

Work in Paris, of which Dr. René Sand was the able secretary. In August I read a paper at an International Anti-Alcohol Congress at Antwerp on the present position of the temperance problem.

1929.—I began my international survey for the Milbank Fund of medical practice as related to preventive medicine. Particulars are given in Chapters XXXVIII and XXXIX.

1929–32 was occupied with the above indicated special work. This work was summarised in *Medicine and the State*, published in April 1932.

1932.—Visit to Soviet Russia (U.S.S.R.), followed by the joint publication by Dr. J. A. Kingsbury and myself of *Red Medicine*.

CHAPTER XXVII

WILLIAM HENRY WELCH

BEFORE outlining my two years' life in Baltimore, I wish, following the same course as in my account of my English official life, to make appreciative and grateful reference to American hygienists with whom I came into fairly intimate contact. With few exceptions I propose to mention only those who have died. Two living colleagues at Baltimore I must specially mention with admiration and respect. With Professor W. H. Howell, the great American physiologist, and Professor Wade Hampton Frost, its leading epidemiologist, I had the happiness to work during my two years' connection with the new School of Hygiene of the Johns Hopkins University.

But so much of my experience of American life is closely related to Dr. Welch, then Director of the School of Hygiene, as to render it convenient to cluster some of my recollections at Baltimore around an outline of my acquaintance with him. This is the more fitting in that of all the Americans I have known, none, I think, has had so great an influence as he in enlarging the scope of pathology in its application to medicine, and in extending the teaching of the science of medicine, especially of preventive medicine.

Stout in figure, of a build under middle height, Welch's large head and good-humoured countenance correctly interpreted his mental power and equable character.

I first met him at Budapest, in 1894, when he described to the International Congress of Hygiene and Demography the early application of bacteriology in America to the diagnosis of diphtheria. Welch always regarded the use of the laboratory, in which Hermann Biggs led the way, as America's most outstanding contribution to advance in public health administration. Our next meeting was in Washington, in 1908, at the International Congress on Tuberculosis; and later during the War at my own table in Ashley Gardens, Westminster, when I had arranged for him to meet, among others, some London public health teachers, and we discussed his plans for the new school of hygiene at Baltimore, under the endowment from the Rockefeller Foundation for that purpose.

On this occasion we discussed *inter alia* the name of the proposed school, the name eventually chosen by Welch being that of "School of Hygiene and Public Health."

My next meeting with him was at Cannes, as stated in Chapter xxv, and it was then that I was invited to undertake a course of lectures on Public Health Administration at the new school. There followed a year and then a second year, which I regard as among the most interesting and useful in my life. My experience among University professors and teachers and other men and women of culture in diverse walks of life forms still a happy memory.

Welch was a universal favourite, a great smoother-out of the difficulties of human contacts. As I remarked at a dinner at which my wife and I were entertained at the end of our sojourn at Baltimore, had Welch not been the most beloved physician in America, he might easily have been among the foremost of the world's diplomatists.

Welch belonged to a family of doctors. Born in 1850 he lived to be 84 years old. He graduated early from Yale, and after being a teacher for about a year, trained for the medical profession. Microscopic work and pathology early attracted him and he spent a couple of years in Germany. In 1877 he was working with Cohnheim at Breslau; and he has told me how one day a young provincial practitioner, Robert Koch, came to the laboratory and demonstrated to Cohnheim the exact steps by which he had discovered the life history of the bacillus of anthrax. It was Cohnheim who in 1877 recommended Welch for the new chair of Pathology at the Johns Hopkins University and thus started the work which has had profound influence on the history of medicine in America. The University at Baltimore, on its medical side, was then in its earliest stage and Welch at once became its leader. Ere long he was joined by Osler, Kelly, and Halstead, and this "great four" raised the teaching of medicine to a high level. Their close companionship had its lighter side, and sometimes their fun was Puck-like. Let me give one instance. For many years Welch, always a bachelor, lived at No. 807 St. Paul's Street, though he was to be found chiefly at the Maryland Club, where he was a princely host. One morning, when Osler knew that Welch was out, he called and inquired if Welch was at home. The faithful housekeeper's answer was negative. *Osler:* Is Mrs. Welch at home? *Housekeeper:* But you know there is no Mrs Welch. *Osler:* Oh. Haven't you heard? And he retreated before further questioning was possible.

Probably this was a counter-stroke to some previous joke by Welch at Osler's expense.

Welch moulded medical teaching in his adopted University and indirectly throughout America; he was Chairman of the Maryland State Board of Health for many years, and he was a trusted adviser when, anywhere in the States, University or similar appointments were about to be made. His advice was in frequent demand on the epidemiological and sanitary work of the Rockefeller and Milbank Foundations.

His seventieth birthday was celebrated by the publication of three large volumes of his various contributions.

In later years he devoted much attention to the social and administrative side of medical practice, and I recall with pleasure his interest in the Wesley M. Carpenter lecture given by me on October 2, 1919, before the New York Academy of Medicine on "The Increasing Socialisation of Medicine." As a result of this and subsequent events, Welch had a share in recommending the Milbank Memorial Fund to arrange for me to undertake the *International Studies on the relation between the private and official practice of Medicine with special reference to Public Health,* which were embodied in three volumes, and in a final volume on *Medicine and the State* (see p. 348), to which Dr. Welch wrote a long foreword.

This interest in Social Medicine was shown even more decisively in letters written to Mr. Kingsbury and myself when we gave a joint supplementary account in *Red Medicine,* published in 1933, of Soviet Russia's system of complete State Medicine. The dedication of that volume as given on page 24 is further indication of Welch's interest in the subject.

In 1916 Welch resigned his University chair of Bacteriology and Pathology at the age of sixty-six, and devoted himself to the great work of organising the new School of Hygiene of the University. In doing so he said:

I am trying to stress the humanistic aspect of Medicine because in the past the whole emphasis was, in my case, and I think the times demanded that emphasis, upon the purely scientific side.

Alongside this statement, which might suggest that Welch had not long been interested in the human and social side of Medicine, should be placed the following testimony to Welch by Dr. Thayer, who succeeded Osler in the chair of Medicine at Johns Hopkins University:

Your greatest work lies in the personal example which you have set your students. . . . You have taught us a religion of earnestness and simplicity and directness—a religion of character and self-restraint, a religion of work, not of words.

Welch was gifted with a marvellous memory, of which there are many stories. I remember his reciting one evening one of Robert Herrick's poems, which, he said, had come back to him after sixty years that morning while he was shaving.

In 1920 I had received from him the mission, while in England after a first year's work at the School of Hygiene, to collect books for the school dealing with the history of all phases of public health work. It was a charming mission to wander through Britain collecting rarities, where possible, at every town I drove through; and later on it was a delight to go over my purchases with Welch. Among these I remember were books by John Howard and John Hunter, each with the author's inscription.

The most pleasing period in my professional life was that spent with Welch and his medical colleagues. He was America's greatest pioneer in modern pathology, and he, with Sedgwick and his co-workers and Hermann Biggs in Public Health Administration, gave America a foremost place in the world in the application of science, in the form of public health laboratories, to the prevention of disease.

Although Welch was indefatigable in encouraging and organising research in the medical sciences, he never missed an opportunity to emphasise the need for greater effort to

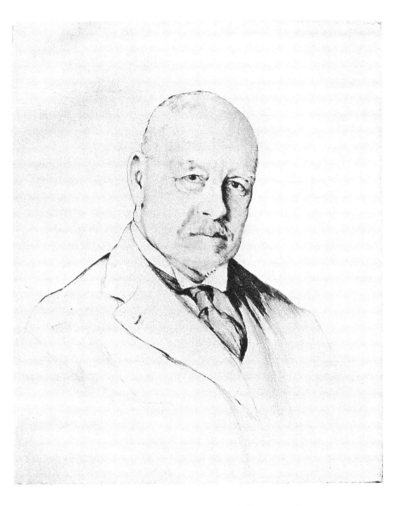

WILLIAM HENRY WELCH (1850–1934)
(*Etching on the occasion of his 80th Birthday*)

secure the application of science already available for preventive work. The lag between science and its application was a favourite subject with him. He made frequent use of the classical instance of scurvy in the British Navy, the controllability of which by the use of fresh vegetables had been known for two hundred years before a compulsory ration of lemon-juice was adopted in 1796.

Welch's help to workers in every branch of Medicine and Hygiene was given freely and to an extent which is almost unbelievable. He was always prepared to suggest investigations and methods of teaching for the guidance of those consulting him, while he remained in the background. Like Warwick he was satisfied with the role of king-maker, when often he was the king.

Welch's physical health was marvellously good until near the end. Of his physical competence when an octogenarian I had embarrassing evidence during a motoring trip we took together in the West of England.

About 1 p.m. we reached Old Sarum after a strenuous morning of sight-seeing in Wells, Glastonbury, and Stonehenge. At that time the only means of approaching the ruins of the old city was by many wooden steps into the fosse, and the ascent of an equal number of steps. I suggested we should not attempt it; but, of course, we had to do it and I admired but regretted the physical vigour of my older fellow-traveller.

At the age of eighty Welch was the recipient of most remarkable and unexampled testimony to his international distinction. The proceedings, organised by Mr. Kingsbury with exquisite skill, included a public meeting at Washington, over which President Hoover presided. The record has been published in a beautiful volume produced by the Milbank Foundation and the speeches at this meeting were broadcast to Europe and other parts of the world. Meetings were held in many cities to celebrate the occasion. The portrait shown here is a copy of an admirable engraving made at the time of the celebrations of his eightieth birthday.

I must content myself with citing the universally true statement made on that occasion by Dr. Livingston Farrand, the President of Cornell University, that Welch showed "constant solicitude for the inconspicuous man who has yet

I

rendered service." To my imperfect appreciation of one of the biggest men I have known should be added Welch's own words, when he responded on his eightieth birthday at the Washington meeting:

It is my inclination, even at fourscore years, to look forward rather than backward. . . . While nothing can be more hazardous than to predict the direction of future discovery and progress in the biological and medical sciences, it requires no prophetic gift to be confident that with the widening of the boundaries of knowledge will come increased power to relieve human suffering, to control disease, to improve health and thereby add to the sum of human happiness and well-being.

When Welch at the age of eighty had resigned his position as Director of the School of Hygiene, the General Education Board of the Rockefeller Foundation, knowing his devotion to the study of the history of Medicine, appropriated the sum of $200,000 to endow a professorship of the History of Medicine in Johns Hopkins University, Welch to be the first professor. The Rockefeller Foundation furthermore appropriated $1,000,000 towards the construction of a great medical library and an income to maintain it. This was opened two years later. It is known as the

William Henry Welch Medical Library,

and one of Welch's latest tasks in the two years prior to its opening was that of collecting in Europe all books that could worthily find a home in this great library. To this library my friend Colonel F. H. Garrison, the author of the standard *History of Medicine,* was worthily appointed librarian, but he too has passed on.

FIELDING H. GARRISON

At the time of his death, Colonel Garrison was Director of the Welch Medical Library and Lecturer at the Institute of the History of Medicine at Baltimore, and it is appropriate to add a note as to his great work as a medical historian. We met at not infrequent intervals when Garrison was Assistant Librarian at the Surgeon-General's Library in Washington. He worked with and succeeded Billings, and while holding his post, raised the library to an eminence which was almost unique. It was especially rich in rare pamphlets and in works bearing on the History of Medicine. Garrison's *Introduction to the History of Medicine* was first published in 1913 and its marvellous conciseness of statement and fulness of detail on every phase of medicine made it indispensable to all students. Three subsequent editions were published in recent years and these increased Garrison's great reputation. This was not his only claim to fame. He was co-editor of the *Index Medicus* 1903–12 and its editor 1912–22.

Such work was only possible to a prodigious worker with an amazing memory. These qualities were shown in many special brochures on the history of special departments of medicine.

He died at the age of sixty-four in April 1935, and many, like myself, will remember him with gratitude for the friendship and help he gave. An untiring worker, he found occasional relaxation in music, which he loved profoundly. A sensitive man, honest and outspoken, he sometimes gave offence in criticism, but to the real student he was always kind and helpful.

For some years, in accordance with military conditions, he was stationed in Manila and removed from his library work, and his stay in the Philippines left him in impaired health. But he returned to the library later, and although we seldom met he was a good correspondent. I have before me a letter from him, dated August 16, 1925, in which he unnecessarily defends himself for a somewhat long silence by saying "I have had so much work to do and so many worries to contend with that . . . I forget things as a kind of defensive reaction." In the same letter he told me of three books he had written since his return from Manila, a little history of artistic anatomy, a history of neurology, and a translation of a volume of essays from the German. His history of pediatrics is well known. To one of his books he prefixed a quotation of a Latin device formerly inscribed on the graduating dissertations of Russian Medical students:

FECI QUOD POTUI; FACIANT MELIORA POTENTES

which fits his entire life-work, though in accomplishment his work deserved a still higher eulogy than this.

CHAPTER XXVIII

OTHER AMERICAN PIONEERS IN PUBLIC HEALTH

CONFINING myself in the main to those whom I have met in the flesh, but who are no longer with us, I can only allude briefly to some of the great men of America who have influenced the course of public health history.

HERMANN M. BIGGS

First among these comes Dr. Hermann M. Biggs. In my *Fifty Years in Public Health* (pages 190, 244, and 259), and on page 288 of this volume, I have testified to his courage in administration, the swift vision with which he seized on possible openings for public health advance, and to the immense influence which his example exercised in expediting reform, and I do not therefore give further details in this chapter (but see p. 361). I recommend the reading of Professor Winslow's biography of Biggs, which does justice to its subject and forms also a history of Public Health during Biggs's lifetime.

WILLIAM T. SEDGWICK

I consider it one of the privileges of my life to have known William T. Sedgwick, PH.D. I travelled with him across the Atlantic and have been fortunate enough to see him on this side, as well as in his Boston home, where he and his wife were devoted comrades in all good enterprises and in the activation of good work in pupils, colleagues, and friends.

Sedgwick was born in 1855, and died soon after he had returned in 1920 from Leeds and Cambridge which he had visited as exchange professor. He began his scientific training at Harvard Medical School in 1877, but found that his chief interests lay in chemistry and biology, and after study at Johns Hopkins University in the latter subject, he was called in 1883 to the staff of the Massachusetts Institute of Technology, where his life-work as teacher and investigator was done. Although this was primarily an engineering school, he gradually established biology and bacteriology as an essential part of its

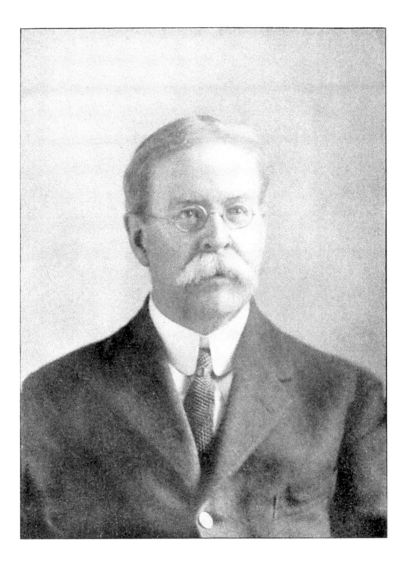

WILLIAM T. SEDGWICK (1855–1921)

training, and he was engaged by the Massachusetts Board of Health to undertake investigations on methods of filtration and sterilisation of water. This led to one of the chief interests of his life, the connection of water with disease, which he studied exhaustively in the field and historically. In the latter aspect he spent time in the Bodleian Library at Oxford, studying the original accounts of William Snow's investigation on Cholera and Water. I have often advised students to read Sedgwick's *Principles of Sanitary Science and Public Health* on its high general merits and because in it was the best account of Snow's early investigation.

At the Lawrence experimental station of the Massachusetts State Board of Health, Sedgwick and his colleagues, particularly Professor S. C. Prescott, did work of great national value. A roster of Sedgwick's pupils would include many of America's leaders in public health and sanitation.

Throughout Sedgwick's writings ran an ethical thread which helps to explain his great influence on the men trained by him. His quotation of R. L. Stevenson to the effect that "the world must return some day to the word Duty and be done with the word Reward" will be regarded by all who knew Sedgwick as exemplified in his own life. See also page 274.

CHARLES V. CHAPIN, M.D. (OF PROVIDENCE, R.I.)

Although Dr. Chapin is still with us, I cannot refrain from placing him in this chapter among the chief of American Public Health pioneers. As I write I have letters before me from him written in October 1935. One of them expresses the sentiment often felt by me that "one of the comforts of advancing years is to know that one is still remembered by old friends and fellow-workers." He goes on to remark that "We had both of us been very happy in our life-work, which was very fortunate for ourselves and for our work too." In the same letter he mentions the fact that, just as Dr. Charles Murchison had greatly influenced the course of my life, so Dr. Austin Flint had influenced Chapin when the latter was an intern at Bellevue Hospital, New York. Flint was scientifically minded and practical, and his influence was backed by that of Dr. Edward G. Janeway, "the most brilliant and accurate diagnostician in

New York," who was "completely permeated with the scientific spirit" and did more than all his other teachers "to infuse some of this spirit" into Chapin.

At his present advanced age, it is interesting to find Chapin singing a paean on behalf of field epidemiology, so much less easy than laboratory work. In his letter he congratulates me on having escaped laboratory work, which at one time seemed my possible fate.

I quote here a letter from Chapin to a mutual friend, after receipt of a copy of my *Medicine and the State*, 1932, in which he makes the following comment significant as to his view of the American outlook: "The axiom (laid down in this volume) is that no sick human being must be allowed to lack all that is practicable and really necessary for his skilful and humane treatment and for his expeditious return to health," and goes on to say that although I had assumed that this axiom was universally accepted, it might not be true among some important classes in the United States.

Chapin's book on the *Sources and Modes of Infection* (1910) brushed aside the current beliefs on aerial convection of infection and the exaggerated belief in the influence of intermediate *things* (not being *persons*) in spreading infection, and thus helped to make our efforts to control the spread of disease more exact and less wasteful. Providence in 1905 was the first city to give up terminal fumigation after infectious diseases. In one sentence in his *The Fetish of Disinfection* he inveighs against those who religiously practise official disinfection, as for instance "after a case of tuberculosis, when for years there may have been no attempt on the part of the patient to prevent the infection of others." Chapin's report on State Public Health work (*A Survey of State Boards of Health*, 1915) showed how a valuable step from the qualitative to the quantitative could be taken by a system of marking for different points in administration, which would assess the relative administrative merit of an area.

Chapin was emphatic in deprecating the survival of the crude generalisation that *Dirt makes Disease*. There was force in his objection to this undiscriminating statement, notwithstanding its having been the slogan crystallising in words the aim of earlier British sanitary improvements. Probably he was influ-

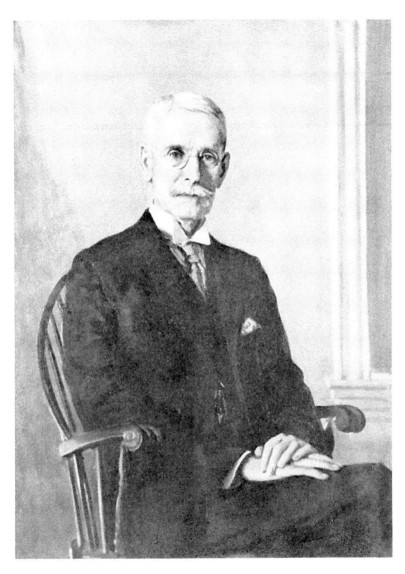

CHARLES V. CHAPIN, M.D., OF PROVIDENCE

enced by the fact that in modern sanitary administration he, like many other medical officers of health, had to concern himself with the removal of many nuisances which, however objectionable, had no direct effect on health. That has now nearly righted itself. His best illustration was the vast sums of money ineffectually spent in cleansing Havana, in order to destroy yellow fever, when specific action directed to prevent the bite of a particular mosquito was the one and only thing necessary. But the crude generalisation of the old sanitarians had led to the provision of clean water supplies; and it might be argued that cleansing operations in tropical cities, if intelligently directed, would interfere with the life-history of the stegomyia.

Into Chapin's important work in tracing the course of *variola minor* I need not enter. But his remarks on *Truth in Publicity* would justify much fuller quotations than I can give. Here are two:

When the publicity man hears something new, he tells it without waiting to learn whether it is true.

Better pay your publicity man for doing nothing than for writing something which is not so.

No history of public health effort, whether voluntary or official, will be complete which does not lay stress on Chapin's work.

CHAPTER XXIX

WORK AND LEISURE AT BALTIMORE

THE SCHOOL OF HYGIENE

I have told how in 1919 I was enlisted by Dr. Welch to give a course of lectures at the new School of Hygiene and Public Health, Johns Hopkins University. The arrangement was to give two lectures and one seminar weekly during the six winter months. There was in addition work with each student, and perhaps this and the seminars—less formal than lectures—were the most useful work I did.

I had a free hand as regards the scope of my lectures; but that Welch took much interest in them was shown by his rather embarrassingly frequent attendance. I was even more regular in attending his weekly lectures on general subjects bearing on pathology and hygiene, and only the other day I turned up some notes which I had taken of these addresses. Their comprehensive scope emphasised that the school was a centre of medical culture and not merely a workshop for training men in the technicalities of various branches of public health work; and this wider outlook was equally evident in the lectures of Dr. William H. Howell, the Professor of Physiology at the school.

The school as a whole was an embodiment of the wider conception of Preventive Medicine. In each department there was laboratory provision, and all training, as far as it could be, was undertaken in the laboratory for each section of work. The professor's time was divided between teaching and investigation, thus giving the student the impetus to regard every piece of public health work as also a problem for investigation. The school was in fact an Institute of Hygiene in the best sense of the word. With the work done in the laboratories of zoology, entomology, immunology, chemistry, and physiology I had frequent contacts, and realised (as can be seen in the annual reprints of investigation) how much was being done at the school to extend the borders of knowledge. I was especially interested in the laboratories dealing with nutrition, in which the highly important investigations of Dr. McCollum on vitamins were proceeding.

The "laboratory" or field work in my own department was difficult to obtain, although the Health Commissioners for Baltimore (Dr. Hampson Jones) and for the State (Dr. J. H. Fulton) were helpful to the extent that was then possible. It was also possible to arrange for demonstrations on midwifery work (Professor Whitridge Williams), on child hygiene (Professor Howland), and some others. Among workers not immediately associated with the school I was indebted to Dr. Mason Knox, a distinguished pediatrician who subsequently took charge of the child welfare work of the State, and to Dr. Dunham who demonstrated his work on defective children. His thoughtful book, *An Approach to Social Medicine* (Williams and Wilkins), is not so well known as it should be. Since my time more complete practical facilities have been arranged for training public health students, Dr. Huntington Williams, now Health Commissioner of Baltimore—at that time a student in my class—taking an important part in this. My students included those about to work in other countries under the International Health Board, several men already in public health work, and students from Canada, and from the Army and Navy Medical Department. Some of these are now outstanding and distinguished workers in the public health field in the States and in other countries.

Dr. Welch consulted frequently as to the subjects to be included in my course and was astonished when I claimed such subjects as tuberculosis, venereal disease, maternity, and child welfare work and school medicine as within my net. But this wider view pleased him, especially as I welcomed supplementary lectures by experts in each of the subjects. We agreed that no logical separation was possible between the study of administration and of causation, and that a statement of the nature of each problem was needed if rational preventive measures were to be described. Paraphrasing Wesley's description of his sphere of labour: the world of medicine was my parish.

Happily this was also the view taken by Dr. Wade Frost, my able colleague, the Professor of Epidemiology at the school.

I*

We had already agreed that epidemiology and administration must both present very similar problems and that any overlapping in teaching was to the student's advantage.

The interest Dr. Welch took in my course was indicated in a lecture on Puerperal Sepsis and Semmelweiss, in which inadvertently I had not adequately stated Oliver Wendell Holmes's contribution to this problem. With complete courtesy he supplemented my lecture by remarks in which his fellow-countryman was restored to his independent pinnacle.

My lectures and especially the weekly seminars were a great personal pleasure. The reviewing of old and new problems, the opportunities given for discussion and the unexpected outlooks of younger minds—more than twenty of them—were stimulating and valuable. I relearnt the lesson acquired when, as a young doctor, I taught physiology and hygiene to science teachers, that teaching—even more than writing—because of the interchange of thought—is the best method to promote accuracy and precision of statement. A useful practice which I initiated was to have in a convenient place a locked-up box for insertion of anonymous queries. This proved especially valuable in eliciting students' difficulties and in promoting valuable discussion at the weekly seminars. The box was unlocked at each seminar.

I have already mentioned opportunities for practical demonstration. Some were supplied by the numerous voluntary societies (milk charities, infant welfare, etc.) of the city; but it was sometimes difficult to utilise these satisfactorily when one did not feel free to criticise their arrangements, and especially their segregation from the local public health service. I was, as will be clear to the reader of this volume, possessed by the conviction that the best voluntary work is that which is carried on in a municipal framework.

During my second year at the school, a useful innovation was an intensive course of lectures and demonstrations for those already engaged in public health work. A large group of workers came from many American States and they contributed much, as did also, I think, the demonstrations, to our common stock of knowledge.

SOCIAL LIFE AT BALTIMORE

I am painfully aware of the incompleteness of my description of the work of the School of Hygiene and Public Health at Baltimore.

I realise also that I have written little of the surpassingly interesting social life my wife and I enjoyed in this University centre.

Baltimore is a port and a large commercial city; and it has two Universities, the Maryland University and the Johns Hopkins University, in which was my temporary work. Baltimore is not very unlike an English town, but there is a foreign vivacity in its people, the voices of women have a southern softness which is charming, and their hospitality could scarcely be equalled. Its merchant princes are among the governors of the Johns Hopkins University and took part in its activities; and we came into frequent relationship with University professors in extra-medical departments, and met the many foreign professors who came from time to time to lecture at the University. Dr. W. H. Welch was a magnet for the heads of Universities and for research and social workers from other parts of America, and at his famous club, the Maryland, hospitality was given on a princely scale.

Religious and social activities in Baltimore were also very interesting. Sunday afternoon addresses were popular. I shall not forget an address I gave to a negro audience during a tuberculosis "drive." To stand before an audience of some hundreds of eager upturned dark faces showing a large area of white sclerotics and equally white teeth was a new experience, as was also the unusual vocal support of my remarks as they proceeded.

The scenery around Baltimore is most attractive, and we could drive in Henrietta to Washington, D.C., to visit friends, or to consult the Congressional Library or that of the Surgeon General, where our friend, Colonel Garrison, was always helpful.

THE SOCIETY OF THE ARK AND THE DOVE

One incident, occurring in 1921 near the end of our two years in Baltimore, fortunately I can narrate in full, as I have before me the relevant correspondence. It displays sympathetically the warm-hearted feelings of many Marylanders for England.

"The Ark" and "The Dove" were the two small sailing vessels in which the original founders of the State of Maryland landed in Chesapeake Bay during the reign of Charles I. The leaders of the expedition were of the family of Calvert (Lord Baltimore). They were Roman Catholics, and in the formation of this colony, complete religious freedom was accorded to all. In this respect the position compared favourably with that in New England, in which orthodoxy as prescribed by the Independents for many years was a condition of citizenship. The warrant for the founding of the Maryland colony was subject to a charter, one condition of which is indicated in the following copy of an actual receipt dated Tuesday after Easter in 1633, in the reign of Charles I.

It sets out that on that day

Lord Baltimore, by the hands of his servant John Langford, had left within the castle of Windsor two Indian arrows for one year's rent to the King's Majesty this present day for a territory or continent of land called Maryland in America, granted by His Majesty under the great seal of England to the said Lord Baltimore for the yearly rent aforesaid. . . .

The Society of the Ark and the Dove was founded in Baltimore to keep alive the memory of this charter between Maryland and the Old Country; and each year a dinner meeting is held at which an oration is delivered. We were both invited to the annual dinner of Easter Tuesday, 1921, Rev. Dr. Magruder, a Protestant Episcopal clergyman, being the President of the Society and our host. He was a great antiquarian and student of colonial history.

In toasting his guests, he referred to my wife, who had "not Baltimorean scalps, but the hearts of all" who knew her attached to her girdle!

Then I was drawn in to undertake to convey a special message to King George V, as will be seen from the following letter written in August 1922.

There had been delay in preparing the large case with its

suitable inscription, a photograph of the original charter of Charles I, and two large arrows, befeathered, and with sharp flints at the "business end," fixed by reindeer tendon, which tightened the attached flint as the tendon became drier. I wrote to the King's secretary, Lord Stamfordham, setting out the circumstances of the original grant by Charles I, which prescribed that there was to be sent to the English King on Easter Tuesday each year two Indian arrows and "a fixed portion of such silver and gold as had been derived from the mines of Maryland." Apparently this arrangement ceased during the War of Independence. Then I described the Society of the Ark and the Dove, at whose annual meeting an oration was delivered directed towards keeping alive the friendship with the country of origin of the Marylanders; and I added a hope that King George would be graciously pleased to accept the arrows, with an assurance in the Society's words of "the continuing value attached by members of the Society to the links of language, law and religion, as well as of a common language which bind America and Britain together."

In answer to my letter forwarding the "exhibit" I received from Lord Stamfordham a letter asking me "to assure the members of the society of the gratification with which His Majesty received the message of respectful and friendly greeting which you conveyed on their behalf."

The King's courtesy went beyond this, for Lord Stamfordham on August 23, 1922, sent the following letter direct to the head of the Society of the Ark and the Dove.

(*Copy*)   BALMORAL CASTLE,

                                                23rd August, 1922.

DEAR DR. MAGRUDER,

The King has received through Sir Arthur Newsholme the two Indian Arrows which the Society of the Ark and the Dove have been good enough to forward for His Majesty's acceptance.

It gives the King much pleasure to receive this gift, recalling as it does the old link of friendship between the Marylanders and the land of their origin.

His Majesty highly appreciates the Society's message of friendly greeting transmitted to him by Sir Arthur Newsholme and cordially reciprocates the sentiments to which it gives expression.

Believe me, dear Dr. Magruder,

Yours very truly,

STAMFORDHAM.

The Reverend
Dr. JAMES M. MAGRUDER,
Governor,
Society of the Ark and the Dove.

CHAPTER XXX

THE TRAINING AND TENURE OF OFFICE OF PUBLIC HEALTH OFFICERS

MY invitation to teach Public Health Administration to the students of the School of Hygiene was evidence that an important part of the work of the new school would consist in the training for their future work of public health administrators. But this was not the chief aim of the school at its initiation. It had a wider and even more important intention. Beyond the teaching required for public health work in its multiple branches a greater conception appears to have actuated Dr. Welch and his colleague Dr. Howell at the school's initiation. The school was to be a Research Institute; and during the years when I watched its work, it became so most fruitfully, for research bulked very largely in its total activities. This was so in the department of immunology (under Dr. Bull), in those of dietetics (under Dr. McCollum), of parasitology (under Dr. Hegner) and so on.

The research work of the school was especially pronounced in the department of physiology under Dr. Howell, his talented daughter, Dr. Janet Clark, being his chief associate; and I had the opportunity of watching important investigations on problems of fatigue, of dust and ventilation problems, of the effect of light on susceptibility to infection and so on.

Such work as is imperfectly indicated above gave a special cachet to the school and I had abundant proof, while at the school, of the value of this association of research and training for the student's life-work.

In particular, physiological and dietetic investigations with their associated teaching, emphasised that the maintenance of health is even more important than the attempt to cure illness, though, in present world circumstances, more time is necessarily occupied in remedial than in preventive measures, even in the special world of public health administration.

It is, I think, a fundamental pedagogic mistake to separate the teaching of physiological hygiene from that of hygiene as applied in public health. To do this is to cut out from the student's impressions the promising if difficult matter of controlling our environment and habits of living so as to prevent the loss of good health.

But my own work at the school was concerned with public health administration, especially with the subjects in which a medical officer of health is concerned. It should be added that at the school some students were in training for work in statistical appointments and in laboratories, chemical, bacteriological, and parasitological, especially as bearing on tropical diseases, and in these laboratories research and teaching were closely related.

In occasional discussions with Dr. Welch, I stressed what I regarded as the two chief difficulties in America in attracting public health students, and in enabling these students afterwards to make a life-career of public health. These difficulties were:

(1) the general absence of any regulation insisting that the applicant for a post as M.O.H. should present evidence of an adequate training for the post, and

(2) the absence of reasonable security of tenure of his appointment, when once made.

TRAINING OF MEDICAL OFFICERS OF HEALTH

I have often represented to American friends that were these two difficulties removed, American Schools of Hygiene would soon have many students in this applied part of their training, and the general standard of sanitary administration would be raised. The training given would not need to be so strictly vocational as to imply the loss of the wider culture given, for instance, at the Johns Hopkins School of Hygiene. In Britain a diploma in public health is only given to medical practitioners already fully qualified to practise medicine who undergo one or two years' additional special training, but in most American States this is not legally obligatory. In the vast majority of cities and States health commissioners or officers are, however, medical practitioners.

As an old examiner for public health diplomas in England, I have found that the laboratory-taught student, who has done

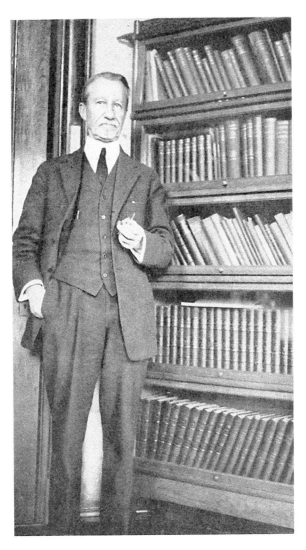

PROFESSOR WILLIAM H. HOWELL

little or no field work, sometimes pins his faith chiefly to laboratory methods of investigation, as for instance when an outbreak of illness occurs. During examination work I have received absurd answers, such as the following:

Question : What action would you take if five notifications of enteric fever were received by you as M.O.H. on a particular morning? *Answer :* I would at once proceed to have a bacteriological examination made of the water supply.

In Britain itself there is need of modification of the conditions laid down by the General Medical Council for obtaining the D.P.H. There should, as now, be a year's training in laboratory procedures; but the second year's training for the student (who it will be recalled is already a qualified medical practitioner) should be spent is assisting in the actual work of a M.O.H. under the supervision of a health officer as his chief. It would not be impracticable to adopt a scheme, somewhat like that already adopted in some great towns for health visitors, in which the nurse during a year receives a small salary while doing useful work under supervision. A like system is indicated for future medical officers of health and for midwives.

It is the privilege of age to reminisce and I yield to the temptation to hark back to several years' experience on this point in my early years as M.O.H. of Brighton. I held also the position of physician to its Fever Hospital; no resident doctor was provided for its 80–100 beds, some of whose occupants were suffering from diphtheria and typhoid fever, and this often necessitated evening visits by me. I had applications from young doctors wishing to come to be trained for public health work; and impelled by the strain of too much evening work as well as by other considerations I proposed to the Sanitary Committee of the Town Council that I should be allowed to secure an unpaid resident house-physician at the hospital, it being understood that after my daily visit to the hospital he should (without any fee being received by me) accompany me in my daily work at my office and in visiting houses and sick persons. The plan was approved; and looking back, it appears to me that no better system of training is practicable for a young doctor than to sit beside the M.O.H. while he interviews persons or discusses procedure with the sanitary inspectors, or goes over the records of infectious diseases and discusses their possible interrelations, or to help the M.O.H. to compile his statistical returns, and to accompany him when he makes investigation, especially where a case of typhoid fever or tuberculosis is concerned, or when the question of condemning a house unfit for human habitation arises.

It is pleasant to recall that I had with me in those early years, in the above capacity the late Dr. C. J. MacFadden, C.B., who preceded me on the staff of the Local Government Board and did outstanding work in Food Hygiene, and Dr. J. P. Candler, who is mentioned on page 163. Among others were Dr. Barrett Heggs, now Health Commissioner in Baghdad, and the late Dr. T. H. C. Stevenson, C.B.E., who did some important statistical work while with me, and who subsequently occupied Farr's chair at the General Register Office with great distinction.

SHOULD A DIPLOMATE IN PUBLIC HEALTH BE FIRST A QUALIFIED PHYSICIAN?

At the School of Hygiene, Baltimore, and at other Universities in America, the degree of doctor in public health (DR.P.H.) is given after two years' training. It is restricted to those already possessing a medical qualification. A D.SC. in Public Health is also given without this restriction. In some other Universities a D.P.H. or DR.P.H. is not restricted to qualified physicians. A few commissioners of health (health officers) who are not physicians are heads of municipal health departments. In Britain this is legally prohibited. Among those in the United States who, while not physicians, have done the best public health work are men who in the past have graduated from the Massachusetts Institute of Technology, after having received their training under Professor Sedgwick and his colleagues. My first meeting with Professor Sedgwick, PH.D., who was then the Director of this School of Public Health, was interesting. It was on December 29, 1919, when the events of the Great War were still vividly in our memories. I was a guest of Professor Sedgwick at the annual dinner of the Society of Bacteriologists, the chair being taken by Professor S. C. Prescott, Dean of Science of the Institute. After a good dinner, Professor Prescott gravely announced that every dish we had eaten was prepared from foods that had been dehydrated for a considerable time. Dr. Prescott had made us the subject of an experiment bearing on his war-time investigations; but none of us had discovered that each excellent dish of the dinner had been preserved.

Sedgwick himself was greatly beloved by his students and colleagues, and the writings he left give but a faint idea of the influence he exercised in several branches of environmental hygiene (see also p. 260).

On this occasion and several times afterwards Sedgwick discussed with me his proposal to limit the technical training of future public health officials on its medical side to the first half of the future physician's training, which is concerned with the preliminary sciences, and to omit much or most of the clinical side of medicine; and although I could not agree with him, in view of the extent to which in Britain clinical knowledge was indispensable in public health work, his views undoubtedly represented one phase of truth. They were set out completely in 1921 in his article on "Modern Medicine and the Public Health" which appeared in *Public Health Reports*, Vol. 36, No. 4. But, already in Britain, as I knew, having been in part responsible for it, purely medical and largely clinical work had crept into English public health practice as shown in official schemes for maternity and child welfare work, and for the treatment of tuberculosis and venereal diseases. Since then the clinical responsibilities of medical officers of health or their specialised assistant officers have still further increased; and there are not wanting those who fear that "pure" preventive medicine and public health may become engulfed by these vast clinical responsibilities.

I have no such fear; there may be temporary loss of perspective, but sooner or later clinical work will become increasingly work in preventive medicine and eventually the ruling conception and practice in the whole of medicine will become that of Public Health.

TENURE OF OFFICE

In more recent years some advance has been made in improving the tenure of office of American health commissioners (medical officers of health). Past practice in cities was that when a new mayor was elected at the end of two or four years he appointed his own staff, all important official posts being vacated and then filled by the mayor's political supporters, too often entirely irrespective of their professional competence. "Spoils to the Conquerors." Sometimes a good M.O.H. was retained; oftener he knew that at the end of three or four years he would have to resume private practice. Under such chopping and changing continuously good work was almost ruled out. This was so in Britain until the later years of last century, with the following important difference. In Britain, appointments, which had been made for a short term of years, were never filled up according to the whim of a single person—the mayor—but were made by a majority vote of the elected local governing municipal councillors. Now in Britain each M.O.H. has security of tenure of office, so long as he remains efficient; and he cannot be dismissed without the consent of the Ministry of Health. The ability of Biggs to do exceptionally fine public health work in New York was due in part to special professional circumstances. Biggs was physician at one time to an all-powerful "boss" and thus he had not only secure tenure of office in New York City, but also irresistible backing from Tammany for his chief medical proposals. When in his later years he became head of the Health Department of New York State his prestige made him equally invulnerable. Until recent years, except partially in New York State, medical officers of health in America have not had reasonably secure tenure of office, nor have they been required to possess a special qualification for public health work.

I am indebted to Dr. Huntington Williams, the Health Commissioner of Baltimore, Maryland, for particulars as to the tenure of office and qualifications required in respect of the appointment now held by him. His appointment is for a period of six years, which prevents direct interference with his office by a new mayor elected at shorter intervals than this.

A six-year tenure has very seldom been previously given and in one instance, that of New York State, the law to this end was discontinued after three terms of office. In Baltimore the change was made by the public-spirited mayor for both supervisors of City Charities and for the Commissioner of Health. It represents a valuable step towards security of tenure, subject to continued competence.

Baltimore also, not more than two years ago, in its City Charter amendment, required that for the future: the Commissioner of Health of Baltimore shall be "trained in public work with at least five years' actual experience in public health performed in departments of Federal, State, or Municipal governments." Prior to this the only requirement had been that the Commissioner of Health "shall be a physician of five years' experience and in active practice at the time of his appointment." The medical requirement has been removed from the qualifications for Commissioner of Health of Baltimore, although it had been legally required for many decades up to 1934. But local tradition makes it improbable that a non-medical health officer will be appointed. In actual fact the medical requirement is almost universal in the United States. All excepting a few of the forty-eight State health officers are physicians. For city health officers there is great variety in regard to conditions of appointment, some enforcing no conditions, some coming up to the standard of Baltimore.

The New York State Sanitary Code, 1934, in conformity with existing law requires a local health officer (of a city, county, or town) to be a physician, licensed to practise in the State or eligible for examination for such licence, and to have as additional qualifications experience or special training or both of one of two grades, Grade I being required for all counties and all cities with a population over 50,000; Grade II for smaller communities. For Grade I at least four years' full-time experience and/or special training in public health, and for Grade II four years' part-time experience of public health, or completion of a course of public health of not less than one academic year, is required.

Evidently important steps have been taken here and there which, we may hope, will culminate ere long in making it the universal practice in the United States for each M.O.H. to have special training in his work and to have indefinite security of tenure of office so long as his health and efficiency continue. To this will also, one can anticipate, be added similar right to a pension on retirement. This is already usually, but not everywhere, accorded in Britain. In British local health service the pension is "contributory," the M.O.H. and the local authority both contributing to the annual payments ensuring the pension.

CHAPTER XXXI

AMERICAN PUBLIC HEALTH AS RELATED TO FEDERAL AND STATE GOVERNMENT

IN Part I of this volume I have discussed some of the defects and difficulties of central and local government in Great Britain as related to Public Health; and have attempted to indicate the gradual evolution of improved methods and standards. It is more difficult for "an outsider" to attempt, as I propose to do in this chapter, the parallel task of commenting on Federal and State organisations in relation to American problems of Public Health; for whereas I have been concerned day by day during several decades in local and central health administration in England, I have been only an observer in a few centres of American administration for relatively short periods. Perhaps I may plead that former experience may have increased my ability to observe and discriminate.

The history of American government presents features of exceptional interest, for this government began as a democracy, it has continued to be democratic for nearly three half centuries, and—if we leave Soviet Russia in a class by itself—the United States has grown to be the largest of the nations that live under self-governing institutions.

It began with a fierce passion for civil liberty, after the long struggle with Britain; and its eagerness for liberty may still be an element tending to occasional lawlessness, the intemperance of liberty. All power in the United States came from the people, and this Sovereignty of the people carried with it the further fundamental principle of equality. It is not for me to follow out the consequences of these two principles; but when the Federation of the constituent States was ratified in 1787–89, there was at once implied the need for a constitution setting out the machinery and respective scope of Federal and State government. In this way, as Bryce has pointed out, the principle of self-restraint followed close on that of Liberty, and the constitution in substance made it clear that a majority of votes is not always right, and rules and checks were formulated imposing impediments to hasty decision.

When the United States cut the cable connecting them with Britain they were thirteen more or less isolated colonies, and they found it necessary to "hang together," although each of them appears to have objected to a powerful central government common to them all.

The history of these thirteen and the subsequently added States embodies the story of a persistent struggle between the forces of centralisation and of State Home Rule.

From its commencement the new Federal Government was limited in its working by judicial interpretation of the Supreme Court as to whether any given Federal or State legislation was in accord with the binding terms of the American Constitution.

This Constitution in fact set up "a superior paramount law," which enabled a majority of the nine members of the Supreme Court to decide that any "legislative act contrary to the Constitution is not law," but is void. The intention of the conservatively drafted Constitution was to prevent invasion by the Federal Government of the rights retained by the States, when they were not specifically delegated to the Federal Government in the Constitution. Thus despotism or dictatorship was to be made impossible. The despotism which apparently was most feared was that of a casual majority of either a State or a Federal legislature which would bring about undesirable changes.

The Constitution was designed to prevent the possibility of rapid changes in law and in administration. Thus as it has been said:

Democracy has been afraid of itself and *of its own chosen officials* and has *hedged them about with so many restrictions that genuine efficiency has been wellnigh impossible,*

and Woodrow Wilson in his *An Old Master and other Political Essays* states that when the American Government was formed

we deemed ourselves rank democrats, whereas we were in fact only progressive Englishmen.

The government when we formed it . . . was simply an adoption of English constitutional government.

Democratic institutions are never done; they are like living tissue, always a-making.

The English have transferred their Crown into a Ministry, and in doing so have recognised both the supremacy of Parliament and the role of leadership in legislation properly belonging to a responsible executive.

We have left our executive separate, as the Constitution made it. . . .

Congress . . . deprived of such leadership (i.e. of the President and his executives) becomes a legislative mass meeting instead of a responsible co-operative member of a well-organised government.

The executive of the Federal Government, except when inter-State matters were concerned, until recently has contented itself in the main in public health matters with advisory and consultant services and medical research; for, apart from the Veterans' Bureau, Federal activities have related chiefly to quarantine, to the leper problem, to vital statistics, to the care of the personnel of the Army, Navy, and Mercantile Marine, with some further powers when health problems definitely affected inter-State relationships. They have exercised valuable advisory functions, and the Federal Government within the last year has been endowed with money on a great scale, which will give great power in promoting public health progress in each State. The Federal Government also organised some years ago under Dr. Lumsden of the United States Public Health Service a system of help—by lending health officers or otherwise—in the carrying out of public health administration in rural areas.

Each of the forty eight States is a Sovereign State, independent so far as its internal policies are concerned; and this explains the multiplicity of medical and public health organisations and of taxation, for each State has its own legislation and special methods of administration. This position creates one advantage which does not, however, count greatly against the disadvantages of the "Sovereign State"; there are, so to speak, forty-eight laboratories or experimental stations in which novel procedures can be tested and tried out. But there are also, it must be added, a vast number of laws and regulations which have been enacted light-heartedly, often at the bidding of social agitators or log-rollers, but which remain almost a dead letter. As one Senator is reported to have said: "I have no objection to legislation, so long as it is not enforced."

This multiplicity of laws and regulations interests the visitor to America; it also puzzles him; and in regard to criminal law he is horrified at the many legal loopholes for criminals and the occasional failure and frequently the almost incredible delay in enforcing the punishment of the guilty.

But I am concerned chiefly with the public health services in America. The Federal Public Health Service, notwithstanding its legal shackles, has increasingly become a centre of public health guidance and information, though without power except in matters affecting inter-State and international hygiene.

The Sheppard-Towner Act enabled the Federal Children's Bureau to give grants in aid of child welfare work in each State; a very few of the States refused the grants as infringing on their sovereign position. In 1935 similar difficulty arises in the Federal Social Security Act concerned primarily with insurance for provision during unemployment and in old age. The contributory old-age insurance scheme is National in scope and Federal in authority. The (non-contributory) old-age assistance or pensions and the unemployment compensation provisions must be made by the State, but the Federal Government are prepared to subsidise on a large scale any State scheme which conforms to stated general conditions. People move from State to State, and how this difficulty in administration will be overcome remains to be seen. Difficulties must arise, owing to differences between the conditions of assistance or insurance in various States.

The Social Security Act (1935) also included appropriations for (preventive) public health work as the first measures against insecurity caused by illness. The U.S. Public Health Service receives under this Act not only new funds for research, also substantial sums to be allotted to the State Health Departments to assist them in their work. The U.S. Children's Bureau also receives such funds for similar work in respect to the care of women and children.

The difficulties and obstacles to good work arising owing to the imperfect co-ordination of the functions of the Federal and the State Governments are continued in the relation between the State and its constituent local authorities. One needs to think of each State as though it were England, and of the relationship between each local authority and the Ministry of Health in England as comparable with that between the State legislature and local public health authorities within the individual State. The analogy is only partial. In England the activities of local authorities are exercised within the limits of the powers conferred by national legislation and local bye-laws and regulations which are consistent with this legislation. These bye-laws and regulations, furthermore, must receive the approval of the department of the central government concerned. Furthermore, county boroughs (usually having a population exceeding 100,000) are totally independent of the government of the county in which the county borough is situate.

In American cities this independence is only partial, though in special matters it is made complete for most purposes, if the State legislature passes a law to this effect.

The State legislatures, which are bicameral, have not had a good reputation. James (Lord) Bryce, writing in his *Modern Democracy* as recently as 1921, gives a somewhat gloomy account, and as he was a great friend of America, I cite the summary which he gives, with the proviso that in 1936 the facts of 1921 do not fully apply. He states that the legislatures do not enjoy the confidence of the people; their civil service is unequal to its tasks, their judiciary is unsatisfactory and the administration of criminal justice is slow, while the laws are often not enforced. "The Government of cities and especially of the largest cities has been incompetent, wasteful and corrupt" (Vol. II., *op. cit.*, p. 155): party organisations "have become selfish and oligarchic" and are worked by professional "politicians"; finally the power of wealth is too great. The average quality of legislators is low and they are not respected, and the civil service is recruited largely on the "spoils system," without regard to competence. Party machines have become a Juggernaut which unscrupulously crushes opposition, and the vast masses of ignorant foreign immigrants have been used, along with other corrupt persons, to maintain the power of the party machine.

This pessimistic summary happily is now partially, though not completely, out of date.

The "better elements" in American society have feared and eschewed democracy *as it is worked*, and have refused to take part in democratic government. The more socially minded among them could not conscientiously remain indifferent, and so vast voluntary organisations have been created which, throughout America, are doing a large, sometimes a preponderant, share of the social work which official local governing bodies ought to do.

Even in the sphere of official administration, the creation of multiple authorities, independently concerned with different branches of public work, has resulted in wholesale inefficiency and confusion. The practice of creating *ad hoc* authorities may have originated in England, where until recently Poor Law Guardians and sanitary authorities were separate from each other and not, as now, constituent parts of the one Local Parliament, which carries out every branch of public administration in its own area. (Non-county sanitary authorities remain a partial exception to this rule, and the separate local administration of National Insurance still remains.)

Public opinion in the United States is rapidly growing in favour of county instead of small units for local government, and in New York State the Milbank Fund, by its rural demonstration (p. 301), has helped to promote this. It is only when adequately large units of government exist that skilled officials, with secure tenure of office for competent men, are likely to be engaged. It may be hoped that ere many years have passed the objectionable system of direct election of mayor, coroner, sheriff, etc., by the collected votes of all taxpayers will cease. This will happen when the mass of the people realise that good government is only obtainable if the taxpayer shares in it by electing trustworthy representatives on governing bodies; and, having taken his part in electing these representatives, entrusts them with the appointment of trained officials on their professional merits.

My justification for discussing American methods of government, even to this limited extent, is in its bearing on my own recollections of experience in the States and I propose therefore in the next chapter to limit myself to certain aspects of city government.

CHAPTER XXXII

CITY ADMINISTRATION IN THE UNITED STATES

JAMES BRYCE many years ago described the failure of its city governments as "the one conspicuous failure of the American people." Since then vast improvements have occurred, though it cannot be said that inefficiency and corruption in city government are now rare. This is especially so for the concessions or franchises granted to private companies or corporations ready to provide the public with such services as gas, electricity, tramcars, etc. In the creation of these monopolies city and State control are intermingled, and there has been vast scope for the machinations of corrupt politicians.

In public health matters, these machinations probably are on a relatively small scale, but there has been much "starving" of essential health services, while lavish expenditure has been incurred in other directions.

Various attempts have been made to escape from inefficiency and corruption in city government. Public opinion has been roused, and a reforming mayor and council have been elected, but reform has been only spasmodic and the "politicians" have got back to their "hunting ground." Three special lines of action have been tried:

(a) There has been direct democracy of the English pattern, in which the elected representatives of the public supervise, through committees of their number, various departments of local administration by means of a permanent staff of secretarial, legal, and technical officers competent to advise them and to carry out executive work.

This is the English method. In the States it has been largely abandoned, apparently in despair, because it has not functioned efficiently in American life. It has been replaced either by:

(b) a city manager, directly elected by the taxpayers, or, in public health matters, by

(c) a health commission, consisting of a health officer associated with two or three others.

The plan of having a city manager, who during his tenure of

office has autocratic power, has been adopted by over a hundred cities within ten years. It is preferable to the alternative plan of having a number of city commissions largely independent of each other, and often with separate power of imposing public taxation.

But both methods imply a partial abandonment by the representatives of the taxpayers on the city council of their inherent responsibility for good government. These plans are more German than English, for they subordinate the public and their elected representatives to the expert. In view of what I have written in several chapters in Part I of this volume, I regard this as not completely democratic, and as not ultimately conducive to continued efficiency of government. The expert's role in part is that of an educator of his authority, and reform is most effective and enduring when sanctioned by the representative authority. The truly democratic method first described may mean disappointing delays, but progress made is solid, not liable to relapse into reaction or opposition. Meanwhile it may be affirmed that many American municipalities have partially stripped themselves of their functions, instead of working with and through their expert technical officers.

RELATION OF CITY TO STATE ADMINISTRATION

As already stated city administration is not so rigidly separated from State administration as is that of county boroughs or cities in Britain from that of the administrative county.

The American situation can be illustrated by the position in Baltimore, Md., and that in New York City.

Baltimore city has an exceptionally long experience of health administration. Its health department was established in 1797, and in 1874 when the Maryland State Health Department was established the City Health Department had already made active progress. A similar history applies to the city of Boston, Mass., for as Dr. Huntington Williams tells me, Paul Revere, whose memory lives as the equestrian of the famous ride from Boston to Concord, and who was a well-known silversmith, served as the first President of the Boston City Board of Health when it was founded in 1799. The Massachusetts State Board was organised in 1869. So also in New York, the City Board of

Health goes back to about 1800, while the State Board of Health was organised in 1880. In Baltimore more than ten years ago a so-called home-rule amendment of State law was passed by the legislature of Maryland, giving Baltimore city the power to pass and enforce local city ordinances, independently of the State legislature.

The description for Baltimore may be extended, as illustrating the greater power entrusted to individual health officers than is ever given in England. A city ordinance commonly delegates to the health commissioner (there is no Board of Health in Baltimore) the power to adopt rules and regulations to carry out the intent of the ordinances; and there is no question of submitting the ordinances passed by the City Council and. signed by the mayor, or the rules and regulations made by the City Commissioner of Health, for approval by the State legislature.

In New York City the position is similar. When, for instance, milk pasteurisation was required, the power of New York City to insist on this was derived from the wider powers granted by the State legislature. This delegation, in specific instances, may be given by *ad hoc* legislation from the State legislature, or in the sanitary codes of the State Board of Health special charters may have been granted by the State to the City. In effect public health administration in New York City is, in general, independent of the New York State Public Health Council, except in matters which specifically affect the entire State. In other respects the public health law of New York State gives powers which relate only to the State outside of New York City.

"BOSS" GOVERNMENT

Preceding remarks apply especially to the problems of public health work. I emphasise that valuable health work is being done in American cities, even where the principles of undiluted democracy are not followed. This certainly is so in the three cities in which I had special opportunities of seeing public health administration, Baltimore, New York, and Chicago. But, in some cities, good work is being done by health commissioners and their staff who are inadequately in touch with the elected members of the municipality. Furthermore, although tenure of office, in America, is becoming less unsatisfactory, these commissioners are usually liable to dismissal when a new mayor is appointed. This ought not to be; and once more I emphasise that the health commissioner should be placed in a position to carry with him in each proposed reform not only the mayor, as at present, but also the municipal council, and not be called on to carry on independent of these during his tenure of office

As I have animadverted on the evils of "boss" government, I will give an instance in which its indirect influence was potent for good.

As is well known, the late Dr. Hermann M. Biggs was never Health Commissioner of the City of New York. His title was General Medical Officer and he had control of all medical matters. He did not give his whole time to his public duties, though his special flair for seizing essential points enabled him for many years to guide the public health policy of the city with success. He was able also to resist the machinations of "boss" government of the city, and whoever was displaced from office, he was retained. This doubtless was due in large measure to his outstanding reputation; but his position was rendered impregnable by the fact that he was the private physician to Murphy, the great Tammany Boss.

In later years Biggs was persuaded to become Health Commissioner of the State of New York and to re-organise its public health service. He did this successfully. A crucial test of his competence and power arose almost immediately after his acceptance of the State appointment. An outbreak of smallpox arose in the City of Niagara Falls, and, as there was a strong anti-vaccination party in the city, vaccination and other precautions were neglected. The local authority adopted the device of denying the existence of smallpox in the city, but the State health department were able to verify a large number of cases. This was in January 1914, and Biggs proceeded to act. He asked the mayor of the City of Niagara to call a conference and publish the facts and pointed out that if prompt and drastic action were not taken it might become necessary to isolate the city from contact with other parts of the State. The city council remained recalcitrant and Biggs proceeded to interview the President of the New York Central Railway, whose trains ran through the city, and obtained his authority to state that no trains should stop at the City of Niagara Falls if in Biggs's view this veto became necessary. Posters were prepared warning people not to stop at the city, and the city authorities were shown the draft of these. A few hours' delay was conceded and before this time had elapsed the opposition to drastic measures had collapsed, in view of the impending merciless publicity.

CORRUPTION IN GOVERNMENT

In previous paragraphs it may have appeared that bribery and corruption are a phenomenon special to American government. This, of course, is not so. The same phenomenon has emerged in all governments, whether democratic, or oligarchic, or autocratic. The corruption in pre-war Russia was especially notorious, but Russia did not stand alone among European countries. Corruption is not special to any form of government. Sir Thomas More (1478–1535) characterised society as a "conspiracy of the rich against the poor, the conspiracy being carried on under the forms of the Law." The difference between corrupt government in Tudor days and now is that venal politicians have learnt to utilise ignorant and poor people to subserve their corrupt ends. The history of England a century ago furnishes illustrations of votes bought and sold in scarcely hidden negotiations, and of sinecures shamelessly awarded for political support. The possibility of this has now almost disappeared.

In America the persistence of the mercenary principle of *vae victis* has ensured the continuance of corrupt government though happily to a decreasing extent. It will disappear or be reduced to insignificance when the American people realise that it is as much their moral and religious duty to take a share in the conduct of government (by voting straight, by constant vigilance over the activities of their representatives, and by themselves taking part in the work of municipalities and other official bodies), as it is to avoid a direct personal breach of one of the ten commandments. When the war against the ward

K

"politicians" and the political "boss" has been won, and mercenary motives in government have thus been enfeebled, it will be possible everywhere to wage successfully the great remaining war, that of more equitable distribution of the overflowing wealth which nature and applied science supply, so that the poor shall no longer dwell in the land.

A vast amount of valuable "social or welfare work"[1] is being done in every American community; and it can confidently be anticipated that this will cease to be chiefly voluntary in character and will become more fully the function of State and City government. Already America sets an example to Britain in the volume and intensity of voluntary social work which has been accomplished, as will be seen in Chapters XXXIII and XXXIV. In some important phases of official public health work, America has advanced more rapidly and further than the older country.

[1] In America "social work" is intended to mean relief or charitable work; but much of it has a valuable preventive side. There is no logical line of distinction between it and public health work.

CHAPTER XXXIII

VOLUNTARY AGENCIES IN PUBLIC HEALTH AND WELFARE WORK IN THE UNITED STATES

In the United States "welfare work" means chiefly charitable work, while public health work is concerned with measures directly concerned with the maintenance of health and the prevention of illness. This distinction is not maintained in Britain, for neither logically nor in administration is it practicable to separate "welfare" from "public health" work without reducing the possibilities of full success of both of them. When monetary allowances or their equivalent in food or lodging are given to the unemployed or otherwise destitute the maximum good is not secured unless attempt is made to ensure that the expenditure shall be associated with circumstances that will conduce to a hygienic life and to social rehabilitation; and the inevitable fusion of welfare and public health work under one general local governing body applies when fully satisfactory provision is made for the placing of deserted or orphan children, for pensions and homes for the aged, for hospital beds or clinics and consultation centres for the sick and poor, and for the many charitable objects promoted in every considerable city.

In America public authorities and voluntary agencies appear to have been less confident in taking this wider view of public health work than in Britain; but the wider view cannot be said to be completely accepted on either side of the Atlantic. Mr. Homer Folks' recent brochure[1] should help to clearer

[1] *Making Relief Respectable*, by Homer Folks (Publication of S.C.A.A., New York City). The following extracts illustrate Mr. Folks' contentions:

"Public relief is something to which each recipient has contributed all his life . . . and will continue to contribute indefinitely."

"Public relief is a two-way business all the way, everybody contributing roughly in proportion to his ability. . . ."

"Investigation as to need may be considerate and adequate."

I am especially glad to quote the following further extract, embodying a truth elsewhere emphasised in this volume:—

"It seems to me wholly clear that we shall need, and on a con-

vision. The next generation will, I trust, act on the conception that what is provided by taxation, whether for instance it be a pension or a hospital, if safeguarded against abuse of the privilege, is potentially the privilege of every citizen, just as much as sanitary and police provision and elementary education.

In the United States voluntary welfare institutions for the sick and the bereaved have been provided extensively, especially in its cities; and voluntary charity has extended in most cities into the region of admittedly public health work, especially in regard to mothers and their infants, and to measures against tuberculosis. Action against tuberculosis (p. 315) by voluntary agencies may be said to have reached the high-water mark of efficiency and success. A similar remark applies, as also in Britain, to the district nursing associations, which are now widespread in both countries. Their work, both in bed-side nursing and in the work of health visitors or public health nurses, is now happily subsidised largely by local authorities.

The proposal to organise a supply of public health nurses under the American Red Cross was ere long abandoned (p. 240), the Red Cross organisation being unwilling to affiliate its nursing work with that of official health authorities; but nursing provision otherwise organised has spread all over the States, and is now one of the most important elements in total public health work.

In both Britain and America, in many branches of social welfare work voluntary workers have anticipated, and thus stimulated, official activity to the same end. This is no new phenomenon. It was so even as regards crime in Britain. In 1839 there were some 500 voluntary societies whose object was the arrest and pursuit of criminals, and not till 1857 did the provision of police became compulsory throughout Britain.

Voluntary organisations for promoting socio-hygienic work, however valuable, have certain drawbacks. They are irresponsible except to their subscribers, and their number is often excessive in proportion to the work effected by them. Efforts at their consolidation and at allocation of spheres of

siderable scale, a rational humane public relief system, and that such a system differs, not fundamentally in kind, but in degree and scope from these other forms of social insurance."

influence are not always successful; and so, to use a military analogy, we may have an army of many regiments, each fighting under its own standard, and with no common plan of campaign. This illustration is only partially relevant; for while the voluntary regiments of social welfare seldom cover the needs of the community, the enthusiasm for work of the members of a small organisation may be more easily maintained than that of a larger and more impersonal body which on paper is more efficient.

There is less difference between voluntary and official organisations than at first sight appears; for in America as in England voluntary societies always, if they are efficient, employ paid officers who do most of the work. To my mind the chief objection to voluntary societies is the fact that each year a large proportion of their total kinetic power may be expended in "drives" to secure the money for their continued existence. There is the further objection, already suggested, that voluntary agencies are supported by the contributions of the charitable few, and the element of almsgiving clings to them; whereas when provision is made at the communal expense, all have contributed, and all when in specific need may rightly share in the provision without hesitation.

The reason why in the States, unlike in Britain, voluntary social work appears to preponderate over the work of official bodies is not far to seek. Not only are local and central government more closely interrelated in Britain than in each of the forty-eight American States, but local health authorities in Britain have emerged more absolutely than American from the position in which it is possible to suggest corruption in their expenditure.

In Britain it has become an honour to be elected by the ratepayers as their representative on the local Council; and to be elected Chairman or Mayor of the Council by the majority vote of the Councillors is an eagerly sought distinction, which stands not far below that of a Member of Parliament. And yet the English Chairman or Mayor, in whose person is focussed the dignity of the Council, has no such power of appointment and dismissal of officials of the Council as are possessed by an American Mayor.

The persistent American disparagement and neglect of official work and of the men who undertake it will, I believe, disappear: but meanwhile its existence explains why so many Americans have resorted to independent social effort. In both countries official bodies are more closely limited than voluntary societies in their work by legal restrictions, voluntary societies being freer to adopt new and experimental procedures: and, although the initiative has not always come from them, voluntary workers have oft-times started important advances in public health work, especially on its personal side, which have been subsequently adopted and extended by public health authorities. The two forms of help have always closely co-existed in English-speaking countries and this will, I think, continue. In two special varieties of social help, the provision of sick-nurses and of hospitals, private charity has been especially successful, but even in respect of these private charity has ceased to be adequate, and taxes are being increasingly called on to make further provision.

Of the American voluntary health organisations probably the majority concern themselves with child hygiene, with the provision of milk, or with tuberculosis, but there are many others. There is similar work in Britain on a large scale. But speaking broadly it is more closely linked up with official work than in America.

My personal preference is for those forms of voluntary medico-hygienic work which remedy defaults and failures of the governing bodies and which, so far as possible, tend to stimulate increased activity or new activity by these official bodies.

A few notes are added here as to voluntary societies, some not chiefly charitable, with which I have had personal contact.

THE PRUDENTIAL LIFE INSURANCE COMPANY

First I should mention the medical statistics which have issued for a long series of years from the American Prudential Life Insurance Co., Newark, N.J., by my old friend Dr. Frederic Hoffman, its consultant statistician. I remember paying a pilgrimage to his unrivalled library of medical and statistical pamphlets at the head office of the Prudential Company; and

I yield to no one in appreciation of the steady stream of Hoffman's contributions to medical statistics for a long series of years. He has made an unequalled contribution to international cancer statistics. The figures naturally vary in their value and Dr. Hoffman knows as well as anyone that corrections for age, sex, etc., will need, when possible, to be made. But, though this is so, the existence of the statistics means the beginning of an international record of the prevalence of malignant disease.

THE METROPOLITAN LIFE INSURANCE COMPANY

Another Insurance Society, the Metropolitan Life Insurance Company, for many years, month by month, has made valuable contributions to American vital statistics. Its monthly statistical bulletins have included articles and paragraphs on various phases of public health, while giving the current medical history of its enormous clientele of insured persons. The Metropolitan Life Insurance Company has also been a pioneer in welfare work for its insured members. I have frequently discussed with Dr. Louis I. Dublin his statistical reports and with the late Dr. Lee K. Frankel the valuable social work for the insured which he initiated and developed on a continental scale. As early as 1871 the company compiled *Health Hints* for its policy-holders. Gradually work of a public health character extended and the formation of the welfare division of the company in 1909 led to widened activities. This work included nursing care for sick policy-holders and its vast staff of agents was utilised to pass on to all policy-holders accurate hygienic knowledge. In this programme of nursing and counsel all existing local public and private health agencies are utilised. The nursing work has been done by employing and paying the nurses of local visiting nurse associations all over the country. Between 1909 and 1934 nearly eleven million cases of sickness were nursed, on an average between six and seven visits being made to each patient. The help given by the Metropolitan Company in organising and in contributing to researches in preventive medicine can only be mentioned (p. 318). And I must not describe the Company's arrangement with the Life

Extension Institute for some of its insured to have free medical overhauls at intervals, the opportunity being taken to give appropriate advice as to the examinee's mode of life. Dr. Dublin's figures of this experience show an apparent lower average incidence of sickness among those thus examined, justifying continuance of the experiment.

The wide use of commercial life insurance for promoting personal hygiene is a valuable indication of what could be accomplished under our English system of sickness insurance, if its organisation were extended and rationalised. This is practicable; its realisation has already been too long delayed.

S.C.A.A.

Among the voluntary associations in America which appear to me to have an ideal relationship to official organisations first place should, I think, be given to the *New York State Charities Aid Association* which needs its abbreviated alphabetical title of S.C.A.A. Its full title has the virtue of describing the scope of the society's work. In 1933 it celebrated sixty-one years of effort to aid and promote effective public administration of health and welfare services in New York State. Its primary intention was to aid official work, that is work paid for out of State taxation; and in accomplishing this it has "utilised citizen interest and scientific progress." In carrying out its work the S.C.A.A. has some 10,000 voluntary citizen workers in the State and runs 171 committees, one or more in every county in the State.

One of the chief fields of work of the society has been to promote legislation for the promotion of social welfare and public health in the New York State Legislature at Albany. All legislative proposals are subjected to examination and the reasons for supporting or rejecting a given proposal are forcibly pressed on the notice of the members of the legislature. Pressure is also systematically brought to bear through the public Press, and thus the society has become an educator for the entire community. Along with the giving of official aid the S.C.A.A. is engaged in multifarious direct work. The following heads extracted from the annual report of the society illustrate the many ways in which voluntary outside workers can give valuable aid in improving the efficiency of both voluntary and statutory bodies:

Public Relief;
Tuberculosis and Public Health;
Mental Hygiene;
Child placing and adoption Agency;
County Children's Agencies;
Mothers' and Babies' Agency;
New York City Visiting Committee;
Welfare Legislation Information Bureau.

The S.C.A.A. is guided in its work by a committee of distinguished citizens, and throughout most of its career has had the services of Mr. Homer Folks, its secretary and director, who is the soul of the organisation. The S.C.A.A. is an admirable illustration of the best possible relation between voluntary and official workers in the public interest.

MILBANK MEMORIAL FUND

The public health work of the Milbank Memorial Fund, with which until recently is inseparably associated the record of its secretary and director, Mr. J. A. Kingsbury, has been another great and beneficent example of joint working of official and voluntary bodies; for the Milbank Fund has been largely concerned during its career in demonstrating the value—by its aid and guidance in finance and personnel—of increased expenditure in staff and in money, in raising the standard of official public health administration in the State.

I do not attempt to describe the work of other American voluntary associations concerned in health work, of which the American Social Hygiene Association and the National Tuberculosis Association are outstanding. With many of the workers in each of these societies I have had frequent contacts and appreciate the important influence each society has had in advancing education for public health work. (On these see also pp. 369 and 315).

K*

CHAPTER XXXIV

ENDOWED FOUNDATIONS AND SOCIO-HYGIENIC WORK IN AMERICA

IN advancing social welfare and public health not only have the national and regional health associations already mentioned borne an important part, but even more far-reaching has been the role of a number of social foundations endowed by rich American philanthropists. I cannot mention all these endowments, but must limit myself to those about whose work I have some personal knowledge. These foundations have not only contributed valuable help to the direct promotion of public health and social work; they have also initiated and promoted measures for the training of personnel, a much needed help; they have undertaken valuable consultative services in sanitary areas; and they have promoted investigations having in view greater control of disease, and improved methods of health administration.

According to a statement by Mr. Pierce H. F. Williams, formerly of the Association of Community Chests, the seven chief of the many foundations in America in 1927 had a combined endowment of 500,000,000 dollars with an aggregate income that year of 28½ million dollars.

All these foundations agree on one point; no charity is given to individuals and, apart from war exigencies, and such great calamities as earthquake and flood and recent unemployment in America, emergency measures of relief are outside their scope. In particular they avoid giving money which will relieve communities from their responsibility as regards everyday charitable work. The Russell Sage Foundation is concerned chiefly with consultative and reference work.

Other foundations do a vast amount of social work, but chiefly as temporary partners with other voluntary and with official organisations, thus stimulating and promoting great extension of their work.

THE ROCKEFELLER GROUP

The Rockefeller Foundation was established by John D.

Rockefeller in 1913. Its Foundation Principal Fund in December 1933 exceeded 153 million dollars and the balance available to meet appropriations, pledges, and authorisations at the same date exceeded 40 million dollars. The object of the Foundation was "the well-being of mankind throughout the world," and in pursuance of this object the Foundation has devoted a large part of its vast capital and income to the promotion of public health.

The Foundation has trained a corps of qualified health administrators and has given generous grants, not only in supporting students of many nations during their training for public health work, but still more has created and endowed institutions at which this training is carried out. Of these the most important are the Schools of Hygiene in Johns Hopkins University, Baltimore, Md., in Harvard University, Boston, Mass., and in London, England. Important grants have been given in aid of medical education in many parts of the world, the object kept in view being to "permeate the curriculum with the preventive idea." In fostering this ideal the teaching of the pre-medical sciences, biology, chemistry, and physics, has been aided; and, on the medical side, important endowments have been given to promote the training of nurses, especially public health nurses.

The earlier work of the Rockefeller endowment was devoted to the subjugation of Hookworm Disease in the southern States of America and in other lands. The romantic story of the great international work accomplished in this special field of public health is outlined in Chapter XXXVII. It was organised in 1909 by the *International Health Board*, the forerunner of the Foundation, and the success of its work led to the endowment of the more extensive work of the Rockefeller Foundation in May 1913.

During and after the Great War the Rockefeller Foundation did much to promote improved health administration, especially as affecting children, and the prevention of tuberculosis in various countries of Europe. In visiting continental cities I had the privilege in the year 1924 of meeting American medical officers of the Rockefeller Foundation, who were engaged year by year in this work in Paris, Montpelier, and other French towns, and in Prague, Warsaw, and some other European cities. Some particulars of their work are given in my *International Studies on the Relation between the Private and Official Practice of Medicine* (1928).

In the year 1934, the Rockefeller Foundation revised its programme of work and in an earlier year, 1929, it had, while continuing its work in public health, laid increasing stress on assisting, without particular limitation, "the advancement of knowledge in the fields of medical science, natural science, social science, and the humanities." A smaller proportion of its total funds began to be appropriated for medical research and more "to the advancement of certain definite sub-fields of knowledge" for which there seemed to be special need. Public health work is being continued, both by its field and laboratory staffs, and assistance for the control of disease, including assistance to governmental activities and for the training of personnel, is being continued. A major interest is now taken in the support of research concerning mental health. Evidently the Board of the Foundation is being attracted also to fundamental economic problems; and as a member of the Board of Governors of the London School of Economics I have witnessed the valuable aid given to economic and allied research undertaken by members of the staff of that school.

But from the strictly public health point of view, the work of the Rockefeller Foundation in the prevention of hookworm disease, of malaria, and of yellow fever has been especially important (see Chapters XXXVI and XXXVII).

THE MILBANK MEMORIAL FUND

As during several years I spent much time in studying and reporting on the special work of the Milbank Fund, I give a rather fuller account of its activities.

The Milbank Fund soon after the War had an endowment bringing in an annual income of about 500,000 dollars, which was being spent largely in "public health demonstrations." Its work up to April 1935 was under the able leadership of its general secretary, Mr. John A. Kingsbury, LL.D., whose driving power and skill in securing collaboration from distinguished physicians, hygienists, and social leaders brought rapid success to the tasks that were undertaken. The Milbank Fund has been concerned with social pioneering, and this meant not only blazing trails for extended work in the promotion of human health and welfare, but also much investigation directed to the extension of the borderland of knowledge. By this combined attack on specific problems, not only has the volume of ordinary administrative public health work been increased but also the possibility of new work to the same end has been created.

Up to 1929, the 25th Anniversary Year of its work, the Milbank Fund had aided some 131 organisations and projects, over two-thirds of the money expended having been in the field of public health. Nearly two million dollars at that date had been spent in maintaining and extending public health programmes in the three New York State communities which had been selected as demonstration centres.

The special work which characterised the Fund during a series of years consisted in the establishment of "Demonstrations" of improved public health work in certain selected towns and rural areas. Hermann M. Biggs, William H. Welch, and other distinguished men shared in the framing of schemes for this programme, and the general principle of action was that there should be initiated a partnership for five years or longer between the Fund and the selected public health authorities, the Fund furnishing monetary aid and an increased staff when required, so that in each selected area relatively complete public health work might be initiated and continued. The hope, fulfilled in the selected areas, was that the local authorities concerned would, when the partnership terminated, continue their improved and extended public health administration without external financial help.

Of the three demonstration areas, one was in a city in the central part of the State, Syracuse, one in a rural district, Cattaraugus County, and one in a special district of New York City. My observations in this chapter relate to my visits to the two first-named centres. In 1926, midway in the first five years of experimental work, I was asked to visit these centres and report on their work. I described the fourfold intent of each demonstration as being

1. To raise the local standard of public health administration to the highest degree of efficiency practicable:
2. By local experimentation in different aspects of administrative work to "test out" the methods which will secure the maximum effect for a given expenditure of money, time, and human effort:
3. To demonstrate to the local authorities concerned, and to the general public represented by them, the benefits which accrue from efficient and complete sanitary work; and, incidentally,
4. Thus to stimulate more rapid development of similar work in other cities and counties and even more widely than this.

The local authorities were the willing partners of the extended local work, and the chief responsibility for its success rested with them.

All previous demonstrations of American Foundations, so far as I know, had been concerned with the promotion of special items of public health work, as the prevention of tuberculosis, malaria, hookworm disease, etc. The programme of the Milbank demonstrations embraced the whole of local health administration, and was carried out in intimate affiliation with existing local official and voluntary effort having the same aim. Each demonstration operated in a setting of official agencies, and was so organised as to strengthen and not to supersede these.

The method adopted was gradually to increase staff and agencies in the light of advancing experience, thus increasing the probability that the local official and voluntary agencies would continue on an extended scale. The Cattaraugus work was pioneer in New York State, this county being the first in a rural area in that State in which a full-time unit of professionally qualified personnel was appointed. Previously such officers had been limited to a few cities in the State. The comprehensive scope of the demonstrations I regarded as specially commendable, for, to quote my report, "no branch of public health work can be satisfactorily executed without aid from collateral branches of public health work."

I revisited these two provincial demonstrations in May 1928, and then reported on the advances made during the two years' interval between my visits.

For the reason set out in a following paragraph I need not further describe the important work done at Syracuse by Dr. H. G. Weiskotten, Dean of the Medical School of Syracuse University, and then by Dr. G. C. Ruhland, who were successively Health Commissioners of Syracuse, or that done in Cattaraugus County by Dr. R. M. Attwater, its chief medical officer, and that of their coadjutors.

When, after ten years, the demonstrations ceased, a complete survey was undertaken of accomplishments in Syracuse and in Cattaraugus by Professor C. E. A. Winslow and a staff of expert collaborators. This is described in two volumes, *A City on a Hill* (Doubleday), and *Health on the Farm and in the Village* (Macmillan Co.), which give full particulars of the work accomplished.

MEDICAL PRACTITIONERS AND THE CATTARAUGUS
    DEMONSTRATION

But I must refer to the cloud which arose from the objection of a few medical practitioners to the giving of medical advice by official doctors; for my comments on this subject were among the factors which led the Milbank Fund in a later year to invite me to undertake a wider investigation of the relation between the private and the public practice of medicine, which is described in Chapters XXXIX to XLV. When I made my second visit to Cattaraugus in May 1928, I heard both sides of a controversy which had arisen, threatening the success of part of the work of the demonstration. The circumstances of this controversy are fully set out in Professor Winslow's volume. It did not seriously affect the work of the demonstration. I was able to recommend that the Milbank Fund should ignore the attacks made in the public Press in various parts of New York State, inspired by local associations run by small groups of disgruntled medical practitioners. This course was followed, and the demonstration successfully completed its ten years' work. At the time I remember making the remark in private conversation that sometimes physicians engaged in private practice were the chief enemies of public health progress on its personal side. My past experience had occasionally illustrated this one-sided truth, and the controversy in Cattaraugus County confirmed it, though my later experience had shown how in Britain this difficulty had largely disappeared. (See for instance pp. 365 and 366.) In the United States the earlier British difficulty was being exemplified in 1928. Two grievances emerged in this localised "storm in a teacup." There was objection to "dictation of lay bodies"; and in this respect the fundamental difference between general administration and the actual technique of medical care was being ignored. (On this see p. 373.) Then there was the cry of encroachment on the sphere of private medical practice, although there had been scrupulous care to avoid this. It had appeared to me that caution in this respect had been excessive.

This temporary disturbance, as I have said, played a part in determining the laborious task of survey of medical work in various European countries (see p. 347) which occupied me during several successive years, and this circumstance makes the comment written at this point an appropriate introduction to Part III of this volume.

CHAPTER XXXV

THE STORY OF "PROHIBITION" IN THE UNITED STATES OF AMERICA

IN other chapters it is my pleasant task to tell my experiences of some important branches of public health administration in which the United States have led the way for other countries, and to describe my memories of American leaders in Preventive Medicine, who have passed to the great majority, or who, like myself, are near the margin of terrestrial life. I have also tried to outline faithfully some defects of American government. Among these a leading place must be given to the legislation securing "prohibition" throughout the States and the lamentable failure in its enforcement, through lack of support of the same public who had voted for it. After this failure, cancellation of the national action previously taken with deliberation appeared to be the only practicable action, and this course was adopted. The alternative of persistent Federal attempt to make prohibition effective, in the face of active or passive opposition on the part of many, if not most, of the governing bodies of the forty-eight "sovereign" States, was outside the range of practicability.

It is commonly assumed that prohibition was hastily enforced under the influence of the emotions of war; but, after detailed examination of the obstacles which had to be encountered in securing prohibition, I came to the conclusion that it was the deliberate and slowly-arrived-at determination of the vast mass of the American people, so far as this is represented in those elected as its representatives on the State legislatures.

Indeed I wrote (for reference see p. 306):

> For Americans prohibition is a means to secure liberation from a great slavery; and if the will of the people remains constant, then America will have successfully carried through a bold and momentous experiment in social reform.

But when resolutions and enactments needed to be transformed into executive action for their enforcement, it became clear that the majority of the people had agreed to prohibition only in the spirit of the legislator who was willing to pass laws, but drew the line at having them enforced.

The whole story is worth re-telling in a condensed form. It emphasises the distinction, too often forgotten, between consenting to what was in some measure emotional law-making, and in large measure concession to the persistent pressure of active and almost fanatical prohibitionists: this on the one hand; and on the other hand willingness to keep the promises registered in personal votes.

Let me first summarise the action which led to prohibition.

The following particulars are taken from my brochure which was published by P. S. King & Son, London, in 1921, entitled *Prohibition in America and its Relation to the Problem of Public Control*, 1921. This had a large sale and was reprinted in 1922. It had been given in a shortened form as the Norman Kerr lecture before the Society for the Study of Inebriety in October 1921.

It must be generally agreed that alcoholic excess has been and, to a less extent, still is a national curse in most Western countries, and I remind the reader that in nearly all these countries various measures intended to restrict the sale of alcoholic drinks are enforced. Britain is one of the best examples of considerable success in measures of restriction, by high taxation, by limiting hours of sale of these drinks, and by restricting the number of public-houses or saloons at which they are sold.

The practical question for social well-wishers is, therefore, not whether there should be restrictions or prohibitions, but how far restrictive measures should go.

For many years the movement in America in favour of voluntary total abstinence had been very strong, but early in the abstinence campaign its advocacy had passed beyond the stage of the educational efforts of various societies, and there had been engrafted on it the determination to shut up saloons. These, it was notorious, were centres of drunkenness and other forms of vice, and were the local headquarters of corrupt "politics." Britain, sharing largely America's abhorrence of excessive facilities for drinking, has, as indicated above, slowly adopted coercive measures of an indirect kind, but American reformers were not content with these—they did not try them very generally—and the evils of excessive drinking remained rampant, much more so than in Britain, though in the latter country there still continues much excessive drinking in some sections of society. The States could not easily follow Britain's example of increasing taxation and of restriction of facilities for the sale of drink; for there are forty-eight Sovereign States, each a law unto itself, each with its own separate system of taxation.

Individual States, however, decided in favour of total prohibition of the sale of alcoholic drinks within their borders, the first being Maine in 1846. Other States slowly followed. Under the compulsion of public opinion, State after State tried prohibition, sometimes first for limited areas and then for the entire State. Some of these States revoked prohibition after a trial period and some of them resumed it after a lapse.

As I stated in 1921:

Prohibition has for some eighty years been the policy of a section of the American public; this policy has found favour with a steadily increasing proportion of the total population; and it has eventually culminated in the National Prohibition Act of 1920.

When this Act was passed, nearly half the total population of the United States was living under local or State prohibition, and prohibition was enforced in sections of a large number of additional States. Thus America had already travelled far on the way to national prohibition. The Great War undoubtedly hastened nationalisation of American prohibition by the only possible immediate method, namely by an amendment to the Federal Constitution. Looking back one may regret that the slow process of conversion of community after community and State after State to prohibition was not allowed to continue; for each additional State converted to prohibition must have reduced to that extent the smuggling and transmission of liquor by post which continued to make State prohibition an imperfect means of prohibition.

The hastened national movement was doubtless expedited by the Great War, and by the example of anti-alcoholic action in Europe. The sale of absinthe had been prohibited in France from the beginning of the War; a few weeks later the sale of vodka had been prohibited in Russia, and gradually in Britain the consumption of alcoholic liquors became extremely restricted, by methods which I have described elsewhere.[1]

The American steps to secure prohibition by Federal action were as follows:

At Washington the House of Representatives in December 1914 took the initial step to secure an amendment to the Constitution without which no Federal action was possible. They decided that a resolution proposing a prohibition amendment of the Constitution should be submitted (as required by the American Constitution) to the vote of each State, and in August 1917 this was agreed to by the Upper House (the Federal Senate). This initial step was secured under the stress of energetic lobbying on the part of prohibitionists, who were more importunate than the scriptural widow. The resolution may have accorded with the convictions of the majority in the two Federal Legislatures, or it may be that they were "passing the buck" to the State Legislatures, in the hope that these would refuse the necessary majority for an amendment of the Constitution. To enable the proposal to come back (in accordance with the Constitution) to the Federal Congress and Senate, three-fourths of the forty-eight State Legislatures (two Chambers in each of them) must ratify it. Within fourteen months forty-five out of the forty-eight States had formally approved, nearly always by very large majorities. These included a vast majority of the total population of the United States. Note, there was nothing precipitate in these stages. The provisions of the Constitution amply provided against hurried or fevered action. In accordance with constitutional procedure the proposal was returned to the Federal House of Representatives, which passed the National Prohibition Act in July 1919 by 287 to 100; and in September of the same year it was passed by the Senate without a roll-call.

President Wilson favoured local option and he vetoed the

---

[1] See chapter on "The Story of Alcoholic Control in Great Britain" in my *Public Health Problems in Organised Society* (P. S. King & Son, 1927).

Bill, but the two Federal Houses by large majorities forthwith passed the measure over the President's veto. The facts do not support the view that prohibition became law solely as the result of an hysterical attack of temporary duration, though this element was present.

I was in Balitmore at the time of the Presidential election of 1921, and heard both Harding and Cox, the two Presidential candidates, address public meetings. Each of them pledged himself, if elected, to enforce the new 18th amendment to the Constitution. This could scarcely have happened had the majority of the people been opposed to its principle. The elected candidate, Senator Harding, went so far as to say:

> In another generation I believe that liquor will have disappeared not merely from our politics but from our memories.

Already the abolition of the saloon had shattered its power as a vote-getting and vote-influencing agency.

It is only by remembering these historical facts that one can judge the sinister significance of subsequent events.

At first there was a wonderful moral transformation, seen best in great cities like New York. I can remember being conducted around empty wards of the largest municipal New York hospital reserved for "week-end drunks." These in previous years had been filled with patients with delirium tremens and the like. Arrests for drunkenness dramatically declined and the traffic in drink, which had been described by the United States Supreme Court as "the most prolific source of insanity, pauperism, vice and crime," became for a while a subterranean dribble in contrast to the vast stream of previous years. I need not give detailed evidence: the facts are beyond doubt.

Many influences had combined to bring about National Prohibition. Foremost came the activities of the Anti-Saloon League in each State. The militant propagandism of this body was pushed to an extreme, and I think to an unjustified extent. As happened in England with the militant methods of Female Suffragists, some politicians were doubtless unwillingly induced to support prohibition.

An energetic minority can turn an election on almost any

social problem, if this minority is determined to sacrifice every other to this one consideration. Such lopsided mentalities constitute a menace to steadily successful democratic government.

I do not suggest that a minority vote carried prohibition; but it may be that the will of such a minority coerced the will of a large proportion of the total population.

Other factors conduced to the same end. For many years anti-alcoholic teaching had been given in elementary schools, and the desire for "clean politics" uninfluenced by saloons led many to vote for prohibition who were only actively concerned to get rid of saloons, which

corrupted elections, debauched voters, and debased many legislatures and their officials.

The American Medical Association helped by passing a resolution that not only did they oppose the use of alcohol as a beverage, but discouraged the use of alcohol as a therapeutic agent. The desire for increased industrial efficiency for employers of labour was a powerful motive in favour of prohibition; and Southern States were influenced in favour of it by the desire "to save white women from negroes inflamed by drink." The partial failure of prohibition in individual States, owing to smuggling of spirits from other States, was a further further motive for making prohibition nation-wide.

I cannot detail the stages of decline in the efficiency of prohibition. There was rapidly organised a gigantic system of smuggling spirits across the vast continental borders of the States, and from overseas. Vast numbers of people, who must have voted for prohibition, employed a "bootlegger" to supply them with drink. They had wished to apply prohibition to others, but for themselves the bootlegger.

At one time the spirits supplied often contained methyl alcohol and many people were permanently blinded or were killed by this vile stuff.

Wherever one went, after the two first years of prohibition, one saw evidence of illicit supplies of whiskey and wines and beer of high alcoholic content. In some circles it became "good form" to break the law. Students at some Universities carried flasks and young ladies going to balls were expected, it was said, to carry a flask for their beaux.

Attempts to enforce the law were largely ineffectual. Sometimes State officials refused to help and only Federal prosecution was possible. It was worth while to corrupt police agents and this was done by bootleggers on a gigantic scale. Reputable members of the community, including many legislators who had voted for prohibition, connived at breaking the law and thus a spirit of lawlessness not only in regard to smuggling of drink, but also as to the law in general became very widely prevalent.

LAWLESSNESS IN U.S.A.

It would, however, be erroneous to ascribe the widespread lawlessness in America solely to the evil influence of anti-prohibition. Vast moral injury was inflicted on the community by the law-breaking, bribery, corruption and actual crime which went with bootlegging; but it is fair to remember that Americans had, so to speak, habituated themselves to legislation on various subjects which was seldom enforced, or in connection with which the process of enforcement when attempted was hopelessly slow and uncertain.

Much of America's failure to secure orderly and general compliance with laws is of old-standing. In its pioneer days people living in remote parts had to "take the law into their own hands." Like the rebuilders of Jerusalem they required to hold a sword in one hand and a trowel or an axe or a spade in the other. And in mining camps, lynch law was sometimes the only available form of justice. It had the drawback that the wrong person might be hanged: and this applies still more to the occasional occurrence, even now, in certain States of lynching of negroes. In the latter case lynching is merely a manifestation of mob fury, anticipating and sometimes thwarting the course of available justice. The only flimsy excuse for it which can sometimes be advanced is the uncertainty and terrible delays in legal processes.

The abuses of local and central government by interested persons, seeking concessions and monopolies, which will enable them to "bleed" the suffering public by legalised means, are too well known to need description. These abuses are not special to any one country: in the past they have prevailed in England; and wherever they occur they can only be controlled by constant vigilance and action on the part of the honest majority of the community. These past abuses and corruption in public life cannot be disconnected from the racketeering which has been rampant in recent years in American city life. Bootlegging extended to an indefinite extent the possibilities of racketeering: it vastly increased the possibilities of ungodly gain. But racketeering existed prior to bootlegging; and apart from deep-seated and extensive reform it will continue, even were the taxation on alcoholic drinks reduced almost to nil and the profits of bootlegging were correspondingly reduced. With bootlegging commonly goes racketeering in other trades. It is terrible to think that, in some cities, a milk vendor or other trader may only be able to pay his way and continue his trade if he gives a monthly or quarterly sum to the racketeer who monopolises to himself that particular district or trade. By this means the tradesman is insured against interference in his reduced earnings. Occasionally the curtain is lifted and one discovers that two racketeers have quarrelled over their respective territories and have settled their differences by means of machine guns.

So in attributing blame to prohibition it becomes necessary to remember that, while prohibition gave greatly increased temptations and opportunities for lawlessness and violence, it did not originate these evils.

It can, I think, be contended justifiably that a large part of America and its population are still in the pioneer stage of development. America has been described as a "melting-pot" of the nations and the melting is still incomplete.

I give no statistics; but one cannot visit the great cities of the States without learning that they have, usually in segregated sections, thousands and tens of thousands of European immigrants and their children, who still speak Italian, Polish, Czech, Hungarian, Russian, Yiddish, and other languages. This is in addition to the large German and Scandinavian sections of America. These immigrants have their own newspapers; most of them have never enjoyed freedom and a representative government in their country of origin. As soon as possible, they are made American citizens by the active help of political ward "bosses," they are shepherded to the polling booths, instructed how to vote, and it is made "worth their while" by the giving of jobs or charitable help at the public expense, after the ward "boss" has himself received his greater political reward in the shape of a job or in cash.

To complete the story, it should be stated that prohibition was repealed by a like procedure culminating in the 21st Amendment to the Constitution (December 5, 1933). This reversal of policy does not imply that in the forty-eight States alcoholic drinks can now be sold or purchased. A State which remains "dry" by its own independent action is protected against the importation of intoxicating liquors from "wet" areas; but postal and other possibilities make this protection imperfect. The position has reverted to what held good before the introduction of Federal Prohibition in 1920. Various modified systems of restriction of sales are being tried in different States.

In the preceding pages I have refrained from discussing the underlying objection on the part of many to prohibition. This would be embodied in a negative answer to the following question:

Is Compulsion justifiable as regards Personal Habits?

I have discussed this problem in my brochure on *Prohibition in America* (P. S. King & Son, 1921), and perhaps with greater exactitude in three chapters of my *Health Problems in Organised Society* (P. S. King & Son, 1924), entitled:

The Relative Roles of Compulsion and Education in Public Health Work;
Consideration on the Relation between Government and Conduct;
The Limitations of Liberty in Communal Life;

also part of the chapter in the same volume on "Compulsory Insurance against Life's Contingencies" bears on the same problem.

In modern insurance schemes in many European countries, a large proportion of the total population are now compelled to make provision week by week for the contingencies of sickness, unemployment, old age, and for pensions for dependents.

We may agree that the end of all government is to make government superfluous, but this ideal will only be attained when every single person is imbued with the spirit of the two Great Commandments.

In the modern world views of liberty have necessarily been modified, as aggregation in communities has increased; and, in particular, compulsion has been exercised to protect women and children, the tenants of insanitary houses, those engaged in dangerous occupations, sick persons, etc. In these and like respects, as I have said

it becomes possible to realise that coercion may be and often is a channel or avenue to greater liberty, to liberation from bondage, whether economic, social, family, or personal.

Whether these considerations justified the temporary enforcement of prohibition in the States is still debatable, but that a large measure of compulsion is called for in regard to alcoholic restrictions is shown by the experience of restrictive enactments in most civilised countries. I may conclude this imperfect sketch of an important subject by an extract from page 123 of my *Health Problems in Organised Society*, 1927.

During the Great War in England the amount of drink was severely rationed, its alcoholic content was greatly reduced, the hours during which it could be bought or consumed in public houses were reduced and the intervals lengthened; and, furthermore, treating became illegal; and the result was seen in a remarkable reduction in the number of deaths from alcoholism in women and in offences due to drunkenness. *Once for all* it was *demonstrated that a country can be made sober by Act of Parliament.* Since the War these restrictions have been reduced, with increase of drunkenness and disease. . . .

PERSONAL CONTRIBUTIONS

Those wishing to "hear further" concerning Prohibition and the general problem of Compulsion in Communal Life can consult the volumes already mentioned in this chapter. The following further contributions by me are noted.

New Light on the Drink Problem. (*Contemporary Review*, April 1924.)
The Social Aspects of the Alcohol Problem. (*Revue Internationale contre l'Alcoolisme*, 1925, and *Practitioner*, October 1924.)

CHAPTER XXXVI

OUTSTANDING AMERICAN ACHIEVEMENTS IN PUBLIC HEALTH

IT is impracticable for me to describe each of the aspects of advanced public health administration in which America excels. I must content myself with three illustrations. Did not considerations of space forbid, I should write further, for instance, on the great work accomplished in safeguarding public water supplies, the early and extended use of laboratory aids to diagnosis and prevention of disease, the extensive employment of public health nurses, the success in reducing infant mortality, and the (I think) unexampled extent to which in American cities the hospital care of childbirth and of total disease is being employed.

In this chapter I give three examples of American pioneer public health work and in the next chapter three examples of similar work directed to the prevention of great scourges—one, Texas fever in cattle, and two, yellow fever and hookworm disease, equally serious for mankind.

TUBERCULOSIS

In the space at my disposal I cannot hope to do justice to the remarkable success of the anti-tuberculosis campaign in the United States, and can only indicate some outstanding points.

There are striking differences between the organisation of preventive measures against tuberculosis in Britain and in the United States. In both of them voluntary efforts have taken an important part in the initiation of this work, but these voluntary efforts have always occupied a less important place in Britain than official work, while in the States the converse has been true. This is true even when we bear in mind the pioneer official work of Hermann Biggs in New York, and recall the voluntary efforts of a number of tuberculosis dispensaries in England and Scotland, before these were taken over by local authorities. In the United States no such rapid supersession of voluntary by official dispensary and sanatorium work occurred. Each of its forty-eight States is a law to itself; State and still more federal control is limited in extent; and one realises with admiration the persistence and national extent of the great work which the American National Tuberculosis Association has accomplished. This does not mean that the leaders of the great voluntary anti-tuberculosis work in America do not realise the need for increased official effort. Thus Dr. Charles J. Hatfield is quoted by Dr. P. P. Jacobs in his work on *The Control of Tuberculosis in the United States* (published by the Nat. Tuberc. Assoc., 1932) as saying:

We must start with complete acceptance of the fact that the duly appointed health officer is the sole agent responsible for the health of the territory he represents. . . .

(But) In most places officials and official action are not yet perfect; the public is not yet thoroughly aroused and educated; and we must admit that any aid toward the desired end is welcome, provided it is worked into the general plan.

The relationship between official and voluntary agencies, and between them and the family doctor, who may be said to occupy a key position, is illustrated in the following further quotations:

The public health department must understand that there is no aspect of public health more important to the community than the marshalling of all forces, lay and medical, public and private, into a single attack on local problems.

This was the testimony of the late Dr. Linsley Williams, who had wide experience of both official and voluntary work; and in the same number of the report of the Milbank Memorial Fund (p. xi, 1929) Mr. John A. Kingsbury, LL.D., then Secretary of the Fund, stated that

no persons and no agencies can take the place of the family physicians . . . (they would) be the last to sanction or to promulgate measures that would threaten the future of the family physician, for by so doing they would defeat their own ends.

I have had the good fortune to meet many of the leaders who have guided anti-tuberculosis work in the States. Trudeau

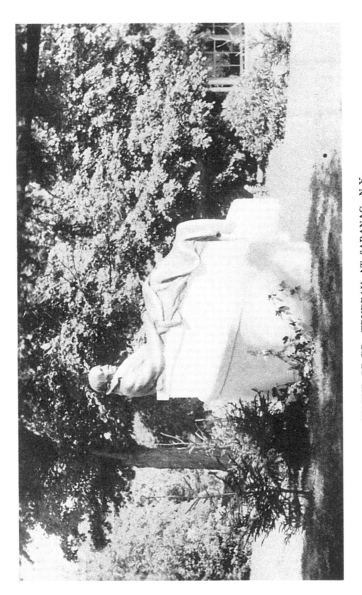

STATUE OF DR. TRUDEAU AT SARANAC, N.Y.

only in public; but Dr. V. Y. Bowditch in Boston where in 1908 I saw one of the earliest State Sanatoria; and Dr. Lawrence F. Flick, when I was conducted by him over the first institute for tuberculosis research in America, the Henry Phipps Institute in Philadelphia.

Nor must I omit to refer to the anti-tuberculosis work of Homer Folks and the State Charities Aid Association of New York. We have reason to be grateful for his frequent public reminder that the mere fact of the tuberculosis death-rate being now not more than a third of what it was, is still consistent with tuberculosis remaining a chief cause of invalidism, death, widows, and orphans, and of social dependence; and that we cannot afford to rest contented until we are in sight of complete conquest over this chief enemy of mankind.

My Baltimore friend Dr. P. P. Jacobs has reminded us that, aided by the Russell Sage Foundation in 1907, Folks was "able to organise under the State Charities Aid Association of New York the first comprehensive State-wide campaign against tuberculosis, setting up a model followed by most of the States of the Union." This tuberculosis campaign has been carried on in close co-operation with both city and State authorities in New York State.

If I do not further detail the educational work of the National Tuberculosis Association it is not for lack of recognition of its value.

On page 245 I mentioned my visit to Saranac. In this mountain village began the earliest sanatorium work in the States. E. C. Trudeau, a young consumptive doctor, was sent to winter in the Adirondacks in 1873. There while enduring the rigour of its winter climate and, when his improved health enabled him, sharing its hunting and out-of-door life, he started a small cottage sanatorium, following the methods of rest in the open air as recommended by Brehmer and Dettweiler. The sanatorium grew in size and reputation, and gradually the whole of the village of Saranac became almost its annexe. Laboratory investigations were undertaken, and under the direction of Baldwin and Lawrason Brown in more recent years these investigations have added much to our knowledge of tuberculosis. A yearly School of Tuberculosis drew many doctors in the summer months, and in 1919 I had the honour of taking a small part in its work (p. 245).

When I met Trudeau in 1908 at Washington his course was nearly run; but it was pleasant to observe, in that great international Tuberculosis Congress, how he was greeted almost with reverence, and the pleasure with which this greeting brightened up his emaciated countenance.

In 1916 a significant experiment under the leadership of Dr. Armstrong was inaugurated in Framingham, a small town in Massachusetts, in the detection of unrecognised cases of tuberculosis and in bringing them to treatment. The expense of the Framingham Demonstration was borne by the Metropolitan Life Insurance Company of New York, and the experiment showed how much good can be achieved when all practising doctors and the general public can be induced to co-operate to this end.

In Cattaraugus County in 1922 I saw similar work being done, aided by grants from the Milbank Memorial Fund. Overlooked cases were found, early diagnosis was facilitated by the free provision of an X-ray service for all practitioners, and incidentally—as everywhere when an effective anti-tuberculosis programme is carried through—general public health work also greatly improved. This has been so wherever tuberculosis work, educational, sanitary, and medical, has succeeded, and not the least gain in the modern tuberculosis campaign lies in this fact.

On the important role in their anti-tuberculosis work played in the States by large-scale efforts to secure the hospital segregation of advanced and bed-ridden consumptives, see page 129. I add here the following additional quotation bearing on this point, as it has autobiographical interest.

Dr. Jacobs (*op. cit.*, p. 21) states that at the International Congress on Tuberculosis, Washington, 1908,

the fundamental elements of the program were derived largely from the work of Biggs and Philip in the preceding two decades; Sir Arthur Newsholme's classical paper at the International Congress, urging the necessity of hospitals for advanced cases as the most immediate step necessary for the reduction of the death-rate, also had great influence.

The conclusion reached by Dr. H. W. Hill (*The Epidemiology of Tuberculosis in the Human*, B.C. Provincial Board of Health, 1931) was to the effect that

the crucial factor in the control of the disease is the prevention of massive infection, a conclusion which, as I have always urged, is fundamentally important in public health administration.

This general conclusion would now, I believe, be accepted by all hygienists, though it is still not universally conceded that the prevention of massive infection has been in past history, as it is now, of primary importance.

IMMUNISATION AGAINST DIPHTHERIA

This is perhaps the most outstanding example of advanced public health work in the United States.

In my *Fifty Years in Public Health* (pp. 189 *et seq.*) I have described how very early practical action was taken in New York and some other American cities to utilise bacteriological means for the diagnosis of diphtheria, and for ascertaining the duration of infectivity in patients convalescent from it.

Hermann M. Biggs and W. H. Park were responsible for the very early work in this connection in New York.

It remains to describe the application of the more recently acquired knowledge as to immunisation against attack by diphtheria. By subcutaneous administration of a carefully adjusted mixture of the toxin and the antitoxin of diphtheria it is possible to produce immunity against an attack of diphtheria comparable to the immunity conferred by an actual attack of this disease. In recent years toxoid or alum-precipitated toxoid has been generally employed. Action on these lines has been pursued with vigour by American public health authorities, and on a scale large enough to produce a remarkable decrease in the total incidence of diphtheria and in deaths from this disease.

Official health authorities have been the chief pioneers in this work, but its large-scale success has been ensured by the active co-operation of various voluntary bodies.

The death-rate from diphtheria in the years 1880 to 1935 in New York City is shown in the chart on p. 320, reproduced from the Statistical Bulletin of the Metropolitan Life Insurance Company for September 1935.

Even if we remind ourselves that some of this steady reduction of the diphtheria death-rate may be due to diminution of imperfectly known factors which, apart from personal infection, favour epidemics or even pandemics of this disease, it cannot be

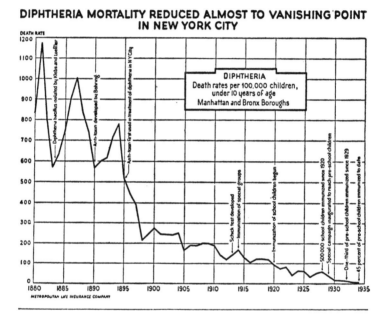

DIPHTHERIA MORTALITY REDUCED ALMOST TO VANISHING POINT IN NEW YORK CITY

seriously doubted that a new factor, that of valuable human intervention, has been the chief reason for the recent reduction of diphtheria in New York almost to vanishing point.

The experimental work by Dr. W. H. Park, first on special groups of children in New York, then more generally among all the school children, was followed in 1929 by the foundation of a Special Diphtheria Prevention Commission, with a view to a more intensive effort to persuade parents to submit their children to artificial immunisation. The campaign was so successful that in 1934 it was estimated that 45 per cent of all pre-school children had received prophylactic injections since the special campaign began. As Dr. Shirley W. Wynne, the then Commissioner of Health for New York City, wrote: "hand in hand with the increase in the proportion of the immunised children there has been a decline in the mortality caused by diphtheria."

The campaign was skilfully arranged and the co-operation of the medical profession was secured. The results in the different boroughs in New York were published in such a way as to excite wholesome rivalry between them. Social agencies, religious groups, the Press, and educational bodies generally were induced to co-operate. Public notices were exhibited in ten different languages. Doctors issued warning slips to their patients, and doctors were paid a fee for each immunisation carried out by them. The total cost of the campaign was about $85,000, half of which came out of the budget of the Health Department, $40,000 was contributed by the Milbank Foundation, and $4,000 by the Metropolitan Life Insurance Company. Dr. Wynne, writing at the end of the campaign, said: "in five years I hope we shall have practically wiped out diphtheria in New York City."

Equally good work had been done in other American cities and I could cite at least six cities, including Syracuse and Salt Lake City, in which in 1934 there was not a single death from diphtheria among children.

Probably the difficulty will be to continue for an indefinite period to secure immunisation of all young children in the first few years of their life. If the effort and fervour illustrated in the above campaign can be maintained in every community diphtheria need never become prevalent. Will this be done?

In Britain there has been similar work, but in no part of this country on a scale to secure the immunisation of so large a proportion of the total children as in some American cities.

(Fuller particulars as to "The History of Diphtheria in New York City" are given by Dr. William H. Park in *American Journal of Diseases of Children*, December 1931.)

SAFEGUARDING OF MILK SUPPLIES

In regard to this elementary hygienic need, it must be confessed that Britain is still behind some other countries, and especially behind the United States, in the protection secured

L

for the milk supplies of its great towns. This is so in each of the problems concerned in this protection to milk at its source, during its importation into large towns and in its final distribution. I have frequently suffered friendly gibes from American friends as regards the sale of "loose" milk in England, and the absence of general regulations for pasteurisation. I have only been able to plead, that although no town in Britain, as yet, possesses legal power to insist on pasteurisation of milk before distribution, this condition in practice is fulfilled, because most of the milk entering large towns is supplied by large collecting and distributing companies, who find it to their advantage to pasteurise the milk collected by them before sending it into the town. I have also asked my American friends whether the admirable safeguards for city milk are practised in the vast rural areas of the American Continent. So far as I can ascertain this is not done to the extent that is desirable.

Gradually hygienists in most countries have arrived at the conclusion that uncooked cow's milk is not a safe food for either adults or children. So far as I know, Chicago, in 1908, acting on the advice of Dr. Evans, its Health Commissioner, was the first American municipality to insist on all milk supplied to its inhabitants being pasteurised, except milk which had been derived from cows proved to be free from tuberculosis.

Nathan Straus in 1893 had organised in New York on voluntary lines the provision of a large amount of sterilised milk for children from milk stations. I cannot detail here the stages of American provisions for safeguarding milk, including the movement initiated by Dr. Coit for certified milk. In 1903 W. H. Park and Emmett Holt published investigations which gave an impetus to the movement in favour of pasteurisation. In 1906 Rosenau's important work was published on the thermal death-point of pathogenic bacteria in milk, and in the same year North suggested the abolition of the "flash method" of pasteurisation of milk and the substitution of the "holding. method." In 1912 New York City adopted milk regulations requiring pasteurisation of milk. (As to legal powers for enforcing this see p. 287.)

I recall being told by Dr. Emmett Holt, I think in 1919, that in his Infants' Hospital the highest grading of milk did not adequately protect infant patients against diarrhoeal and other infections by milk; and that it had been found desirable to pasteurise the high grade milk supplied to patients.

I can only allude in passing to the widespread efforts made in America to eliminate bovine tuberculosis from herds of cattle.

In Baltimore, Md., except for 1·5 per cent of the total supply, which is exempted as of very special quality, the whole of its milk is pasteurised.

The commercially pasteurised milk supply in most cities has improved greatly during the last twenty years, certified pasteurised milk having become not much more desirable than ordinary pasteurised milk. Dr. Huntington Williams, Health Commissioner of Baltimore, informs me that now about thirty-eight American cities by local ordinance require the pasteurisation of all milk sold within the city, with the exception of certified milk. In some small Southern cities the sale of raw milk still continues almost exclusively, and in other places various gradations are found between this and pasteurisation of the entire milk supply.

In England the greater part of the milk supplied to London and the larger towns is pasteurised by the great milk companies which control its distribution. In smaller towns and in country villages of England there is still much unsatisfactory distribution of unprotected milk. Whether this is so in the United States I cannot state.

"MILK SCANDALS"

The enterprise of the public Press is universally, though sometimes ruefully, recognised, and one must give first place to the American Press. Their ability to ferret out scandals is familiar to us all; and it may be that, on balance, this work is both salutary and sanatory. One could desire that zeal were always more intimately associated with accuracy. While I was in the States in 1926 much newspaper writing was devoted to bribery and "milk rackets" in New York. It was alleged that milk inspectors of the city had taken bribes to accept milk coming into the city from unauthorised sources. The matter was exhaustively investigated by Dr. Louis I. Harris, who was then City Health Commissioner. Several employees who had accepted bribes were dismissed and a secretary in the department concerned was sent to prison. Prompt justice was enforced as soon as the evil was discovered. The bribery arose out of the strict regulations of the city. The Department of Health cannot enforce regulations outside the city, but they can embargo milk and milk products on arrival if they have come from dairy farms and plants which have not been approved by the City's Department of Health. These regulations for a short time each winter meant a higher price for approved cream; and in the winters concerned the cream supply ran short, until, using the phrase of Dr. Shirley W. Wynne (formerly Commissioner of Health of the City) in an unpublished letter, "there was a sufficient margin between the price of unapproved cream from the West and approved cream to make it profitable to bootleg."

According to statements made by publicists vast sums of money were made in this way, and even more in racketeering the vendors of milk in the city. These are stated to have been charged a tax of five cents for each forty gallons of milk sold. Of the accuracy of this statement I cannot judge, but publicity did something to "tear the mask from this gang."

These incidents are given here not as reflecting on the executive of the Public Health Department of New York City, but as illustrating the fact that only constant vigilance, including the appointment of well-qualified inspectors with adequate salaries, can minimise the risk of occasional corruption. No public authority can claim to be completely exempt from this danger.

There is a close connection between a safeguarded milk supply and the mortality among young children during the summer months from diarrhoea, and the following figures from the official records of New York City are of interest.

DIARRHOEAL DEATH-RATE PER 10,000 CHILDREN UNDER 5 YEARS OLD

in the three summer months of single years of the periods

1901–10 varied from 107 to 66
1911–15   ,,   ,,   49 ,, 39
1916–20   ,,   ,,   37 ,, 23
1921–25   ,,   ,,   19 ,, 8
In 1927 it was 4

The reader who considers Chapter xxxviii in my *Fifty Years in Public Health* will not need to be reminded that a satisfactory milk supply is not the sole factor concerned in diarrhoeal mortality; but it is a great factor, and the above figures may be taken as an index of the extent to which New York's milk supply is now protected.

CHAPTER XXXVII

AMERICAN ACHIEVEMENTS IN TROPICAL AND SUB-TROPICAL DISEASES

IN Chapter xxxviii I give some particulars of my itinerary in Jamaica and Central America, as bearing on Tropical Medicine. In this chapter I propose to sketch the work of Americans in controlling certain diseases of tropical and sub-tropical climates, viz. Texas Fever in cattle, and Hookworm disease and Yellow Fever, the two last named being human diseases which in past experience have destroyed more health in some parts of America than any other single disease, except Malaria and Tuberculosis.

THEOBALD SMITH'S INVESTIGATIONS

The name of Theobald Smith deserves to be placed alongside that of Walter Reed and his co-workers as standing foremost in the list of American biological investigators. I met Theobald Smith several times on the Board of the Milbank Memorial Fund in and about 1920. He was born in 1859. After studying Koch's method he was employed in the Bureau of Animal Industry at Washington. In 1888 his official chief set him the task of investigating Texas fever, a disease which devastated the herds of cattle in the southern States. Ordinary bacteriological investigation gave a negative result; and then Theobald Smith heard the apparently unlikely story that this disease was carried by a tick which lived on and sucked the blood of the cattle. One is reminded of the story of the milkmaid who told Edward Jenner that she had had cow-pox, and was therefore immune from smallpox, and thus suggested Jenner's experimental investigations with their resultant saving of more lives than any other biological discovery. Theobald Smith's earlier work "on the micro-organism of Texas fever was published in *Public Health Papers and Reports* in 1889. In this article he did not mention the method of transmission. In 1893 he, with F. L. Kilborne, demonstrated the method of transmission, and showed that the protozoal parasite of the disease passed from the tick to its offspring through the ova.

They proved that Texas fever was in fact conveyed by ticks. Female ticks having sucked the blood of a diseased cow drop to the ground and there deposit thousands of eggs, which on their development, some thirty days later, if they are able to migrate to healthy cattle, pass on Texas fever to their hosts.

This was the second occasion in which a protozoon had been suspected of causing animal disease. Laveran in 1880 had described a protozoon in the blood cells of malarious patients and regarded it as causing malaria. But Laveran had not suspected the double life of his protozoon in successive animals. It was Theobald Smith who first proved the existence of this double life cycle in the protozoon of Texas fever, without a knowledge of which practical preventive measures might have continued to be misdirected. It is interesting to note that as early as 1878 Patrick Manson observed micro-filaria in the mosquito, and later observed what he considered to be metamorphosis in the mosquito. In 1894 he published his hypothesis of mosquito carriage of malaria, and in 1897 Ronald Ross traced the life cycle of malaria in birds.

It is not clear that either Manson or Ross knew of Theobald Smith's independent work.

This early discovery is not Theobald Smith's sole claim to scientific immortality. His extensive laboratory studies were largely responsible for recognition of the fact that there are three types of tubercle bacilli—human, bovine, and avian. This distinction has enabled hygienists to prove how immensely more important is human than bovine infection as a source of human tuberculosis, although tuberculosis of bovine origin is also serious, especially for children.

THE PREVENTION OF YELLOW FEVER

Research by American workers rendered possible the completion of the Panama Canal by American engineers. In 1897, Ronald Ross in India had traced the life cycle of malaria in birds, thus demonstrating the truth of Manson's already published hypothesis. Soon afterwards, in 1899, Surgeon (later Assistant Surgeon-General) Henry R. Carter, of the American Public Health Service, made careful field observations proving that a mosquito which has bitten a yellow fever patient cannot by biting another human being infect him until some two to three weeks have passed. In 1901 he put the usual limits of extrinsic incubation at from ten to seventeen days. During this interval, the bite of the yellow-fever-carrying mosquito is harmless, and the inference is that some developmental changes of the microbe of yellow fever occur in the interval. It was also shown that the human patient suffering from yellow fever is only able to communicate the specific virus for a very limited part of his illness. These field observations opened the way for the momentous work of Walter Reed and his colleagues of the American Army Medical Service in 1901, acting as a Government Commission. They demonstrated that it was a particular species of mosquito usually known as stegomyia which is the vector of yellow fever from one patient to another, subject to the epidemiological conditions already ascertained by Dr. Carter.

In 1924 I travelled in Jamaica and Central America with Dr. Carter and his talented daughter and learnt to appreciate his modesty as to his share in the elucidation of the life-history of the contagium of yellow fever.

The above voyage included a stay of several days at Panama, and I could then realise the magnitude of the American achievement in constructing the Panama Canal. General W. C. Gorgas's task would have been impossible if action on the scientific discoveries just indicated had not made the canal zone habitable to white workers.

In the city of Panama itself, although I was there in August, no mosquitoes were encountered and there were fewer domestic flies than are found in an ordinary middle-class English home. I was personally conducted along the streams leading into the canal and shown how every possibility likely to aid the breeding of the larvae of mosquitos was being controlled. Any householder, whether in large houses or in native huts who was found to have kept within his curtilage a broken bottle or a tin can which would hold water, and serve for depositing mosquito eggs, was at once fined, and the arrangements as to privies and refuse heaps were of military severity.

This is a convenient point for further mentioning my visit to New Orleans in October 1919, on the occasion of an American

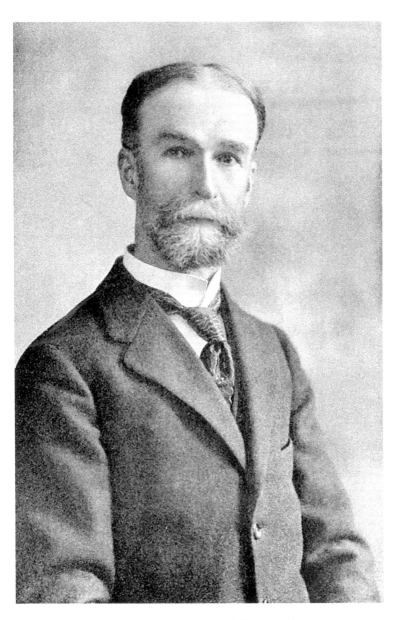

DR. THEOBALD SMITH (1859–1934)

Public Health Congress. This city was formerly a centre of endemic yellow fever and vast sums were spent on main drainage and on a public water supply, in the hope of stopping this. The city is below the river level and by constant pumping is prevented from becoming water-logged. So effectual has been this pumping, I was told, that the ilex trees have languished owing to the removal of the ground water. A visit to the older cemeteries of New Orleans was significant. Instead of tombstones over graves in the ground, various forms of mausoleum were erected above ground-level.

The story of the disappearance of yellow fever from New Orleans has much epidemiological interest. The first great efforts to this end were drainage of the subsoil and the introduction of a complete municipal water supply. But outbreaks of fever continued. Then it was found that the old domestic water-cisterns belonging to the former intermittent water service had been retained in the houses. With the removal of these cisterns yellow fever disappeared. It is now well known that the stegomyia is a "domestic" mosquito. It frequents dwelling-houses so long as breeding-places for its larvae exist. Hence the efficacy of action against domestic storage of water and of the provision of covers preventing access of the mosquito to any temporary store of water.

During my residence in Baltimore I met General Gorgas several times and heard him lecture at the School of Hygiene. As in the case of General Carter, who also lectured at the school, I was impressed by the modesty and restraint of these two distinguished men. General Gorgas died in Europe and a public memorial service was held at St. Paul's Cathedral, probably unique in the history of preventive medicine. It was worthily accorded, for the construction of the Panama Canal is America's greatest accomplishment in the sphere of applied public health. I represented Johns Hopkins University at this impressive ceremony.

THE CONTROL OF HOOKWORM DISEASE

The control of this disease forms an important chapter of the history of American Public Health Administration. This control has been in part the work of the American Public

L*

Health Service, in part of the local authorities, and perhaps chiefly of the International Health Board of the Rockefeller Foundation. For some readers a short preliminary account of this disease is perhaps needed.

The hookworm is a small intestinal parasite, the disease caused by it being known scientifically as Ankylostomiasis. The minute worms, of which there may be some thousands attached to a single victim's small intestines, greedily absorb blood from the small wounds which they make in his mucous membrane. The females produce a multitude of eggs, only visible under the microscope, which are discharged with the faeces of the host. The eggs in warm moist soil very soon become minute larvae, which on coming into contact with human skin (usually the ankle or the foot) penetrate into the blood, circulate with it, escape from the lungs into the mouth, are then swallowed and finally attach themselves to the intestinal mucous membrane of the new host and then develop into adult worms and commence their life of blood-sucking. The method of invasion by the skin was discovered in Egypt by Looss in 1895. One or other variety of ankylostomiasis had been found in many countries. It has occurred once or twice in Cornish tin mines and it was serious during the tunnelling through the St. Gothard. But the larvae do not hatch out below 50° F., and Western Europe is nearly free from hook-worm disease, which flourishes chiefly in the southern States of America, in the West Indian Islands, as well as in India.

The importance of man's infestation by this worm lies in its wide prevalence and the serious illness caused by it. It produces profound anaemia and weakness and symptoms of toxaemia. Physiological growth is delayed and diminished. I have seen boys and girls approaching adult life who were like children of ten years old, stunted in growth and often correspondingly stunted in mentality, as the result of the slow blood-sucking.

Two stories told me when I was in Jamaica in 1924 illustrate its effects, my informant being Dr. Washburn, then Rocke-feller director of hookworm work in that island.

(1) The doctor received a letter from a former patient to the following effect: "Your treatment has caused me great

trouble. I was mild and sweet in disposition and very patient. Now I have been fighting and am threatened with the law."

(2) An East-Indian was seen by the doctor being conveyed to the local poor-house to die. The doctor suspected the real diagnosis and offered to keep the man while he was treating him for hookworm. His sole apparel was then a loin-cloth. In a few days the patient appeared with a shirt, a week later with a hat, soon also he had trousers, in the fourth week he had shoes, and in the fifth he had changed his name and was in future to be known as Mr. Christopher Padmore.

The treatment of this disease consists in ridding the patient of his parasites by an efficient vermifuge. The physical and mental improvement which follows is almost beyond belief. The severity of symptoms varies with the degree of infestation.

But treatment alone gives only temporary benefit. It is essential to prevent re-infestation. As the larvae penetrate through the skin, the wearing of shoes and gaiters greatly diminishes this risk; and I have occasionally used this fact as illustrating that preventive medicine may sometimes necessitate the provision of foot-wear, perhaps at the public expense. The essential remedy is elementary sanitation. Dr. J. A. Ferrell, of the International Health Board, stated that in 1920 sample observations in 236 rural areas of the southern part of the United States showed that over 5 per cent of the houses had no privy accommodation and that in nearly 10 per cent this accommodation was unsatisfactory. In Jamaica I found that treatment for hookworm very properly was only begun when a satisfactory privy had been provided according to a simple specification, with a fly-proof trench.

On the official side Colonel Charles W. Stiles was a pioneer in the prevention of hookworm disease. He proved that the hookworm chiefly responsible for the disease in southern United States was the *Necator Americanus*, and his work was primarily responsible for the campaign organised by the International Health Board both in the States and internationally for the control of this plague. This campaign was begun under the leadership of the late Mr. Wickliff Rose, who though not a professional hygienist was a great educator and an admirable organiser. He gathered a staff of medical officers and organised measures of control in a large number of centres. First, surveys were undertaken of a given population to ascertain the degree of infestation, and then followed sanitary reform combined with treatment of individual patients. Investigation soon showed the Rockefeller workers and also the local governing bodies in each area in which demonstration work was carried out, that in tropical and sub-tropical regions the problem of an improved standard of health for the people consisted primarily in curing and preventing hookworm infection. Next to this in importance was the reduction of the incidence of malaria.

CHAPTER XXXVIII

HEALTH PROBLEMS IN TROPICAL MEDICINE

IN 1924 I was asked to take part in an International Conference on Health Problems in Tropical America, and the notes of the experiences of my wife and myself during the tour of Central America and Jamaica which was combined with the Conference, present features of general interest, which I jot down in this chapter.

The recollections would, I confess, be more interesting were it practicable to incorporate much of what my wife wrote in her diary; but in adhering to my self-imposed restriction I limit myself to items having socio-hygienic interest.

My recollections take the form of a running commentary based chiefly on our two diaries, supplemented by items from the official volume in which the proceedings of the week's Conference held in Jamaica, July 22 to August 1, 1924, are recorded.

The Conference was called by the American Fruit Company, and was presided over by Dr. W. E. Deeks, the chief medical adviser to the Company. In the words of Professor Rosenau of Harvard its object was

to consider sanitary and administrative questions, to discuss tropical diseases, to standardise practice and to promote preventive medicine and hygiene in tropical lands.

The meetings of the Conference were held at the Myrtle Bank Hotel, Kingston. The Conference was intended, in the first instance, for the superintendents of the admirable hospitals of the Fruit Company, erected by them for their employees, as a necessary part of the outfit of each of their banana plantations. It had been extended by invitations sent to a large group of American and of British hygienists and experts in tropical medicine. One thing was demonstrated during our subsequent tour of these hospitals, that the United Fruit Company were pioneers and leaders among great corporations in their regard for the health of their employees. This can be affirmed after critical visits by a large contingent of foreign hygienists to the hospitals of the Company in Honduras, Guatemala, Costa Rica, and Panama, as well as Jamaica.

Our voyage from Avonmouth to Kingston was most pleasant. The company included among tropical authorities, Sir Leonard Rogers, Dr. Thomson of the London School of Hygiene, Dr. Patterson of Kenya, Dr. W. J. Stephens of the Liverpool School of Tropical Medicine, Professor Fülleborn of Hamburg, and others. The chief excitement during the voyage was the receipt of two wireless messages. One of these was from a ship of the same Company on its way to Hamburg. It was wonderful to observe how, directed by wireless messages, we met the ship in question without difficulty and a couple of doctors from our ship went on board, found that the captain was suffering from gall-stones, but that he could continue the voyage to Europe. A further wireless message was received during the voyage from the American contingent on their way from New York to the Conference, conveying greetings from the New to the Old World.

We sat at table with Sir Thomas Oliver, the distinguished industrial hygienist, and Mr. W., a mining engineer returning to Columbia. Naturally stories, "chestnuts" and others, formed a staple of amusements on board. I heard a variation of an old joke. The best illustration of perpetual motion is a Scotsman pursuing a Jew for a sixpenny debt. Sir Thomas told us of Pavlov's experiments on dogs, illustrating the inheritance of feats acquired by teaching. Mr. W. capped this by the story of a young dog. It had been whipped for some misdemeanour, and shortly returned, wagging his front paw to be shaken. It was ascertained that the mother of this pup had been taught the same trick, though the pup had never seen this action of his mother.

Next to watching the sea, the flying fishes and many other attractions, a chief interest of the voyage consisted in talks with fellow-passengers. Sir Thomas Oliver I have already mentioned. One of his stories I must tell. At Verdun a French fort was long defended, though surrounded by Germans. At night pigeons were sent out and a pigeon returning with messages would alight on a wire which rang a bell. One pigeon arrived, a feeble ring was heard and the pigeon was discovered minus one leg. It only survived to give the message. Now it is preserved and figures in Napoleon's tomb, with the Legion of Honour on its chest. Mr. W., who served in a Scottish division in the War, then told of his division being sent to the French part of the Front in an emergency. Later they were told of a stone monument erected on the spot where many had fallen, with the inscription "Here the glorious thistle will for ever flourish among the roses of France."

Several talks with Dr. Patterson, of the Colonial Government Service in Kenya, have a general interest. The black rat in recent years had superseded a small local rat, and with its invasion came also the plague. It was the inverse story of England in its Hanoverian invasion by the brown non-domestic rat. Dr. Patterson emphasised the possible relative neglect of general public health problems when emphasising the measures for the prevention of individual diseases. In Kenya they were having problems resembling those of industrial England in the early part of the eighteenth century. A great problem was how to prevent the creation of slums. One great difficulty in preventing this in Bombasa was that the Arabs possessed small patches of land, preventing satisfactory schemes of town development. The Arabs in Kenya had been deprived of their chief occupation by the destruction of the slave trade. Dr. Patterson deprecated the separation in the Colonial Medical Service of clinical from preventive medicine. He told me of the prevalence of yaws and of the avidity with which a crowd of children in one room submitted one after another to gluteal injections of salvarsan, having witnessed the spectacular improvement effected by it in others. This naturally pleased me and I told my analogous experience in securing voluntary notification of cases of tuberculosis when this was accompanied by the offer of sanatorium treatment.

One of the most interesting passengers was Professor Fülleborn, Director of the School of Tropical Medicine at Hamburg. He held himself at first somewhat proudly aloof, but when he realised one's friendliness, his conversation was full of interest. His protozoal researches are well known. We discussed artificial control of conception and he gave instances of its ancient practice. The Maori sub-penal operation appeared not to be related to anti-conception, for it was practised before the connection between coitus and pregnancy was known.

Fülleborn was clear that the North European races were being superseded by those of the South European type, who were largely Jewish. This in view of the more recent anti-Jewish national movement in Germany is interesting, for it gives a semi-scientific colouring to the present suicidal policy in Germany. Fülleborn thought that later would come the preponderance of the Eastern races. He was doubtful whether the Chinese would adopt birth-control. They have a philosophy rather than a religion which consists in ancestor worship.

Sir Leonard Rogers was a member of our party and I heard much of his work. We had a common interest in the study of the decline of leprosy and we both read papers on this at the subsequent Jamaica Conference. My paper consisted chiefly of what is stated as to the Norwegian experience in my *Prevention of Tuberculosis*, 1908. Rogers gave me the even more striking instance of Iceland. He was of opinion that sodium morrhuate and the sodium salt extracted from chaulmoogra oil might be as specific a remedy for leprosy as is emetin for dysentery of the amoebic type. I mention here our visit on July 22nd to a leper asylum in Jamaica where there were some fifty patients, men, women, and children. One leprous woman had a child aged six months apparently well. Somewhat belated arrangements were being made for the child's removal. In connection with this visit Rogers addressed the members of the Conference on the new methods of treatment, which were inducing patients to reveal their condition, because great amelioration, if not also cure, was being experienced. Dispensary treatment was being organised and differential segregation secured, but only for those with open sores.

Among others in our company going to the same Conference was Sir Arbuthnot Lane. His views on health and disease generally are well known. He has a gift of insight, but his views on certain points are extreme. This is illustrated by a paper he read on cancer at the Jamaica Conference. His contention was that most people are "constipated for twenty-four hours" and that if they would revert to the habit of "three motions daily" many diseases, really due in his view to toxaemia from intestinal stasis, would cease. To avoid constipation daily doses of medicinal paraffin were recommended. One can surmise, as I said in the discussion on Lane's paper, that intestinal stasis may favour malignant disease of the alimentary canal, but excessive imagination is required to believe that this is important, for instance, in the causation of the two chief cancers in woman, in the breast and the womb.

The Conference at the Myrtle Bank Hotel proved interesting. Dr. Deekes's inaugural address emphasised how in the Western hemisphere tropical diseases were retarding industrial and commercial development; in particular malaria and yellow fever, hookworm disease, and dysentery were blocking the way. Happily amoebic dysentery was curable by emetin.

I had already learnt during a long talk I had in 1919 with ex-President Taft that the importance of dysentery in preventing Philippine development and progress was being realised by the American people (p. 244).

At this point I may mention my meeting Dr. A. Agramonte, who was one of the group of Army doctors led by Major Walter Reed, who "changed Finlay's theory as to the role of a mosquito in producing yellow fever" into a doctrinal certainty. Noguchi, the distinguished Japanese bacteriologist, of the Rockefeller Institute, was also present, a modest man then busily engaged in important investigations.

Dr. G. E. Vincent, at that time President of the Rockefeller Foundation, gave an eloquent evening lecture, in which he emphasised that an efficient medical service was a necessary part of commercial enterprise in the tropics, and then described (see p. 299) the vast extent to which the International Health Board had helped to secure this.

The veteran Dr. H. R. Carter dwelt on the importance of going beyond the usual aim of curing the individual attacked by malaria to further systematic efforts to prevent infection on a large scale.

I have already described hookworm disease (p. 329), but I must here mention my meeting with Dr. Bailey K. Ashford, whose autobiography *A Soldier in Science*, 1934, I have recently read with much interest. Therein is given an account of his important work for the control of hookworm disease in Puerto Rico.

A few words about Jamaica itself. It is a beautiful island and nothing but distance, I think, can prevent it from becoming an important winter resort. Even at the end of July one can secure in Jamaica great variations of temperature. With several colleagues we took a two-days' independent excursion to Mandeville, which owing to its height has very cool nights. I do not attempt to describe the great variations of scenery and cultivation.

The trade winds in Jamaica blow so hard every afternoon and evening—they are called "the doctor"—that the sea is squally and tree palms are in active motion.

My description of visits made to the United Fruit Company's banana plantations and to their hospitals for workmen and staff must be very short. Unquestionably the development of these plantations in Jamaica and still more in the Central American countries next visited by us have been great agents in advancing civilisation among the natives. They receive wages many times higher than those current in these countries, and their standard of living is thus improved. The Company provide schools for their children and even build chapels for their people, according to their desires. The hospital treatment seen in all the hospitals visited by us was of high standard. Medical Superintendents of experience and skill are assisted by a junior medical staff, and the Company have made it a rule not to limit treatment strictly to their employees and their wives and children. I must not attempt to describe these banana plantations, except to state that they may be more than ten miles long, running through low-lying, perhaps water-logged, areas granted to them by the Government of the country. This fact implies that drainage operations are carried out and the incidence of malaria is reduced.

On Saturday, August 2nd, we went on board s.s. *Zacapa*, next morning arriving at Puerto Castillo on the north coast of Honduras. We there visited a beautifully appointed hospital of the Company. Malaria and dysentery are the two most common diseases, but 30–40 per cent of the patients are said to be venereal. Honduras is on the borders of civilisation, and here we first saw the machete used in hacking through the jungle and sometimes also when drunken quarrels arise. We were told there were about ten "killings" a month at the hospital.

Thence we went on to Tela, also in Honduras, which was found in the throes of a local revolution. In Central American Republics suffrage is farcical, for the votes always give a majority to the President in power. A revolution takes the place of a general election and commonly the President is assassinated. This occurred in Guatemala some months after our visit.

From Tela we went on to Puerto Cortez, where Cortez first landed in Central America, and on August 6th we crossed the harbour to Omaa, saw an old Spanish fort, unsuccessfully attacked by Drake, but subsequently captured by the British.

Later on we crossed by s.s. *Zacapa* to Barrios, whence we started for Guatemala. We entrained at 6 a.m. on August 7th, and travelled until 11 a.m. through lush jungle country. A visit was made on horseback to Quinigua, where are remains of the old Maya civilisation. Many stones still stand erect, with elaborate inscriptions giving evidence of a very old civilisation.

Why it was wiped out is doubtful. Perhaps plague or some other great pestilence caused its abandonment by the survivors.

We lunched elaborately at the Company's hospital *en route*, 350 feet above sea-level, but in sight of mountains some approaching 10,000 feet high. Then train again, climbing to the city of Guatemala. We were met at railway stations by local bands, playing patriotic tunes and shouting vivas. We reached the Palace Hotel at Guatemala at 10 p.m.

Next morning we visited the local hospital and church, recently much damaged by earthquake; went to the market and bought Indian shawls. In the afternoon we were received by the President, General Orellano, at a *thé dansant* where wines followed by sweets and tea were given. The President gave an address of welcome and it was my task to respond for the visitors. As I could not speak Spanish, I arranged for Colonel Ashford of our party to sit next to me, and my speech was given sentence by sentence, each sentence being translated by the

Colonel before I proceeded. According to Colonel Ashford, who has amusingly described the scene in his book (p. 337), the speeches were a success. After tea my wife was escorted by the President to a roof garden and we all followed, and there dancing began, the national instrument, the *zarimba*, being used. It provides an entire orchestra in itself. The wood is cedar- or satin-wood, similar to that used for old violins. Our cards of invitation showed a quarter coat of arms, in which the *quetzal*, the mythological bird of the Aztecs, appears. We had seen the same bird depicted in the Maya stones.

From the roof garden one could see the smoke or steam of a neighbouring volcano. Much of the damage done by former earthquakes, I was informed by the Dutch Consul, who had lived here fifty-four years, was due more to bad building, to rotten woodwork, and to wilful damage than to actual earthquake.

Next day we drove in two and a half hours to Antigua along zig-zagging mountain roads. Looking back we could see the city of Guatemala, 4,500 feet above the sea, and *en route* to Antigua we ascended much higher. But I must not enlarge on what can be more fully read in other books.

On the 10th we left Guatemala at 6.30 a.m. and arrived at Barrios in the evening and went on board ship. On the 13th we arrived at Cristobal and thence were driven to view the locks of the Panama canal at Gatun. Their working was demonstrated. Returning to Colon we went on board s.s. *Tolua*. From the deck, as we sailed, we could see the points on the coast immortalised by Columbus, Drake, Morgan, and others.

· Next day, the 14th, we reached Port Simon and then by train to San José. After skirting the coast for twenty-four miles, we began our ascent by train, often very steep. This is a region where the annual rainfall is 220 inches. Near the highest point of the railway is the town of Cartago. As we travelled we saw telegraph posts that had sprouted and some had branches. Arriving at San José, which is on the Pacific side of the divide of the mountains, we saw much evidence of volcanic activity. In the evening the party was entertained to dinner, the chair being occupied by Dr. S. Munez, who was formerly in my class at the School of Hygiene, Baltimore. I must here again not yield to the temptation of giving further local detail, except as to social talks I had with a highly intelligent American living in San José (see p. 342).

On the second day we returned late to s.s. *Tolua* and had a disturbed and terribly hot night while the vessel was being loaded with bananas. I refrain from copying my notes on the difficulties and romance of banana cultivation.

We arrived back in Colon on the 17th, went on board s.s. *Heredia*, and in the morning disembarked at Almirante. After various visits during the day, my wife and I were accommodated at the manager's house, thus escaping a night on board ship while in dock. In our bedroom I failed to find the switch for one electric light which lighted a cupboard. Next morning our hostess explained that it would have been serious had I switched off this light as boots and clothing would have become mildewed.

August 20th we arrived again at Colon and took train across the peninsula for Panama. Next morning I visited the Ancon Hospital. It has some 130 beds and is most elaborately and scientifically equipped. At dinner with Dr. James, the chief American physician, I was entertained by incidents illustrating attempts of the Roman Catholic Church to prevent civil marriages, and was taken afterwards to a Masonic Lodge, although my recollection of its ritual had become somewhat sketchy.

As references to Panama are made in other chapters and as our visit to the Great American canal was our last chief visit, it is convenient to end my account of our visit to Central America at this point, except for concluding paragraphs on two subjects.

SYPHILIS AS A TROPICAL DISEASE

In our visits to the various hospitals of the United Fruit Company we had with us Dr. (now Sir Aldo) Castellani, whose knowledge of tropical diseases is perhaps unsurpassed. At each hospital the medical officers had collected cases, especially skin cases, of doubtful diagnosis and I was impressed by the large proportion pronounced by Dr. Castellani to be manifestations of syphilis. This disease, in fact, is one of the greatest human scourges in the tropics. In Honduras, as already seen, the proportion of total cases that were syphilitic was very high and I doubt if this experience was exceptional.

In Jamaica more exact information was available. Promiscuity is stated to be almost general; and perhaps the story told me of a negro mother who took her son aged sixteen to a doctor is not exaggerated. Said the mother to the doctor: "There must be something wrong with the lad, for he has not yet had the gentleman's complaint."

Doubtless this wide promiscuity is in part a survival of the former slave traffic which destroyed family life.

Several influential citizens doubted the possibility of early improvement in this respect. Another animadverted on the practice of many white people of having an "inside" and an "outside" family. With better economic conditions and improved education, especially on ethical lines, slow improvement is likely.

SOCIAL CONDITIONS OF COLOURED PEOPLE

I was much impressed by conversations at San José with Mr. K., an experienced American resident. He contrasted Costa Rica's former self-independent position with its present condition, dependent economically on France and England and still more on the United States. This dependence implies dangerous lowering of the standard of life for its people by competition. The people's welfare has been sacrificed to international commerce. True the older civilisation was of a somewhat low order, but exploitation was avoided and the people were not merely drawers of water and hewers of wood for the rest of the world. A similar condition was I was assured widespread in British colonies, and world-wide competition could, in his view, only be avoided by a policy of Imperial preference. The fact that labourers are brought from one tropical country to another makes competition keener and sometimes leads to a condition approaching slavery. Trade Unions have always failed in the tropics. According to Mr. K. the fertility of the tropics has been overrated. In fact, the struggle with nature is more intense than in the temperate zone. All the time destructive forces are overtaking the constructive; and weeds soon gain the victory. He held, further, that the real enemy of mankind is the "machine," namely international competition. The conditions of production in the tropics will continue to have some of the characteristics of slave labour unless wages are greatly raised, and this is only possible when the forces of competition are reduced.

I have no adequate knowledge to assess the exact value of the above-quoted comments; but I think they deserve record and study by those competent to judge.

PART III
THE INCREASING SOCIALISATION OF MEDICINE

CHAPTER XXXIX

EUROPEAN INQUIRIES ON MEDICAL WORK

THE circumstances which led to this investigation are stated on page 304.

A preliminary note may be made on my travels.

As it was important to come into touch not only with private and public physicians in each country and town visited by me, but also with as many other people as possible who were affected by insurance or other measures of medical help, I decided to travel by road. I had a competent chauffeur, whose skill was severely tried, as for instance in the Maritime Alps, in travelling from Trieste to Zagreb, and from Breslau to Posen and Warsaw. We had with us a lady secretary and typist. By this method of travelling we came into personal contact with more of the people than would have been otherwise possible. I wish I could enliven my pages with extracts from our domestic diary, but must refrain, as in the main these extracts would be irrelevant to my quasi-medical record.

We left England on March 14, 1929, and the first week was spent in Paris and its vicinity, interviewing Red Cross officials, seeing public health centres, and visiting hospitals and some official departments. Then we journeyed to Geneva, and on to Berne and Bâle, where similar visits were made. Thence we motored to Montpelier in South France and afterwards I spent a few days at Menton, writing up the information already collected.

Next came an interesting tour of the Italian Maritime Alps and somewhat detailed inquiries in Genoa, Florence, and Milan. The last-named city is a centre of active medical work and I was especially impressed with its work in school hygiene.

Crossing the Apennines, after visits to Trieste and Fiume, we arrived in Zagreb, which I made the centre for observing the medico-hygienic work of Yugoslavia.

From thence we journeyed to Budapest, in which, notwithstanding national impoverishment, valuable work is being done; then to Vienna and Prague, each illustrating important sanitary and medical work; and thence to Breslau. This was our starting-point for a difficult but fascinating travel across the plains of Poland, calling at Lodz on our way to Warsaw, and at Posen on our way back from Warsaw to Berlin. The intense patriotism in the eastern countries was most striking, as was also the enormous expenditure on military forces, when money was badly needed to succour the poor and reduce their misery.

My inquiries in Holland and Belgium were made in separate visits preceding this wider tour, and Scandinavian countries I visited later, when I had the advantage of Mr. Kingsbury's company. I saw much medical work in Hamburg, and then we flew to Copenhagen, and travelled to a number of centres in Norway and Sweden.

I give here a few notes on my European inquiries. A fuller summary is given in my *Medicine and the State* (George Allen & Unwin, 1924) and a complete statement in the three volumes of my *International Studies* (same publisher). In following chapters is given a comparison of the experience of the two English-speaking countries, Great Britain and the United States.

MEDICAL ATTENDANCE ON THE INDIGENT

It is universally accepted that the indigent ought to be cared for at the expense of the community, and in theory at least it is agreed that no person or family shall be allowed to die or suffer serious harm through lack of shelter or food or medical care. The extent to which this universally accepted principle is realised in practice varies enormously in different countries and even in different parts of the same country. Nowhere is the position of medical care for the poor such that the hygienist and practical public health administrator can regard it as nearly satisfactory. In the Netherlands medical assistance is not regarded as a State responsibility, but is limited to instances in which voluntary organisations do not suffice.

In Scandinavian countries district medical officers (as also in Ireland) provide a large share of the total medical needs of the community, at the community's expense.

In Germany and Austria local arrangements vary, but usually

there is official provision. So also in Switzerland, Belgium, and France. In Italy and in Hungary there is little private practice, each district having a communal doctor.

For non-domiciliary treatment all countries provide gratuitous beds for the indigent, but to a very varying extent and of very varying medical quality.

HOSPITAL TREATMENT AND CONSULTATIONS

Ireland approaches more nearly to general free domiciliary and hospital treatment than Great Britain, though the average quality of the Irish provision has been less satisfactory than that in Great Britain. In the Netherlands municipalities provide for the necessitous. In Denmark and Sweden, and largely also in Norway, each country is admirably served by official hospitals. German hospitals are in part supported from taxation, in part from insurance funds. In other European countries tax-supported hospitals and hospitals to which insurance funds contribute are the rule and voluntary hospitals are exceptional.

The degree to which treatment is given in hospitals instead of at home varies greatly; but the trend to increased hospital treatment is obvious. The reasons for this are well known.

Consultation centres for patients not admitted to hospitals are common in nearly all European countries. In some of the countries visited by me it appeared that, in connection with their national insurance schemes, the use of these centres had become excessive and that the treatment there given was not always in satisfactory relation to the work of the patient's chosen doctor.

INSURANCE MEDICAL CARE

The various sickness insurance schemes in Europe determine in large measure the extent to which the medical needs of different European countries are being met and the quality of the treatment that is being given. Around my notes under this heading can be grouped what needs to be written on the medical aspect of our tour.

In the first place every scheme of sickness insurance in Europe is now obligatory so far as concerns wage-earners, or in American phrasing, persons on a "pay-roll." Denmark was a partial exception to this rule until 1933, and yet in 1928 some 65 per cent of the population over fifteen years of age were members of State-recognised sickness clubs. Even in Denmark there was indirect social pressure, tending to make insurance general, for an uninsured person could not claim public assistance, nor could he marry without special official consent. For particulars I must refer the reader to the books already cited.

Each insured person is required to pay periodically for future financial and medical benefits during sickness. In Britain the employer of the insured person pays weekly as much as his employee and the Government contributes a large fraction to the total cost. In other countries the employer may or may not share the cost, and the proportion of total cost borne by the Government is less in European countries than in Britain. On the other hand European insurance schemes, unlike the British, include institutional as well as home treatment and the terms on which insured patients are admitted to hospital are far below the actual cost of hospital treatment.

In Chapter XIII I have given rather full details concerning sickness insurance in Britain. The initial scheme of medical care under insurance was rigorously opposed by medical practitioners through their Association, but as eventually adopted and since modified from time to time it is now regarded very favourably by them, and they have recommended that it be extended with modifications to the dependents of those already insured. This, were it adopted, would mean that more than three-fourths of the British population would be medically attended under insurance arrangements, to the extent to which a general practitioner can be reasonably expected to supply this service. Already three-fourths of all the medical practitioners in Britain, possibly more, are taking part in this contract medical work. The proportion varies in different parts of the country. In industrial areas this insurance medical work is undertaken by nearly every doctor, while in residential districts the proportion of doctors undertaking it may be small.

The method of remuneration in operation is that of capitation fees, 9s. per annum for each insured person placing his or her name on a doctor's list, and this sum is paid by the insurance authorities to the doctor whether medical care is needed during the year or not.

I cannot detail here the varying defects and virtues of continental insurance schemes. They give more nearly complete treatment than is given under the British system; but the conditions of medical service are more irksome. In regard to the conditions of his medical work the British doctor, who negotiates only with the Government and a partly medical committee, is in a specially favourable position. In some European capitals I saw evidence of over-development of specialised medical work for the insured, and of unchecked consultations with specialists, without the knowledge of the private practitioner.

CHAPTER XL

THE COSTS OF MEDICAL CARE IN
THE UNITED STATES

IN this and the next chapter I give some further discussion of medical work in the United States as compared with Britain, as the contents of these chapters have an essential connection with the remainder of Part III of this volume.

The report of the American Committee on the above-named subject gives me an appropriate peg on which to hang an attempt to outline my own observations and reflections on the position as regards the growth of socialisation of medicine in the United States.

The formation in 1927 of the Committee on the costs of medical care showed that many physicians, social workers, and others realised how unsatisfactory are present conditions of medical practice in the States. The final report of this Committee (University of Chicago Press) was issued in 1932, and from it can be culled the facts required for a study of American conditions. The introduction to this report written by Dr. Ray Lyman Wilbur, the President of Leland Stanford University, contains the following explicit statement, which defines the position:

> As a result of our failure to utilise fully the results of scientific research, the people are not getting the service which they need—first because in many cases its cost is beyond their reach, and second, because in many parts of the country it is not available.

Appreciation of the position led to a meeting of fifteen leaders in the fields of medicine, public health, and the social sciences in Washington in April 1926, with a view to the formation of a Committee for investigation of the problem. After preliminary inquiries and consultations, at a further meeting of sixty representative persons in Washington in May 1927, the nucleus of the Committee on the costs of medical care was formed, and an Executive Committee was appointed. There followed a five-year programme of investigation, resulting in the issue of a series of special reports, which I read as they appeared. The membership of the Committee included men and women representing private medical practice, public health, various institutions, the social sciences, and the general public. A staff of expert investigators was employed. These were given freedom in their expressions of personal opinion and some twenty-six special studies were published. The total cost of the Committee and its collaborating agencies was over a million dollars. Like so much advanced social investigation in America, it was rendered possible by the financial support of eight social foundations, among these the Rockefeller Foundation and the Milbank Fund.

The final work of the Committee in formulating its Report must have been formidable, and its accomplishment redounds to the credit of the Committee and of its executive Chairman, Professor C. E. A. Winslow, who showed remarkable appreciation of the medical point of view. But, even so, with such a large team, representing not only very diverse points of view but also interests apparently incompatible with agreement, it is not surprising that the final Report of the forty-eight members then constituting the Committee consisted of a Majority Report with many individual reservations on particular points; a Minority Report signed by nine members (with some individual points of reservation); a second Minority Report signed by two members; a very searching separate statement by Professor W. H. Hamilton; and a short statement by Mr. Edgar Sydenstricker to the effect that he could not sign the final Report of the Committee, as in his opinion it did not "deal adequately with the fundamental economic question which the Committee was formed primarily to study and consider."

I cannot attempt here an adequate discussion of this Report. Unanimity of conclusions was from the first obviously out of the question for, as already indicated, the Committee was a voluntary aggregation of persons of diverse social views and interests. The Committee's inquiries and its Report became public at a time of unparalleled economic depression, and this gave much added importance to the clear and convincing statement of facts as to the unsatisfied medical needs of the

M

American people. I have already quoted Dr. Wilbur on this. Here is a further statement from the Majority Report, p. 2.

The problem of providing satisfactory medical service to all the people of the United States at costs which they can meet is a pressing one. At the present time, many persons do not receive service which is adequate either in quantity or quality, and the costs of service are inequably distributed.

The chief Minority Report does not appear to dispute the accuracy of the above quoted statements, and it very justly recommends better medical provision by the State for the actually necessitous, instead of leaving the burden of their care, as largely it now is left, to the charity of private doctors.. Some of the Minority recommendations are criticised later.

My chief difficulty in weighing the contents of the Report of the Committee on the Costs of Medical Care has been that it is almost completely static or contemporaneous in its survey. Furthermore, even so far as contemporaneous conditions are concerned, while a clear picture is given of present deficiencies, we are left partially in the dark as to the exact position and relation to each other of the medical services, official and non-official, which are already available. Doubtless these facts were familiar to members of the Committee and their special investigators, but for others, who like myself have only partial knowledge of the position throughout the United States, a succinct but comprehensive statement of official and non-official provision already existing (beyond private medical practice) would have placed the conclusions of the Committee in a more satisfactory setting. So much for the position now. But we need to know also how the present position has evolved, as well as to have a clear picture of what now exists, if future reforms are to have within them the prospect of continuity and success. My experience of progressive movements is that they succeed best when vitally related to what already exists. New developments may be lop-sided, one or other subject receiving undue attention; but with further growth, still related to the living past, lop-sidedness disappears, and permanent advance is secured without loss of what is already provided.

The relative obscurity in the Committee's Report as to this

vital connection with total medical work is regrettable. Consider the position.

In America as in Great Britain a vast proportion of total medical work is already socialised, officially and unofficially. The amount of hospital provision in America, official and voluntary, is colossal, some of it under the control of popularly elected State representatives and a smaller part under the control of voluntary Committees representing the donors of the hospital funds. In either case this hospital work is divorced in large measure from the private practice of fee-charging doctors. This is true, in part at least, for "paying patients," who pay their doctors directly. It is true even more for the vast numbers of health centres and of tuberculosis and other special clinics, which are found in every considerable centre of population. Let us see how these are to be related to the proposals of the Majority Report.

(1) It is recommended that medical service shall be furnished largely "by organised groups of physicians, dentists, and other associated personnel," self-organised preferably around a hospital. Thus it is intended to give a better service of specialists and consultants for the sick and be advantageous in other respects.

(2) It is recommended that all "basic public health services" shall be made generally available according to need. Here exactitude of statement is urgently needed; for in Britain, and also largely in America, much medical care is given at the public expense at welfare centres, and in tuberculosis and venereal disease clinics, and in large part without much if any reference to the financial position of applicants for advice. The Committee's view apparently is that these should become or remain public health problems when they "cannot be solved effectively by the other available medical and health agencies." To act on this somewhat ambiguous dictum in Britain would necessitate lamentable retrogression of important work; and in America it would also, I think, mean abandonment of much valuable medical and hygienic work, which is unlikely for some decades, if ever, to be carried on effectively by "organised groups of physicians."

One can hope that it will become possible to restore much

of the non-specialist work now being done at child welfare centres, in special clinics, in school clinics and so on, to private medical practitioners who have been entrusted by the head of a family with the family's medical care, if this is made conditional on adequate use of consultative facilities by these practitioners. But, if in the absence of a system of prepayment by each family on an insurance basis, payment for medical care continues as at present, this will remain an unrealised aspiration. Much of the official work done at these clinics by public health and school authorities is, however, specialised help, requiring doctors of consultative rank; and it is futile to suggest that the rapidly growing work at public clinics shall be superseded until an effective and equally available substitute is in being.

The Report of the Majority creates (on paper) a new unnecessary and undesirable doubling of medical provisions, (a) of public health authorities and voluntary agencies doing quasi-official work, and (b) the proposed "organised groups." It is satisfactory to note that in the Report it is realised that—whether the duality be created or not—the costs of medical care, if any payment whatever is exacted, for a large proportion of the total population must be borne "on a group payment basis, through the use of insurance, or taxation, or by both of these methods."

In Britain the work of the various official (and some voluntary) centres for special counsel of mothers and their infants and for specialised clinics is paid for by the municipality and the State. Furthermore, all sickness insurance work is partially subsidised by the State. Indeed, no insurance system hitherto organised has been able to continue its work without State aid. In Britain were hospital treatment included in the medical benefits of sickness insurance, State subsidies would need to be largely increased. In short no complete medical organisation for the entire wage-earning community, on the lines of prepayment by insurance or otherwise, is practicable except as part of a State system, in the sense that a considerable part of its cost must be paid out of public taxation. My statement to this effect appears also to be implied in the Majority Report of the Committee.

The real problem of management of the proposed "Organised

Groups" recommended in the American Committee's Report is left obscure. The groups are not to be official, in any true sense of this word; there is no recognisable machinery for avoiding lamentable competition of rival "groups." Each medical group, we are told, is to "be inspected and graded." But by whom? If county or State authorities are fit to undertake this task—and they alone, it would appear, could secure the statutory authority to enforce their decisions—then *ought they not to be entrusted to form the groups?* If this were done, the position would then be that already partially existing in Great Britain; for there are official group centres for maternity and child welfare work, for tuberculosis and venereal disease clinics, and for school children, and there are the beginnings in the municipal hospitals throughout the country of consultative facilities available on any doubtful case for private practitioners.

Even for insured patients some uniformity of arrangements in each county and county borough is secured by the Local Insurance Committees (chiefly officials, but doctors are represented on them) and there are small beginnings of consultative facilities.

GROUP MEDICAL PRACTICE

The chief Minority Report regards the Majority Report as having given far too much importance to the value of private group clinics, and with this view I have some limited sympathy. It is convenient to discuss this point here.

The need for consultations between private physicians and consultants having some special skill in some department of medicine frequently arises, but in the majority of total illnesses such consultations are not, in my view, a necessary condition of satisfactory medical care. In at least half and probably more of the sickness treated by the family physician consultations are unneeded and not desired either by him or his patient.

In giving this restrictive opinion I am assuming that the private practitioner advises routine dental and similar additional aid as required. The essential condition for a completely satisfactory medical service is that consultations (and when necessary a period of observation or treatment in a hospital) shall be available for the sick, whether rich or poor, and that these consultative and institutional services shall furthermore be available at the request of the patient, even when the family physician may not consider them necessary, subject always to reasonable and practicable regulations to avoid abuse of this privilege. I have already alluded to the excessive use of consultative and hospital services (p. 351) in some countries. Sound administration, based on medical considerations, can be made to prevent this abuse, when services for consultations and for residential hospital treatment as needed are made universally accessible.

The chief Minority Report in effect is in the main obstructive to practicable reform. It concludes that the formation or community medical centres would not accomplish "what ought to be the first object of this Committee," the lessening of the costs of medical care. Perhaps we may infer that in the opinion of the Minority as well as of the Majority reduction of these personal costs is needed.

The main point of the Minority Report is embodied in the following sentence:

The Minority recommend that Government competition in the practice of medicine be discontinued and that its activities be restricted to the care of the indigent.

They add that in their opinion State activities in this field (apart from services for soldiers, veterans, etc.) should be restricted to "the promotion of public health work." Obvious fallacies lurk in the definition of "indigence" and of "public health work" which public health workers and those responsible for the Minority Report would respectively give. The public health worker will necessarily contend that "indigence" may be limited to inability to obtain the specific treatment needed for present needs, and yet external help for this end is called for; and he will rightly claim that improved medical care, general and specific, clinical and hygienic, are all needed in the promotion of the public health and come within the legitimate scope of public health administration, carried out by the authorities elected democratically by the community.

Most wage-earners and many others are at times indigent in some specific particular. Speaking logically every insured person is indigent, inasmuch as in no European country has it been found practicable to supply adequate medical aid for "pay-roll" workers when sick, without calling for State subsidies for a very considerable part of the cost.

The Minority Report objects to "the adoption by medicine of the technique of big business, that is, mass production"; and to what it, with much probability, describes as the inevitable "destructive competition between individuals or groups concerned with these movements." It makes a protest against the degradation of the medical profession "through unfair competition or inadequate compensation" with which one can sympathise; and although its objections to group medical practice are overstated, I have already indicated that they are not entirely unbased. The statement in the Minority Report that the "supposedly rosy path of insurance" is the shortest road to "the commercialisation of medicine" is contradicted by national experience in Britain, and it is not confirmed by my inquiries and observations in many European countries. In all these countries the position, as regards medical care, of the insured is greatly improved, as compared with the past; and such defects of insurance medical care as exist are slowly diminishing.

From my incomplete statement it will be seen that the recommendations of the Majority Report are not in the true line of evolutionary development, in so far as they adumbrate the establishment and extension of duplicated medical arrangements, official in part and "organised groups" in part, but both involving the expenditure of money derived from taxation, one of them with no visible prospect of satisfactory control of this expenditure, or its satisfactory relationship to other organisations for promoting clinical and preventive medical work.

The many interesting conclusions of the several Reports of the Committee on costs of Medical Care suggest unlimited discussion; but to pursue this course would mean repetition of much which is more consecutively stated in my *Medicine and the State* (George Allen & Unwin, 1932), written before the publication of the Report of this Committee.

CHAPTER XLI

TWO NATIONAL MEDICAL ASSOCIATIONS:
A CONTRAST

THE views of the medical profession on new proposals of health authorities for changes in medical practice, clinical or preventive, and the action taken by the medical profession in regard to these proposals in Britain and America, constitute a vital part of my recollections of the recent history of medicine and public health; and at this stage some consideration of the medico-hygienic movements of the past thirty years in their political bearings is called for. The contents of the last chapter throw some light on this subject; but it appears to me that, without attempting an all-round review, we can obtain further light on the evolution of opinion and of administrative action by contrasting certain illustrative events, looked at from the point of view of the two great national Medical Associations, British and American, to which a majority of the private medical practitioners in the two countries are affiliated. These professional Associations have great importance, for changes affecting their members cannot hope to succeed permanently unless these changes are approved by a majority of them.

I say "of a majority" advisedly, for in both countries not only are there many doctors who are not members of their national association either from indifference or because they are opposed to its policy; there are even more who, being members, do not take part in determining its policy. In Great Britain the British Medical Association is an active body, led by representative men, and the conclusions of the Council of the Association usually carry with them the willing consent of a majority of the profession. I gather that this statement does not apply to the decisions of the American Medical Association, which sometimes, it is stated, represents only the views of a small political coterie retained in power by the inertia of a vast membership scattered over an entire continent.

Whether this be so or not, there has been during the last thirty years (a) a striking resemblance between the early attitude of the Medical Associations in both countries to some important medico-hygienic reforms; while in more recent years there is (b) a remarkable contrast in this respect between the British and the American Associations. The same statement may be made concerning the medical profession generally in each country. The obstructive policy in certain respects of the American medical profession in recent years can only be explained by believing that the American doctors—as a body— have not realised the medical needs of a large part of the people and therefore, unlike their British colleagues, have not set themselves the task of recommending and aiding social reforms.

THE HESITANCY OF THE PRIVATE PRACTITIONER

A few preliminary remarks are needed on the conservative mentality of so many doctors. It is due in part to the doctor's confidential relationship with the families engaging his services— a relationship much closer in the past than in this day of specialists and hospitals. He regards his position as almost sacred, and resents third-party intervention. It has been found impossible to maintain the integrity of this relation in all circumstances. Thus a doctor can be compelled to give evidence in a court of justice as to medical facts ascertained in his confidential relationship to his patient. A further breach of the secrecy of medical practice occurred within my memory when in the '90's of the last century the notification of many acute infectious diseases was initiated. In England some years elapsed before the entire profession gave way and were brought to realise that they owed it to the public to give prompt informa- tion of each infectious case to the medical officer of health; that, in short, the confidential relationship of doctor and patient could only, in justice to the community, be maintained when the public weal was not thereby endangered.

In my earlier volume I have told of the long struggle we had in securing the compulsory notification of cases of tuber- culosis. Dr. Hermann Biggs was the first to secure in 1893 an enactment for the compulsory notification of this disease in New York, and it is not surprising to learn that his activities in this direction did not meet with the approval of the medical profession. By many of them this "extraordinary missionary work" of the New York Board of Health was regarded as "threatening and ominous," and as possibly leading to interference between patient and physician.

The then Medical Society of the County of New York resolved that

the compulsory reporting of cases of tuberculosis is unnecessary, inexpedient, and unwise.

In commenting on this in the manuscript prepared for a Hermann Biggs Memorial Lecture, 1932, I said:

How often, alas! in the history of medical progress, has the medical profession, in so far as it is voiced by the active minority who attend meetings of medical societies, damned work which is accepted as valuable by their successors, and commonly also by their contemporaries who take no part in medical politics.

Similarly when in 1894 the municipality of New York, guided by Biggs, insisted that the date of release of diphtheria patients from isolation should be determined by the result of examination of convalescent swabs, this was resented by some private practitioners as a form of "official impertinence . . . an interference with personal prerogative." It has always been difficult for some medical practitioners to realise that they have no proprietorship in their patients, and particularly so when their management of their patients runs counter to public health considerations.

I might give further illustrations of infringements of public welfare in the private practice of a minority of medical practitioners, especially on missed opportunities for preventing disease, but will only enumerate without elaborating a few examples.

Failure to secure adequate treatment for syphilis after miscarriages.

Failure to examine contacts with a tuberculous patient and to urge on the patient precautions in coughing and spitting.

Failure to urge immunisation against diphtheria in family practice among children.

Failure to speak out plainly concerning injurious personal habits, and so on.

The fault in these instances lies with the ordinary conditions of private medical practice more than with the doctor himself. The doctor is often called in only when illness has become serious and is expected to cease his visits when continued medical supervision, he knows, would be valuable to the patient. And thus, so long as professional services are paid for on the basis of "professional acts," the doctor is awkwardly placed when he suggests that further medical aid should be paid for.

Valuable initiative work was proposed by Dr. Hermann Biggs in 1920 with a view to securing improved medical services in the rural areas of New York State. In that year I was asked to prepare a statement in favour of Dr. Hermann Biggs's proposals for a health centre plan for the State of New York, then before the State Legislature at Albany. Dr. Biggs's plan was initiated in view of the dearth of doctors in the rural parts of the State. The older medical practitioners in remote districts were not being replenished by younger doctors, who preferred to practise in towns and cities where consultants and hospital beds were available. The plan included the opening of health centres administered by the local health departments under State supervision and aid. At these centres consultant special services would be provided. It was hoped that not only would the total medical service for rural districts be thus improved, but the trend of doctors to the towns would be stayed. The plan was defeated by the Legislature, but its provisions since then have been adopted on a considerable scale. State aid is now given to local communities on a fifty-fifty basis for local health work, including grants for the provision or maintenance of a public hospital, clinic, dispensary or other public health activity subject to the approval of the State Commissioner of Health. In a recent Hermann Biggs Memorial Lecture (*S.C.A.A. News*, May 1935) Dr. Thomas Farran, the New York Health Commissioner (who has now been appointed Surgeon General of the Public Health Service at Washington), has stated his preference for this plan, on which already large expenditure has been incurred, over health insurance for medical purposes. He refers to the fact that growth in medical provision up to now has been haphazard and unco-ordinated and fails to meet current needs, and concludes with the following important statement, showing that in America the same evolution of appreciation of medical necessities as in England is rapidly progressing.

This situation arises from the fact that standards of indigency applicable to the giving of public relief are not applicable to the giving of public medical care. A man may be entirely self-supporting, so far as furnishing himself and his family with food, shelter, and clothing is concerned, yet he may be unable to provide needed care for catastrophic illness.

As illustrations of the attitude and work of the two contrasted Medical Associations, one may instance first the

SCHOOL MEDICAL SERVICE

a service which is of essential national importance in preventing unfitness in the young and still more often in preventing its continuance. For further detail as to this service in England, see my *Fifty Years in Public Health*, pp. 389–99.

Discovery of defects and diseases in school children by school medical officers increased general medical treatment by private doctors, as parents were informed of what needed to be done. Then followed official treatment for conditions such as dental caries, orthopaedic conditions, defective vision and squint, adenoids, and still more for contagious skin complaints, which either required specialist treatment or were otherwise apt to be neglected. The subject is discussed on pp. 196–202 of my *Medicine and the State*, where my conclusion was that "on balance the practitioner has many more patients referred to him as the result of school medical inspection that he loses by the work of school clinics." Private medical practitioners now not infrequently refer special medical defects among their young patients to school doctors, and school medical work is already being conducted with minimum friction between school doctors and private practitioners. This was not so in the early years following 1908, when school medical work on a national scale began. On pages 6, 368–73 of Vol. III of my *International Studies*, I have given an illustration of the extent to which the British Medical Association in 1910 was prepared to carry its strenuous opposition to whole-time school doctors, as well as to their undertaking treatment for school children which required exceptional or specialist skill.

In that instance the medical journals refused to advertise the vacant post for a full-time school medical officer, and the bold doctor who was appointed was ejected from his membership of the British Medical Association. Now whole-time appointments of school doctors are the rule throughout England; and most private practitioners appear to prefer this arrangement to one under which a rival practitioner would examine or even treat the children of their adult patients.

My data are too scanty for me to attempt a corresponding summary of the school medical position in America; but I do not think it wide of the mark to suggest that the treatment secured for school children who need it has hitherto been on a small scale for equal populations as compared with the vast amount accomplished in the British school service. A few American cities may perhaps need to be excluded from this statement. Fear of the American private practitioner is at the back of this suggested contrast.

My next illustration relates to

INFANT AND CHILD WELFARE WORK

The details of British work under this heading are given in Chapters IX-X of Vol. III of my *International Studies*, and I need not now devote more than a few paragraphs to it. British work centres around home visits to parents by nurses specially trained for this branch of public health work. The nurse gives hygienic and quasi-medical advice to mothers, and as her visits are made independently of the family doctor (if there is one), there is need for tact and good judgment. Only exceptionally does difficulty arise with the doctor. As I have elsewhere stated, health visiting as it now functions "does not encroach on medical practice, *as this has existed in the past*, but increases the demand for it, by conducing to early medical attendance in illness, and by creating a demand for hygienic medical guidance." Much of this work might be undertaken by the private doctor, were it not for considerations of cost, and also because there should be economy of medical effort, a doctor not being employed to do work for which a nurse suffices.

The work of the health visitors is complemented by infant consultations at Health Centres conducted normally by a lady doctor, who is a full-time official. Most of this work also might be done by private medical practitioners, were private doctors to devote more attention to infant and child hygiene, and were the system of medical attendance radically changed. At present if this work is not done at these centres, it will remain undone. Much of the centre work again can be better done by the nurse than by a doctor, who would have little patience for the minutiae involved.

There has been considerable complaint in Great Britain as to these infant consultations. I recall in the years 1909–14, when these centres were being organised, being promised— or perhaps threatened—with serious medical and Parliamentary opposition to our proposals. The opposition gradually died down, and here again, as in school medical work, the British Medical Association ere long ceased to press for the appointment of private practitioners as medical officers for the Health Centres. Practitioners who had not been appointed began to object to other practitioners advising *their* patients concerning their children. In my *Medicine and the State* (p. 193) I summed up as follows:

Both health visiting and infant welfare centres have become embodied in public hygienic practice in many European countries, especially in Great Britain. Of their value to the community there can be no doubt; and that they will continue to function, perhaps to an increasing extent, is indubitable. The only possibility of their partial displacement and replacement appears to be through the family doctor reorganising his family work on an insurance basis of annual payment, and becoming—what he should be—the skilled hygienic as well as medical adviser of the families who employ him. Even then, unless the private doctor employs a nurse, he must undertake much work which a nurse would more appropriately carry out. He can best undertake such work when acting in co-operation with a group of doctors.

What is the corresponding position in the United States?

In surveying the work of the special Milbank Demonstrations I found some jealousy of this work, fomented by a small group of private practitioners (p. 303). I cannot state to what extent remedial treatment as well as diagnostic services are provided in most American official child welfare centres. Doubtless it varies in extent in different States. In the United States a multitude of voluntary societies also undertake work bearing on child hygiene; and the States are the special home of public health nurses, their value as missioners of health being realised even more than in England. I have met Miss Lilian Wald, Miss M. Adelaide Nutting, and Miss Mary Beard, whose names come to one's mind in this connection. Their names are associated both with sick nursing and with public health nursing. With child welfare work on a national scale, the names of Julia Lathrop and Grace Abbott (p. 242) will always be associated, also that of their medical colleague, Dr. Anna Rude. I have already mentioned the fine work of the Metropolitan Life Insurance Company in the same field (p. 295).

THE CONTROL OVER VENEREAL DISEASES

The story of work for this control furnishes a remarkable contrast between the American and the British Medical Association. I must not repeat here the story of the highly successful work in Great Britain in the control of these devastating social diseases, given in Chapter XVI of this volume and more fully in Vol. III of my *International Studies*. Important work has also been done by the American Social Hygiene Association, led by its director, Dr. William F. Snow. Here I can only enumerate the main items.

In 1917–18 the Local Government Board issued Regulations making it obligatory on every local authority (County Council or County Borough Council) to establish clinics for the treatment of venereal diseases and to provide pathological facilities for the gratuitous examination of specimens from suspected cases of these diseases.

The clinics and pathological facilities were to be open to all applicants, without any residential limits, and the treatment given was to be strictly confidential between the medical officer of the clinic and his patient.

No charge was to be made for treatment in these clinics and an applicant of any social position could insist on treatment. *The test of monetary ability to pay was entirely abandoned.*

The inducement offered to induce local authorities to start these treatment centres was that three-fourths of the total expenditure would be paid out of the National Exchequer, leaving only a quarter of the expenditure to be borne by local rate-payers.

The reason for this total abandonment of any charge for treatment was that there should be no excuse for evading treatment, and that resort of the patient to a druggist or any unqualified practitioner would thus be greatly reduced. Resort to quacks was rendered impracticable somewhat later by the passing of a general law making unqualified treatment of these diseases subject to severe penalties, and forbidding the advertising or other publication of any offer of remedies for them. The main proposals set out above were sent in draft to the British Medical Association, and were approved by the Council of that Association and afterwards by their representative meeting. The quotation on page 160 states the wise and broad-minded reasoning which led British medical practitioners to adopt this attitude.

This method of attacking venereal diseases, and especially syphilis, was inspired, in large measure, by the urgent need to sterilise the virus in the superficial lesions of each patient by the therapeutic action of arseno-benzol preparations. Prompt treatment minimises infection and curtails its duration. Direct statistical evidence of the effect of these national measures exists.

There has been no enforcement in Great Britain of notification of each case of venereal disease by the doctor in attendance, and I continue to doubt whether it would effect more than is already practicable when a patient comes willingly for confidential gratuitous treatment at an official clinic. At these clinics all acute and communicable stages of both gonorrhoea and syphilis are treated. Later manifestations of venereal disease, when it is still communicable, are still apt to receive inadequate treatment. This applies especially to the syphilitic woman who has had one or more miscarriages, and to children with congenital or directly acquired syphilis. The chief hope in such cases lies (a) in the development of the public health conscience of every private practitioner, and still more (b) in the alteration of the conditions of medical practice for wives and children, following the line of sickness insurance for working men. This has already been urged by the British Medical Association.

The position in the United States is not so clear, though Dr. Snow fortunately has summarised the American position in the *Journal of Social Hygiene*, January 1935. He states:

Now every State and nearly all cities provide such services (laboratories for blood and other examinations for syphilis) . . . ; and to-day the resources of private practice are supplemented by more than eight hundred clinic services, in addition to increased hospital and institutional services. . . .

The U.S. Public Health Service in 1932 reported the receipt of over 400,000 case reports of syphilis and gonococcal infections. . . .

The number of blood examinations was 1,740,000 in 1933.

In America there is also evidence of some decrease in the terrible toll of deaths from syphilis. Thus from general paresis of the insane the death-rate in civil State institutions dropped almost one half. Perhaps the chief progress has been on the educational side of the crusade led by the American Social Hygiene Association. American facilities for free treatment of venereal diseases are still deficient in number and in general availability, for, so far as I can ascertain, they are restricted to poorer people. This restriction has doubtless been found politic in view of the outcry which would be likely to accompany the offer of the free treatment which is given in Britain to all comers; but the restriction is contrary to public policy. These diseases are a national bane, a canker which permeates the entire community; and they are diseases, furthermore, in which the patient hesitates to or refrains from going to a practitioner who knows him, and is apt to go to an unqualified person. Unqualified treatment of venereal diseases, I believe, is not prohibited in any American State, and could not very reasonably be prohibited, unless the British precedent were followed, and free gratuitous skilled treatment at the public expense were first offered to all needing it. Are the members of the American Medical Association educated—as a body—to accept this view? and are they, furthermore, prepared to admit that the treatment of these diseases, perhaps above all others, is a specialist concern, and that a general practitioner who, when a more skilled alternative is available, treats these diseases, may be conniving at the retardation of the cessation of their spread, with calamitous results to personal and family life? It is but fair to recall that the willingness of British medical practitioners to abandon treatment of these diseases—so far as a third of the total adult population is concerned—was favoured by the fact that for insured patients the doctor's responsibility, but not his remuneration, is reduced when he encourages his insured patients to go for treatment to a special clinic. It is well with the State when personal and public health motives coincide in this way.

My last contrast relates to

INSURANCE FOR MEDICAL CARE

The British Position.—Reference is invited to Chapters XII and XIII for an outline of the British system of sickness insurance (financial) and insurance for medical care. It will be noted that this care is limited in the main to such domiciliary treatment of ailments as can reasonably be expected from a medical practitioner of average ability.

When in 1911 legislative proposals for medical attendance on the insured were laid before the medical profession they were strongly opposed. Doctors had suffered badly under forms of contract for medical attendance under the already existing friendly and allied insurance societies, and there was no guarantee that they would not suffer similarly under the Government's proposals. These proposals were altered. Insurance societies were not to be allowed to engage medical practitioners, under the new insurance medical service, but this was to be arranged by special Insurance Committees, on which doctors were represented. Actually the Insurance Department of the Central Government made a uniform national arrangement for payment of medical service on the basis of a capitation fee for each insured person. The fee was much higher than the Government had intended. There was much medical agitation against the revised arrangements, and some attempt to hold out against "contract practice." But wiser counsels prevailed, and—without attempting to describe subsequent modifications counselled by the British Medical Association and adopted, sometimes under pressure, by the Government—the position has developed in such wise that it has now become satisfactory on the whole both to doctors and to their insured patients. In Vol. III of *International Studies* and in Chapter VII of my *Medicine and the State*, full details are given. The outstanding fact now is that the medical profession, as represented by the British Medical Association, have by repeated resolution *endorsed a continuance and extension of insurance for medical treatment on a contract basis.* This is noteworthy, as in the British system (I quote from the last cited volume) "medical payments are made not on the basis of payment for each individual 'medical act,' but on a basis which makes the doctor share the risks of work, which will vary greatly according as sickness and injuries among the insured vary from season to season and from year to year."[1]

It is certain that the British insurance system has greatly improved the financial position of the average medical practitioner, not only by diminishing the amount of unpaid medical work which formerly fell to him, but also by increasing his average remuneration for the total sum of his industrial medical work. The service, as I have stated on page 111 is not altogether satisfactory from a hygienic standpoint, though even in this respect it is better than in the pre-insurance period, and is ready for vast further improvement.

To complete the British story I must allude to the "proposals of the British Medical Association for a General Medical Service for the Nation" (August 1930). The preface to this report states that the scheme is not one which the Association

[1] In a few areas the doctors at first adopted the alternative plan of remuneration according to work done, payment being made out of the total funds available for medical attendance in the area; but this method was abandoned in a few years.

wishes to press on the attention of the Government, but is "simply a record of proposals which the Association is making as to the way in which the medical services of the nation should develop, submitted for the consideration of all who are interested in the matter." The scheme was approved by a large majority at a meeting of the Representative Body of the Association in July 1930.

The scheme proposed to bring all indigent persons and all the dependents of the present insured within the terms of the contract insurance terms arranged under the present Insurance Act, with financial modifications. It proposed also that specialist services be included in medical benefit. From a public health standpoint a very important recommendation was that the present Insurance Committees should be replaced by statutory Committees of the County and County Borough Council. This represents an important change in the policy of the Association, for it was partly due to the opposition of the Association, when in 1911 the Insurance Bill was being discussed, that this most desirable unification was rejected. In this scheme it is claimed rightly that "as regards the control of the purely professional side of the service . . . as much responsibility as possible should be placed on the organised medical profession." In *Medicine and the State* I made the following comment on this scheme, which need not now be expanded:

The scheme shows how far the general medical profession in Britain has travelled in the realisation of the need for State and municipal organisation of medicine, for no scheme can become practicable without a large measure of State and municipal subsidisation. This advance is quite consistent with the continuance of some choice of doctor by the patient. It is consistent also with a part-time service of doctors in ordinary and expert medical practice, and with freedom of doctors from interference in their medical work. But this proposed vast extension of insurance for medical treatment will almost certainly mean that a high proportion of the doctors employed in insurance work will be occupied in this work almost exclusively; and no special foresight is needed to realise that the scheme as it develops may readily progress more and more towards a State service in which the number of full-time medical officers will greatly increase.

Although it would be relevant to the subject of this section, I cannot spare space for comment on the more recently published attitude of the British Medical Association towards the provision of an official municipal midwifery service for the entire country. In their proposals it is suggested that every midwifery case should be attended by a midwife, with a doctor in reserve, who will be called in for any abnormalities that arise either before or during childbirth, or in the immediately following weeks.

The American Position.—The attitude of the American medical profession, to the limited extent to which the American Medical Association can be said to voice it through its Board of Trustees or its House of Representatives, is unlike that of the medical profession in Great Britain. The temporary opposition in Great Britain to insurance for medical treatment was not directed against insurance itself, but against the methods proposed to effect it. The opposition of the American Medical Association appears to be one of objection to any form of medical insurance, except what can be arranged between individual doctors or groups of doctors and groups of prospective patients, without intervention of any external co-ordinating or controlling authority, whether industrial, or private enterprise, or governmental.

Evidently this position implies objection to any compulsory system of insurance; although compulsion, directly or indirectly, is needed if those most in need of the benefits of insurance are to be included.

This position, furthermore, implies distrust of local and central government in the States, and we have seen that there may be historical and sometimes contemporaneous justification for this. But no insurance scheme, on an adequate scale, is possible in which general taxation is not called on for substantial and continued financial support; and if the State contributes it must share the control of expenditure. This does not imply interference with the medical work of insurance, but only some control of the business side of the work involved. Organisation must, in part at least, be a subject of lay control, but the technique and conduct of medical care is for the technician, the doctor, alone.

If then the medical profession in America, as voiced by its politicians, continues to object to governing bodies, whether State or Federal, taking any part in the provision of medical care for the vast masses of people, who cannot possibly make complete direct payment, the profession must face certain stern alternatives. Either these multitudes must be left by the medical profession in suffering and distress, *or* the profession must organise non-official charity on an unprecedented scale, and this must be complete in all geographical and other circumstances, *or* the profession must cease to object to governing bodies taking their share in administering the non-medical side of this work. If—as is probably the case—they have "no confidence in politicians," is it not their bounden duty to join with other citizens in electing and giving continued support to official bodies that can be trusted?

These remarks apply not only to insurance for medical care but also to special child welfare and maternal care and clinics for special diseases, in relation to which these obstructive doctors have no righteous alternative but themselves to supply every medical need *or* to permit and support official governing bodies to join with them in supplying these needs, each taking its appropriate share in this work.

CHAPTER XLII

A VISIT TO SOVIET RUSSIA

INTRODUCTION

My European and American inquiries into methods of provision of medical—including hygienic—care for the community—briefly indicated in preceding chapters—were planned to give a fairly complete picture of what has been already initiated and, in part at least, accomplished to this end. In outlining these provisions in this volume, and in describing them more fully in my *International Studies* and in my *Medicine and the State*, I have been compelled in some chapters to dwell in somewhat fuller detail on the care of the sick than on measures for the prevention of sickness. In a description which was intended to indicate the evolution of these services in my life-time, this stress on sickness and its care was inevitable, for the problem of poverty in the sense of inability to provide needed help has governed the course of events; and the treatment of the sick—thereby curtailing its duration and ofttimes preventing its multiplication—has stood out among the successful methods of minimising poverty and disease. Indeed, it has been in treating sickness and in investigating the circumstances in which it becomes excessive, that a very large part of preventive medicine and its application in public health measures has been revealed and developed. The greater advance in recent decades has been due to the increasing realisation that this is true not only for diseases communicable from person to person, but also for illness of every category. Even the modern discoveries in nutrition have resulted in part from clinical investigation. They have greatly expanded the possibilities of disease prevention and of a higher standard of health. These more physiological aspects of medicine have had a highly successful application in infant and child welfare work in all English-speaking countries and doubtless also in other countries, of which the classical instance is the prevention of rickets (p. 174).

My later investigations in U.S.S.R. now to be outlined illustrate the same points. Clinical medicine is a vital essential part of preventive medicine. In previous chapters I have expressed regret that in poor-law medical work, in hospital work generally, and in domiciliary medical care—including what has been given on an insurance basis—there has been failure to realise the realisable potentialities of clinical work in its entirety as a guide to improved health and to prevention of recurrence of illness. This has been so in Great Britain and in other Western countries. The chief reforms of the future will consist in part in the application of our steadily increasing physiological knowledge, but even more in the use by all those attending the sick of the opportunities given by clinical medicine for securing improvements in environmental circumstances and in the hygienic control of living.

No apology, then, is needed for the stress laid on clinical medicine in my final visit of medical investigation, which is roughly sketched in the following pages. In this investigation I had the collaboration of Dr. J. A. Kingsbury, and the results of our work were embodied in *Red Medicine: Socialised Health in Soviet Russia*, 1933, pp. 324 (Doubleday, New York, and Heinemann, London).

This investigation was made to complete the investigations detailed in the three volumes of *International Studies*, after it had become clear that in the Soviet Union an ambitious and complete system of medical care by the State had been initiated "designed to provide preventive and curative medical care for every man, woman, and child" throughout its vast area. For a detailed description of this organisation as it was seen in 1933, I must refer the reader to our joint volume; and for a detailed description of the entire Soviet regime the two volumes (pp. 1174) of *Soviet Communism: A New Civilisation?* by Sidney and Beatrice Webb (Longmans, London) should be studied. These volumes not only bring our outline of Soviet Medicine up to date with convincing detail, but also set out with marvellous skill and force the entire Soviet philosophy, and not only its bearings on health, with which Dr. Kingsbury and I were chiefly concerned.

Let me first describe the circumstances of our itinerary.

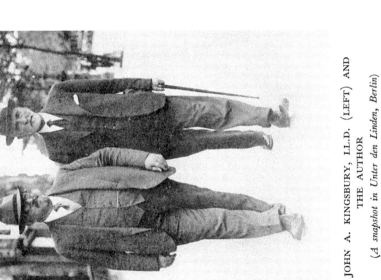

PROFESSOR ORBELI AND THE AUTHOR OUTSIDE
PAVLOV'S LABORATORY, LENINGRAD

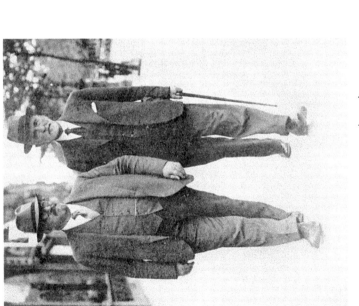

JOHN A. KINGSBURY, LL.D. (LEFT) AND
THE AUTHOR

(*A snapshot in Unter den Linden, Berlin*)

THE ITINERARY

We first travelled to Berlin by train from Bremenhaven. The photograph facing page 376 was taken by a street photo- grapher as we walked in Unter den Linden, and we were begged to let him bring post-card prints to our hotel. Leaving Berlin by train it was discovered on our night journey towards Poland that my passport lacked a Polish visa, and after spending four hours in the night in the waiting-room of a small station, we had to return by train to Berlin, where the necessary visa was obtained by our hotel porter without my presence being required!

Our itinerary after reaching Moscow is shown in the map facing page 378, taken from *Red Medicine* by permission of the Milbank Fund. After a few days in Moscow we travelled by train to Leningrad.[1] We spent busy days in both cities in inter- views and visits which are set out in our account in *Red Medicine*. Next, after a night journey by train we reached Nizhni–Novgorod (now Gorky), the Detroit of Russia, and after visiting great industrial works we took our place for several days on a boat travelling down the Volga. The course taken by the Volga can be seen in the map, and in our slow progress as far south as Stalingrad, we passed eastward to Kazan, an ancient fortress of the Tartars and capital of the Tartar republic. Kazan itself dwells in one's mind as an Oriental city in course of transformation towards Western conditions. The steamer stayed at many intermediate landing stages, and we had vivid glimpses of the excessive mobility of the peasants in search of occupation, crowding on to the boat, loaded with their belongings tied in a shawl or sheet, and with kettles and other utensils tied to these bundles. The crush of landing and embarking was some- times distressing, but the captain and crew were wonderfully patient, and the peasants and their families once aboard were good-tempered and adapted themselves cheerfully to manifold discomforts. It was difficult to walk on board, owing to these family encampments, and in the morning no breakfast was obtainable until our dining-room had been vacated by its

[1] The second photograph facing p. 376 was taken by Dr. Kingsbury outside Pavlov's laboratory, after a long interview with the son of Russia's greatest physiologist. Pavlov himself was absent from Leningrad.

night occupants. Strangely enough we suffered scarcely at all from the parasitic vermin which one anticipated under these conditions.

Passing Ulyanovsk, the birthplace of Lenin, a scene of many battles in the post-revolution civil wars, we came to Samara, the chief town of the Middle Volga region. Late on the third day of our Volga voyage, we reached Saratov, the centre of a district in which some half million Germans live in a semi-autonomous republic, speaking their own language and pre-serving their national characteristics. At the end of four full days we reached Stalingrad, where we left the Volga. On board we had numerous discussions with fellow travellers, and at each chief landing stage we had been met by representative officials, and when time permitted had visited typical institu-tions. Already we had realised how many races and subsidiary republics are included within Soviet Russia, and had seen how complex was the problem of administration of this continental empire. From Stalingrad we took train to Rostov-on-Don, reaching it some twenty hours later. It has a population approaching half a million, and is the chief centre for the northern Caucasus. I will not describe our inspections of factories, socialist farms and medical centres in this and other centres, but merely outline our main movements. More than twenty-four hours after leaving Rostov we arrived at Vladi-kavkaz. Next day we travelled by motor-car some 135 miles through the Caucasus Mountains, reaching Tiflis, the capital of the Trans-Caucasian republic and of the republic of Georgia, a great centre of eastern industry and of education. After interviews with its chief officials and visits to important institu-tions, we visited a State farm and a collective farm. We travelled from Tiflis to Batum on the Black Sea, and were impressed by its sub-tropical trees and shrubs. Here we inspected a splendidly organised large tea farm. From Batum we took a steamer bound via Sochi for Yalta in the Crimea, and enjoyed the restfulness of two days skirting the coast, with views of sub-tropical gardens and the vast snow-capped Caucasus Mountains in the back-ground. On the boat we found medical women and others with whom we discussed Russian hygienic and social problems.

Yalta, where we spent two days, is the workers' paradise.

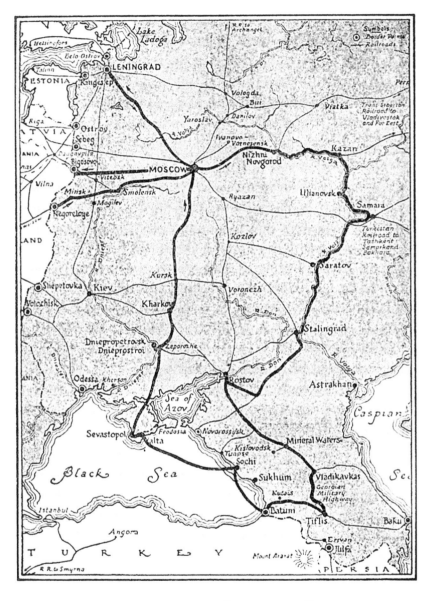

REPRODUCED FROM "RED MEDICINE"

By permission of Messrs. W. Heinemann Ltd., and the Millbank Memorial Fund

Here some tens of thousands of workers are sent on vacation for rest and treatment. They live in palaces, including Livadia, the palace of the former Czar, in which were accommodated some 1,500 workers, who needed special treatment, or who, as "shock-workers," had distinguished themselves by their great output. From Yalta we motored to Sevastopol, and thence took the night train to Kharkov, then the capital of the Ukraine, one of the seven constituent republics of U.S.S.R. Here as in other cities visited by us we found examples of very advanced medical provision, both curative and hygienic. From Kharkov we returned to Moscow by night train, and spent some days there, before my return by air on one day to Berlin, and on the next day to Croydon. This I found far and away the most comfortable and least fatiguing of my travels. In Soviet Russia itself these travels had amounted at least to 9,000 miles.

This bare outline can give but a faint notion of the vast extent of Russia, which embraces a larger area than the United States and Canada combined. It comprises a sixth part of the land surface of the earth, and has a population of some 165 or 170 million people, including a hundred different nations and languages. Our itinerary, shown in the map, includes only a small segment of Russia.

Much less can this outline bring to the surface the intense interest of each visit and of the social and medical inquiries made by us.

CHAPTER XLIII

SOVIET COMMUNISM

So much has been written on Soviet Russia that it is unnecessary to attempt more than a partial outline of the impression
created by the greatest experiment in social administration
of the world's history. Apart from the comments in this chapter
I limit myself to an account of the unique establishment in the
U.S.S.R. of a complete system of socialised State medicine.

The stages of the establishment of socialised communism in
Soviet Russia are outlined in *Red Medicine*, and are given with
authoritative detail and insight in the book of Sidney and
Beatrice Webb already mentioned.

My own impressions of conditions in 1933 were very mixed.
There had been gross injustice in exploitation of private
property, in confiscations, in merciless killing of those who
would not accept the Bolshevist doctrines. As in Germany
and in Italy, where there has been a partially comparable
course of events, a minority seized power, and have since then
been actively engaged in inducing or compelling the majority
of the people to "toe their line." In Soviet Russia the dictatorship has been that of a skilfully organised educational party,
while in Germany and still more in Italy the dictatorship is
chiefly personal. The party in power in Soviet Russia appears
to me to have had much greater success in its efforts to secure a
crowd psychology favourable to it than has been experienced
in either Germany or Italy. The difference in degree of success
is ascribable in part to the fact that in Germany and Italy
changes which appear socialist or semi-socialist in character have
been initiated within a regime which remains capitalistic, and
in which the poor are still exploited. New wine has been put
into old bottles, while in Soviet Russia capitalism[1] is a thing
of the past. In U.S.S.R. motives of ownership and private profit
have been abolished. This contrast is true for great industries
and for the employment of labour; but it is consistent with

[1] That is capitalism beyond what the capitalist can spend himself,
without employing workers.

wages, which have always been differential in U.S.S.R. and are now based more strictly on the wage-earner's achievement; and it is consistent with the fact that many peasants are now to be entitled to possess as their private property bees, three acres of land, and a cow.

Marx demanded possession and control of production and means of production as a necessary condition of a socialist State, and the Soviet State, notwithstanding the above-named concession to the workers' individualism, may be regarded as consistently socialistic in having abolished money profit in its industrial and agricultural communal organisations. These cover almost the entire field of national activity.

It may be worth while to pursue a little further the comparison between Soviet Socialism or Communism and the efforts at collectivism in other countries. There was much consolidation of total national effort in Great Britain and in other countries during the Great War; but this was associated with colossal profiteering at the expense of the nation. The programmes in the American "New Deal" embody a great effort to carry out gigantic schemes in the public interest, while eschewing excessive private profits; and in England similar schemes have been successfully initiated for transport, for the supply of electricity, and for reorganising the coal industry. These promise well, and present the common characteristic that the profits of the producer or the "middle man" will, in part at least, accrue to the consumer. But in Soviet Russia not only have activities such as those named above been carried to a successful issue, the State being the sole employer, but the whole industry of the country, broadly speaking, has been similarly organised. If corruption in management can be eliminated or minimised this success will continue.

The bourgeoisie as a class has been eliminated. In the Soviet philosophy the bourgeois is the hated proprietor. He was partially eliminated from Russian life in the earlier bourgeois revolution of February 1917. The expropriation of land then announced led to troops in multitudes deserting from the front, to take up the confiscated land. Soviets or Councils of workers were formed, and these gradually usurped the place of the Kerensky Government. In September 1917, Russia became a republic, the Bolshevik Government being formed in November.

This was not accomplished by the votes of the general population, in the then circumstances an impossible method; but in accord with the aphorism of Marx that force is the midwife of history, and according to Lenin's formula: "the State is the tyranny of a minority over the majority." They were not alone in this view. Even Kerensky, the head of the Government formed in the early months of 1917, expressed the view that "no self-government is possible for a nation of newly liberated slaves." This meant that the vast mass of the Russian people were incompetent to judge of the merits of their Government, and it thus became necessary to act through a relatively small minority of well-trained men.

I do not propose to dwell on the cruelties preceding and associated with the early struggles to seize and to consolidate communism. Bolshevism was so organised that a small oligarchy controlled the main elements of government, pending the time when the general population would become sufficiently educated for widened responsibility. That this later stage is already partially reached is evidenced by recent events in U.S.S.R. Local and central parliaments are now (1936) to be elected by universal direct and secret voting. The peasants—until now left out partially in the cold—are being given suffrage with secret ballot the same as for town dwellers, and as already stated some measure of private ownership is now allowed. The comparison with Germany and Italy is now to Russia's credit in approach to representative government; while Russia has cast off entirely, unlike the two Western countries, private ownership of land and of means of large-scale profit. Whether this be regarded as good or not, Soviet Russia is placed in a distinctive and separate category from other countries.

The activities of the Tchekha and its successor the Ogpu, the Russian secret police, led to horrors the magnitude of which can only be guessed. In the early years 1918–22, no man's life was safe. The extrusion or "liquidation" of the Kulaks (labour-employing farmers) also meant vast suffering, and agriculture is only now recovering from the privations and incompetence which too rapid socialisation of farming produced. In towns there has been vast progress in industrialisation, hampered all the time by inability to convert peasants quickly into skilled artisans, competent to work the immense factories which have sprung up.

Soviet Communism is actively anti-religious. The type of religious belief in the pre-revolution period, and the conditions in the orthodox Church partially explain this; the Communists have adopted materialism of an intolerant type, and the anti-religion museums which I saw in a number of former churches included revolting caricatures which misrepresented the true spirit of Christianity. It is strange to contrast what one saw in these museums with what one witnessed at the tomb of Lenin, just outside the Kremlin wall in Moscow. As foreign visitors we had not to wait our turn to view the embalmed body of Lenin, along with the multitudes who daily undertake this pilgrimage. Truly the Soviets have almost deified Lenin; and as with them there is no hereafter, they have tried to immortalise his clay. This was so perfectly preserved that I could not refrain from the probably erroneous guess that a wax model must have been substituted for the original corpse.

I must refer any interested reader to the volumes already cited if they wish to fill up the blanks in this hasty sketch. I add a few paragraphs on

SOCIAL LIFE IN SOVIET RUSSIA

One could not fail to be deeply impressed by the momentous changes, effected in a very few years, in home life and in the position of women in the community. The most essential change is the "emancipation" of women. As Beatrice and Sidney Webb express it, scores of millions of peasant or wage-earning women were not only freed from the exploitation of the landlord and the capitalist, but there was also "an immediate release from the authority of the father or the husband." Woman became possessed in all respects of the same status as man. How far this was hastened by the need to abolish sex differences in order to multiply workers in the fevered advance of industrialism I cannot say; but it is far-reaching and momentous in all grades of society. Three-fourths of the medical practitioners are women; women everywhere worked alongside of men in heavy industries and in driving tramcars. Every help was given them to minimise the disabilities of women as workers when maternity intervened. Thus there were industrial crèches, schools for toddlers, even care of children in the evening so that mothers might frequent their clubs.

MARRIAGE

Marriage itself was deprived of its sacredness. It was registered with a minimum of ceremony, and could be officially dissolved at any time by either of the partners, without the knowledge of the other partner. No obloquy attached to living together without marriage, and these irregular unions had equal legal standing with marriage. I must refer to *Red Medicine* for illustrations of the position.

In such circumstances marriages sometimes became a farce, as did also divorce; and desertions of children were frequent. Recently desertion has been severely punished, and the securing of a divorce is being hedged around by conditions.

Families imply family loyalties, just as religion implies higher loyalties. The State is not all in all; and in these regards the leaders of Soviet Russia still suffer from mental and moral myopia.

THE CARE OF MATERNITY

This, at least in cities, is well provided for. Ante-natal care is given, pregnant women receive a supplementary food ration, they have precedence in shops and in street cars, and they are exempted for from twelve to sixteen weeks from their industrial work, their full wage continuing. In cities nine-tenths of confinements occur in maternity hospitals, and even in rural districts this proportion is considerable. Grants for the infant's clothing and food are given, and free crèches are available up to the age of five years.

ABORTION

The official sanctioning and provision of abortion on request is a startling feature of Soviet life. All laws against abortion have been repealed, and the State undertakes to produce it in suitable cases. It should be borne in mind that in many countries, perhaps especially in the United States and in

Germany, as well as in Russia under the past regime, abortion produced by unskilled persons has been extremely common. This, it may be stated in passing, is a chief reason why the crude death-rate from childbirth (including abortion) has failed to show statistical decline, to the exaggerated dismay of amateur statisticians, and of a crowd of sentimentalists, who look only at the crude figures (see p. 222). This problem was investigated in Soviet Russia, and there began active propagandism in favour of conception-control, and propaganda as to the great risks of surreptitious abortions. I visited a museum in Rostov, illustrating this teaching by life-size wax models and pictures of pathological consequences of abortion. It was open to youths of both sexes, and its realism and lack of reserve made one shudder, however desirable was the object. The State hospitals then undertook to produce abortion if asked for within three months of conception, if it were not a first confinement (this condition was not always required) and if after discussion of the position with the doctor, the woman persisted in her request. In the year of my visit abortions exceeded births at term, as they probably do in some Western countries. But in Soviet Russia they are produced with maximum regard for the mother's safety; in other countries they are usually secret and are much more dangerous.[1]

I do not discuss "birth-control" and abortion in these pages. The two can scarcely be separated, for—inasmuch as contraceptive measures, looked on generally with complacency, not infrequently fail—abortion is often sought in many of these birth-control failures. Can we draw a completely defensible ethical line between prevention by contraceptive measures of the union of germ and sperm, and prevention of the continuance to birth at term of the ovum resulting from their union? It is almost certain that in the next few decades younger hygienists and humanists will be pressing forward new arguments against conception-control, and attempting to stay the

---

[1] In 1936 the public policy of u.s.s.r. both as to birth-control and abortion has been profoundly modified. These methods of restricting population are not to be encouraged, except when special reasons for them exist in individual cases. Divorce also is discouraged. Evidently family ties are resuming their essential importance.

progress towards national suicide and preponderant old age which is in progress.

THE CARE OF CHILDREN

The fact that most infants in U.S.S.R. are born in institutions, enhances the initial prospect of the infant's future health. Infant consultations are general, and every mother has access to skilled medical advice. After infancy public nurseries, open air and other schools, and summer camps relieve parents from a large share of their burden in the care of their children, and this is done for nearly the entire population. It is thus that the State provides for the economic equality of women with men. In the Soviet State married women are regarded more as industrialists than as housekeepers! I cannot here describe the Youth Movement in its many branches, all under State control. The movement embraces both sexes and all ages from seven to twenty-five. Most of its work is excellent, but its encouragement of hatred of class enemies and its anti-religious vows are deplorable. It must be added that in all the three States—Russia, Germany, and Italy—already mentioned, one must regard with dismay the drastic methods and the vast success achieved in so influencing and bending the minds of the young that their personality has become very generally a mere repetition of the teaching and enforced example of the small coterie of governors who yield unlimited power.

SOCIAL INSURANCE

The Russian system of social insurance necessarily differs from that of any capitalistic countries, in view of the total abolition of private capital. The State is the sole employer; its employees are State servants, so that to obtain weekly contributions from workers would be merely financial jugglery. There is practically no intentional unemployment in Soviet Russia for workers in towns. Full wages are paid during absence from work because of illness, and of course free medical services are given for the insured as for the rest of the population. There is an immense amount of use of rest homes, sanatoria, and similar institutions for the sick, and for workers during their vacation. The cost of these various benefits is a definite charge on each industry. There is no charitable relief in Russia, the worker being entitled to his allowances when in need of them.

GENERAL COMMENTS

Can I conclude my summary of Soviet Communism with an expression of general approval? In giving my personal view, I must place Soviet Russia's position as regards medical and hygienic care of the community in a distinctive position. In the adventure into completely socialised medicine, as will be seen in the next chapter, U.S.S.R. has rushed impetuously and "bald-headed" into a policy and action towards which nearly every Western country is advancing by slow and stuttering steps. But writing at this point solely on non-medical activities, can one approve of the present position in Soviet Russia? I find it impossible to give a single answer, either affirmative or negative to this question; for, while in many particulars one can admire the singleness of vision which has brought about the greatest social change in the world's history, there is much in the present position which one disapproves, and much more to disapprove in the means by which the present position has been reached.

In the social development of humanity, progress based primarily on coercion, in my view, is unsound, even when the result attained is communally desirable. Is not the evolution of moral sensibility a chief aim in the ascent of man? But rapid reform by revolution and coercion—even though the aim be desirable—appeals mainly to selfish motives, the determination to win out in the struggle for existence and to advance the glory of the State, which is this struggle extended. This may, as in Soviet Russia, succeed; but it then partakes more of the nature of an animal triumph in a titanic struggle than of a spiritual development, and if so it will not benefit humanity as a whole. Such a triumph must eventually collapse, if my diagnosis and prognosis be correct, unless it is propped up by the higher and nobler motive of love for one's neighbour, which is as far apart as the poles from coercion as a driving power. The great danger of Soviet Russia is the lust for power (and possibly graft) of the small group who still direct its future. I mention "graft," for there must be danger that the lust for wealth which has been ejected will return through subterranean channels.

I have already animadverted on the mental and moral coercion employed in the training of the young (p. 386). Small children and youths are constantly indoctrinated in communistic teaching and they must—if they join the youth movement—agree formally to an atheistic belief or rather disbelief. There is no freedom of choice of religious conviction even for adults who desire to be members of the Communist Party or Order. In such an atmosphere moral development is endangered. My hope for u.s.s.r. is that these religious restrictions will be removed, and liberty will be accorded on this side of life comparable to the increasing liberty in other less important respects.

Meanwhile is not the Soviet Government to some extent in the position of the man who could see only what was visible to his earth-directed vision?

> Two men looked out through their prison bars,
> One saw mud, the other Stars.

CHAPTER XLIV

NATIONALISED OR STATE MEDICAL SERVICES IN U.S.S.R.

MEDICAL care in Soviet Russia has been completely "taken over" by the Government. There are no voluntary medical charities, and scarcely any private medical practitioners. Excepting these rare survivals every Russian doctor is a State official, and as such is subject to official regulations. This appears to differ entirely from the position in other countries; but, as will be shown in the next chapter, the difference, however striking, is one of degree more than of kind. In judging the official character of Russian medicine, this point must be borne in mind; as must also the need for banishing from our minds prejudice carried over from possible abhorrence of Soviet Communism or Socialism as a whole. In regard to medical work, we all of us, doctors and the general public alike, in every country in some measure are Socialists in matters of medical or hygienic care.

The facts set out in various chapters of this volume, and the fuller accounts of Russian practice given, for instance, in *Red Medicine*, make the accuracy of this statement abundantly clear. I plead, therefore, for impartial judgment on the degree of Socialism implied in State medical services, apart from any doctrinal position in which we may be personally embedded. Orthodoxy in the shape of consistency is a chief enemy of public weal. Why should we not believe in and practise Socialism (defined as exclusion of private profit, except in the form of wage or salary) in any given particular, and decide against it in other respects, if impartial and thorough inquiry points to the decision reached in each instance?

With this preliminary plea, one can now outline Soviet medicine, in a series of somewhat categorical statements. I refer the reader to the details given in *Red Medicine* and in the more complete statement in Webb's *Soviet Communism*.

(1) Free medical services are almost universal in Soviet Russia. They may not be universally available, but the gaps

which have been serious in Russia's vast rural districts, are being filled up, the number of doctors is increasing each year, and will ere long become adequate for the complete needs of the people.

(2) A corresponding change has been effected in the position of medical practitioners. Monetary motives have ceased to operate in Russian medical practice. "The doctor has been removed from the field of monetary competition" (Red Medicine, p. 266). My own official experience in England has been that the quality of medical work is as high in official as it is in private medical practice under competitive conditions, and all I saw in Russia stengthened my opinion that non-competitive medical care was not inferior to the care under a system which includes competition. The experience of insurance medical practice in this country partially points in the same direction. As I have said elsewhere (Medicine and the State, p. 145):

> For the conscientious insurance doctor it is a great boon to be able to give satisfactory treatment to the persons on his panel, without regard to a future doctor's bill.

I have said "partially," because in insurance medical practice in Western countries, certainly in Britain, the practitioner is selected by the patient and works under competitive conditions. These may sometimes lead to unduly hurried work, if not also occasionally to undue complacency in medical certification of inability to work. I need not repeat what I have said (Red Medicine, p. 268), as to the small measure of importance attaching to financial motives for efficiency in medical work. Professional pride, the desire to excel and to stand well with one's fellows are more important than the monetary inducement; and I am confident that this pride and the satisfaction which comes from serving and helping the suffering, are significant and lasting motives of good work.

(3) Medical aid in Russia although substantially free for all, is made preferentially available to all industrial workers and to the peasant, who form the vast majority of the people. In most other countries this is not so, outside the wide range of medical charity.

(4) It is important to note that there is now in Russia only

one wide channel of medical aid. In each of its republics there is a unit national system for all.

(5) Medical treatment is given gratuitously to those receiving it. Its cost is defrayed by governmental funds, derived in the main from the pursuit of the national monopolistic industries. The few minor exceptions to gratuitous treatment, as in some sanatoria, in the treatment of abortion and in certain clinics and for some non-workers, do not invalidate this general statement.

(6) The unit medical system has been rendered more practicable and more efficient by the extent to which treatment is given in centralised clinics and residential institutions. In all Western countries a similar trend to institutional treatment is visible, but nowhere has it become so complete as in Soviet Russia. I must refer readers to my *Medicine and the State* for further discussion of this subject.

(7) Judging by the numerous examples seen in our travels in Soviet Russia and by its nation-wide schemes which are coming more and more into being, a further characteristic must be added as to its medical service. The different parts of the service are carefully co-ordinated, and in every local organisation visited by us, we were struck with the admirable way in which a complete examination of each patient was made possible, without gaps or overlapping. So far as I know, in no country except Russia—at least in its chief centres of population—could the same statement be made, with so close an approximation to facts.

(8) I have not mentioned special public health work in the foregoing review of Russian medical services. As is well known, pre-revolution Russia had an excessive death-rate and an extremely excessive incidence of infectious diseases, especially typhoid and typhus fevers. Sanitation was imperfect, and overcrowding with its associated evils was almost the rule. Without giving details, it may be said generally that there are many evidences of improvement, and, as we saw, there was being built up a system of sanitary control, the effects of which can, as yet, be only partially seen. By thus beginning almost at zero point, Soviet Russia has one great advantage. Its public health service from the first is part of its general medical

service. Thus personal and communal hygiene can be studied and practised as constituent parts of the same health problem. This is so, especially, in combating the evils of overcrowding. Rapid industrialisation has meant extreme crowding of people in Russia's great towns. Large-scale efforts have been made in building new tenements, but they have not yet overtaken the need. The vast hospitalisation of the sick which has been given, has done much, especially for consumptives, to reduce the maleficent effect of this overcrowding.

It is strange that the unification of public health and general medical work which Russia has attained at a stride, is now only slowly and incompletely being reached in Western countries.[1]

The story of successive stages in unification in Great Britain has been partially told in earlier chapters of this volume. The first attempts at English sanitary reform were on a Poor Law basis, and the isolation and treatment in institutions of cases of infectious disease were carried out by local Boards of Guardians. Then Public Health Authorities were created, and were given similar powers, in addition to their work to ensure sanitation, especially safe water supplies. Mental diseases came to be treated in institutions in part by both sets of local authorities. The scope of the work of public health authorities rapidly widened; but it was not until 1929 in Britain that most of the medical work of Boards of Guardians was transferred to the larger public health authorities. Medical treatment of the third of the total population who are officially insured, occupies an intermediate position. Local health authorities have little or no concern with it. It must be admitted that in Britain there still exists much awkward dichotomy of public health and clinical medicine, which clogs the wheels of completely satisfactory administration.

[1] This is true administratively, but it must be noted that so far as purely environmental or sanitary reform is concerned, Russia is struggling to emerge from what was the English position some seventy years ago.

CHAPTER XLV

NATIONALISED MEDICAL SERVICES IN OTHER COUNTRIES

On page 389 I stated that the medical service of the Soviet State differed from the medical services in Western countries, including America, more in degree than in kind. It is necessary for me to justify this statement. This justification necessitates a brief statement of changes in medical administration which have occurred during the last thirty years. I have watched these changes and in some degree have taken part in them in England, and I begin my hasty review with notes on my own country. Some parts of this review are stated more fully in preceding chapters of this volume.

ENGLAND

In some degree medical care of the destitute sick has been a State responsibility from Elizabethan days. Alongside of religious and other voluntary provision for the sick poor, the State has always been held responsible for their general succour. The course of poor-law organisation to this end may be seen partially in Chapter x. In the latter half of the nineteenth, and still more during the four decades of the twentieth century, the public conscience has been roused to perform this State duty less unsatisfactorily. By the Local Government Act of 1929, the general control of the medical care of the poor was handed over to the public health Committees of the great public health authorities, county councils and county borough councils, and at the same time the official hospitals for the poor were made available for other classes of society, payment for treatment being assessed by hospital almoners in accord with the means of the patient or of the head of his family. It should be added that such payments seldom amount to more than a relatively small part of the cost of lodging and treatment; and most of the cost in these official hospitals for the general public falls on local rates and national taxation.

*

In England, as in America, voluntary (charity) hospitals have been generously provided in most towns of considerable size. Most of them in England were intended originally for the very poor, and have had the solitary advantage over official hospitals that there is no limitation of admission to persons living in the same administrative area. In the past the reputation of these voluntary hospitals has been higher than that of official hospitals. They are staffed by visiting surgeons and physicians, who give their services gratuitously, and any recompense coming to them is in the shape of exceptional experience and of the prestige which brings private practice. These voluntary hospitals, especially in London, are not conveniently distributed for serving different parts of the Metropolis, and they have never been equal to the needs of the poor. In practice they have been obliged to select their patients, preference being given to patients with acute illnesses, or those requiring operations, or cases of special interest. Other patients may, in view of limited accommodation, be passed on to municipal or county hospitals, the executive of which cannot refuse any patient who belongs to the municipal or county area concerned, if the patient is in real need of hospital treatment. No financial conditions are now imposed for admission to these official hospitals, though, as already indicated, some share of the cost can subsequently be claimed. In recent years an increasing proportion of acute, including surgical, patients are being admitted to these official hospitals, and the distinction between voluntary and official hospitals as regards competence of staffs is wearing thin.

Voluntary hospitals now also commonly receive patients who can afford to contribute to the cost of their treatment, and schemes of voluntary insurance for hospital treatment when this becomes necessary are now fairly general. (For details of these see pp. 69–80 of Vol. III of my *International Studies.*) Here again it must be noted that these massed insurance contributions only pay a part of the cost of hospital treatment of those who have had the foresight to insure. The remaining cost is defrayed by subscribers and donors to the hospitals concerned.

The preceding statement brings out this fact, that in actual experience the chief part of the cost of treating sickness and accidents in hospitals, voluntary and official, is defrayed by voluntary charity or by local rates and taxes.

The M.O.H. of the County of London has stated that five-sixths of the institutional treatment of the sick in London is undertaken out of public funds. If provision for the insane be included, the London County Council is now responsible for eight times as many sick beds, as all the metropolitan voluntary hospitals.

The preceding statement by itself, apart from the notes on further official provision of medical aid set out below, supports the general statement (on p. 43 of my *Medicine and the State*) that

as civilisation advances and the public conscience is aroused, not only is public health work in its limited sense increasingly developed, but there is also a corresponding increase in communal effort towards satisfactory and complete medical care of the sick.

This is true in varying degree for all countries.

The British position as regards the treatment of the insane and of persons of defective intellect is that in the main it is carried out at the expense of rates and taxes.

In previous chapters it has been shown that on a very large scale medical and still more hygienic care is undertaken at the expense of the State, including the medico-hygienic care for infants and for school children. The institutional treatment of tuberculous and crippled children and adults is chiefly at the cost of the public; and so, almost entirely is that of venereal diseases.

How much of total care of the sick in institutions is supplied at the public cost cannot be exactly stated; but it must vastly exceed what is paid by patients themselves and their relatives. And during the last thirty years this impersonal payment for institutional treatment by voluntary charity and by rates and taxes has steadily increased. The increase extends beyond the sick to provision for childbirth, which although often otherwise, is a physiological event for most mothers. An increasing proportion of mothers are confined in municipal and other institutions, in part at least at the cost of taxes and of charity. Can it be doubted that charity and taxation (including local rates) are the main source of the funds for all the institutional treatment that is needed? And may we not make a forecast that ere long institutional medical provision will be so generally available for the entire population, that the question as to whether payment for individual treatment of a satisfactory character shall be made by the recipient or indirectly through general taxation, will be a mere point of expediency?

When payment for the cost of hospital treatment is by general taxation, the hospital patient ceases to be a recipient of "charity." He is simply receiving what for years he has insured to receive, by paying his rates and taxes. The main reason for continuing partial payment according to means is that the imperfectly educated and not too conscientious recipient of treatment in this way is made fully cognisant of the value of the social benefit he receives, and of his share in its cost.

But, notwithstanding the enormous growth of treatment of sickness in and at institutions, sickness mostly is treated at the patient's home. For the destitute, salaried doctors provide this in England; for others private medical practitioners, the backbone of the medical profession, give it, the patient choosing his own doctor. But this has proved inadequate and doctors are imperfectly distributed. It has the additional drawback, except for insured persons, that there is the constant inducement—in view of medical charges—to delay treatment, sometimes with calamitous result. The same motive leads to delay or failure to secure the skilled consultations which a given case may require. There is, under present conditions, a vast amount of inco-ordination between the private practitioner and consultative services when the patient has recourse to them.

Insurance for medical care has been practised for many decades by private insurance, including Friendly Societies, and this provision in 1911 became national and compulsory in Britain for a third of the total population, the cost of this being shared between the worker, his employer, and the State. Thus the State intervened to make it obligatory for a third of the total population to insure for their domiciliary medical care as well as for financial benefits when they became sick. They must insure, even though they need not avail themselves of the choice of doctor placed before them. (For details see Chapter XIII.) This may or may not be a socialist measure—it is a question of definition of terms—but it is universally accepted in Britain, and not least enthusiastically by the general medical practitioners in every part of the land, who are the agents for this domiciliary medical service. They indeed have combined to express their desire that a similar system should be extended to all the dependents of the insured, and that it should be made to include also institutional and consultant services. This, and especially the extension of the present insurance service proposed on behalf of the medical profession, would constitute a revolution in the conditions of medical work in Britain, so far as four-fifths of the entire population are concerned. But this revolution in its compulsory extension is consistent with the patient's freedom of choice of doctor, and the doctor's freedom to decline to attend any patient. The medical practice thus carried on is in reality a form of State service: for the State contributes to the cost and imposes regulations, and the employer of the worker is involved in payments, over the spending of which he has no control. But it is a branch of State service in which all the ordinary conditions of private medical work are conserved, except the—to many—objectionable condition of having to send out or receive periodical bills for services rendered.

In the medical service for the highlands and islands of Scotland (see Chapter XXIII, Vol. III of *International Studies*) large sums of money are granted from the national Treasury to ensure an adequate medical service, in parts of Scotland in which owing to distance and inaccessibility satisfactory medical care cannot otherwise be maintained.

This sketch of the travel in Britain towards socialised medicine is far from complete; it is especially incomplete in regard to the vast medical work still undertaken by voluntary hospitals and other organisations for domiciliary medical help for the people. But if, as from a broad standpoint we should, we regard these voluntary efforts as vicarious for the gaps in official services, we gain a complete view of the extent to which British experience has drawn us towards socialised medical aid for the entire population. Its chief difference from the Russian system is that voluntary efforts have not been swept aside, and a complete system for the entire British population has not been initiated. But it is a medical service which is steadily increasing.

U.S.A.

I do not possess detailed information enabling me to describe the extent to which in the United States medicine has already become socialised, in the sense that it is obtained apart from direct individual or family expenditure. In one particular the position is less advanced than in Britain. America hitherto (1936) has no national system of domiciliary medical care imposed by obligatory insurance on a large proportion of the total population. But it has, on a vast scale, hospitals and other official and unofficial arrangements for medical care in which the recipient of aid may pay little or nothing. These provisions, especially hospitals, whether voluntary or official, are oftener on a paying basis than in Britain, though the amount of gratuitous hospital treatment in America is very great. Especially for tuberculosis, gratuitous institutional treatment is given on a scale which is probably even more generous than that in Britain. But notwithstanding what has already been accomplished, the words of the final Majority Report of the American Committee on the Costs of Medical Care (p. 135) truthfully state the inevitable general conclusion:

The one million persons who furnish medical care and the one hundred and twenty-three millions who may receive it should make concerted and carefully planned efforts to meet needs and *to devise remedies for present deficiencies and wastes* (italics mine).
See also page 363 for an account of Biggs' attempt.

The same lessons stand out as have led to extensive socialisation of medicine in Britain. The medical care of the American people can only be made satisfactory by calling in aid some form of obligatory insurance for sickness, or with or without this by following the example of Soviet Russia in providing medical care out of communal funds for all who need it.

OTHER COUNTRIES

I must refer the reader to the volumes already quoted several times, for information as to other European countries. I merely give here a brief statement. In all the larger countries a vast proportion of total medical care of the population is at the expense of the State directly, or is provided in part through compulsory systems of insurance. The universal experience is that only by having recourse to communal funds can the total medical needs of the people be satisfactorily met. The State can do what the majority of its individual members are totally incompetent to accomplish, because the cost of action by the State is distributed over the entire population, and communal provision furthermore is more satisfactory than competitive small-scale undertakings. Medical care when supplied by the State ceases to be a charity, and comes into the same category as municipal or national supply of police, of parks and recreation grounds, of sanitation, of clean water and so on. It is for the community in each country to decide what system of medical aid it will adopt.

For many years in most countries it will continue to be partially a private concern and partially a concern of the State. These countries will hesitate to go as far as U.S.S.R., for they are already deeply involved in complex arrangements. But their future arrangements must be such as will meet the conditions as to efficiency and completeness already indicated; and neither the United States of America nor any other country can fail to reach the conclusion ere long that the problem of adequate medical care has ceased to be one which can be solved for the poorer half of its population by direct family payments. Nor can the consequential inference be evaded that aid from State funds is required, with or without insistence on individual insurance payments, in order that all unnecessary suffering can be avoided, and that the transformation of medicine into preventive medicine can be expedited.

LIST OF PERSONAL CONTRIBUTIONS (1908-35)

[Additional to those enumerated at end of Chapters XV, XVI, and XVIII, and at various points in the text]

Some Conditions of Social Efficiency in Relation to Local Public Administration. (*Public Health*, August 1909.)

The Declining Birth-rate: Its National and International Significance. (Cassell & Co., 1911.)

Epidemic Catarrhs and Influenza. (*Lancet*, November 23, 1918.)

Some Problems of Preventive Medicine of the Immediate Future. (An address to the Toronto Academy of Medicine, *Canadian Practitioner*, August 1919.)

Public Health and Insurance: American Addresses, pp. 270. (Johns Hopkins Press, 1920.)

National Changes in Health and Longevity. (Lecture to Harvey Society of New York, *Quarterly Publication of American Statistical Association*, June 1921.)

The Better use of Vital Statistics in Public Health Administration. Address at a Dinner Meeting of the American Statistical Association in honour of the author. (*Quarterly Publication of the American Statistical Association*, September 1921.)

Humane Slaughtering and the Public Health. (B. W. Richardson Memorial Lecture, October 1923.)

The Measurement of Progress in Public Health. William Farr Memorial Lecture. (*Economica*, November 1923.)

Things that Matter in Public Health. (*Journal Royal Sanitary Institute*, 1923.)

The Ministry of Health, pp. 271. (G. P. Putnam's, 1925.)

Medical Views on Birth Control, edited by Sir James Marchant. (M. Hopkinson & Co., 1926). Chapter VII, "Some Public Health Aspects."

Health Problems in Organised Society, pp. 253. (P. S. King & Son, 1927.)

International Studies on the Relation between the Private and Official Practice of Medicine, with special reference to the Prevention of Disease. (Three volumes, George Allen & Unwin, 1930–31.)

Medicine and the State, pp. 300. (George Allen & Unwin, 1932.)

The Relationship of the Private Medical Practitioner to Preventive Medicine. (*Journal Amer. Med. Assoc.*, May 14, 1932.)

Red Medicine: Socialised Health in Soviet Russia. (With J. A. Kingsbury; Heinemann, 1934.)

Some Anomalies of Local Public Health Administration. Presidential Address to the Royal Sanitary Institute Congress, Sec. I. (*Lancet*, June 20, 1935.)

EPILOGUE

My review of social and medical happenings in my lifetime seems to require some general remarks in conclusion. In many preceding chapters will be found a statement of my judgment on the problem or problems discussed in these chapters, and one need only emphasise here a few points.

In these years there has been a marvellous and unparalleled growth of human knowledge. Furthermore, this knowledge, instead of having the prolonged dormancy characterizing the past, has been speedily applied in practice on a large scale. Increased knowledge brought with it the serious problems of urbanisation and urban crowding, and their many dangers to health and well-being; but it has also brought power to overcome these dangers and to secure higher standards of health and comfort, far surpassing those of the past.

Life has been lengthened, sickness has been curtailed, and leisure and recreation have become more generally distributed. Thus on the physical side of life, vast improvements have occurred, largely as the result of the devoted work of social and public health workers.

Even as regards nutrition of the people, social insurance and other reforms have meant that a smaller proportion of the total population suffers from privation than in past generations. Our standards have risen, and the luxuries of the past are now regarded as indispensable, and are enjoyed by the majority of the population. The nation is determined that the children of the poor shall not continue to be worse nourished than the children of the rich, as is shown by the initial national steps for giving milk to school-children. Large-scale experiments have shown that the height and weight, age for age, of children of the poor, which are less than in the children of the well-to-do, can be increased; and we can confidently anticipate that this public provision of milk will become as universally available as is elementary education itself.

In my lifetime, the improved care of the necessitous whether sick or not, is an outstanding feature; and it is especially noteworthy that this improvement is increasingly on preventive lines, and not merely on lines of immediate relief. We have ceased to be only Good Samaritans; we are concerned also to capture the gangs of thieves who rob us of health and social justice; and, beyond this, we anticipate increased success in converting thieves and exploiters into honest men. But this last necessitates inspiration by the first as well as the second of Christ's great Commandments.

A further lesson learnt in my lifetime is that, in the communal struggle for health and equity, we can abandon fear that efforts to mitigate the struggle of life will lead to moral parasitism. Even in animal life we have examples of honesty, fidelity, mercy, and sympathy, showing that co-operation is more important than competition. The altruism shown by animals is evidence that they "follow the law but know not the doctrine." That man, in theory and partially in fact, has advanced ethically is proved by the fact that the public conscience no longer is content to allow one set of men to enrich themselves by producing the degradation and suffering of others. We aim to fit the many to survive, not only to secure the survival of the fittest.

On page 167 I have emphasised my conviction that the most important, but the most neglected, part of our educational and hygienic work, from the cradle to the university, is the training of Personal Character. The possession of a sensitive conscience in social life will go far to remove remaining neglect of our duty as citizens to help good work in every branch of public administration; and, in individual life, a sensitive conscience and its resultant self-control will lead to rapid decrease of some of our chief social diseases.

Modern psychology is becoming a valuable auxiliary of public health reform. It throws new light on the processes by which habits of self-control can be initiated and fortified; but it is only when this knowledge is vitalised by Christian teaching that its full possibilities can be realised.

It may appear that, at present, self-interest both in national and personal matters is supreme, but we are justified, when comparing the past with the present, in discerning that there has been no general degradation of ideals, but rather that we are slowly learning that a truly happy life is only attainable when we act on the Christian determination that in our individual life we will give more than we receive.

And so, one can share in the confidence that the best is still to come. Browning's words are apposite:

> He said, "What's time? Leave NOW for dogs and apes,
> Man has for ever."

INDEX OF NAMES OF PERSONS

INDEX OF SUBJECTS

(See also headings of chapters and of paragraphs in chapters)

Milton Keynes UK
Ingram Content Group UK Ltd.
UKHW022051141024
449569UK00031B/1597